CLINICAL EPIDEMIOLOGY OF ACUTE LYMPHOBLASTIC LEUKEMIA - FROM THE MOLECULES TO THE CLINIC

Edited by **Juan Manuel Mejia-Arangure**

Clinical Epidemiology of Acute Lymphoblastic Leukemia - From the Molecules to the Clinic
http://dx.doi.org/10.5772/45999
Edited by Juan Manuel Mejia-Arangure

Contributors

Gallegos Martha Patricia, Borgas Cesar, Zùñiga Guillermo, Puebla Ana Maria, Luis Figuera, Garcia Juan Ramon, Haitao Zhu, Dongqing Wang, Shoko Kobayashi, Ezequiel M. Fuentes-Pananá, Abigail Morales-Sanchez, Juan Manuel Mejia-Arangure, David Aldebarán Duarte-Rodríguez, Juan Manuel Mejía-Aranguré, Arturo Fajardo-Gutierrez, Richard McNally, Patricia Perez-Vera, Roman Crazzolara, Maria Luisa Perez-Saldivar, Angélica Rangel-López, Marco Antonio Leyva-Vázquez, Jorge Organista-Nava, Yazmín Gómez-Gómez, Berenice Illades-Aguiar, Alicia Enrico, Jorge Milone, Janet Flores-Lujano, Juan Carlos Nuñez-Enriquez, Alejandra Maldonado-Alcazar, Carlos Alberto García-Ruiz

Published by InTech

Janeza Trdine 9, 51000 Rijeka, Croatia

Copyright © 2013 InTech

Notice

Publishing Process Manager Iva Simcic
Technical Editor InTech DTP team
Cover InTech Design team

Additional hard copies can be obtained from orders@intechopen.com

Clinical Epidemiology of Acute Lymphoblastic Leukemia - From the Molecules to the Clinic, Edited by Juan Manuel Mejia-Arangure
p. cm.
ISBN 978-953-51-0990-7

For EU product safety concerns:
IN TECH d.o.o., Prolaz Marije Krucifikse Kozulić 3, 51000 Rijeka, Croatia,
info@intechopen.com or visit our website at intechopen.com.

Meet the editor

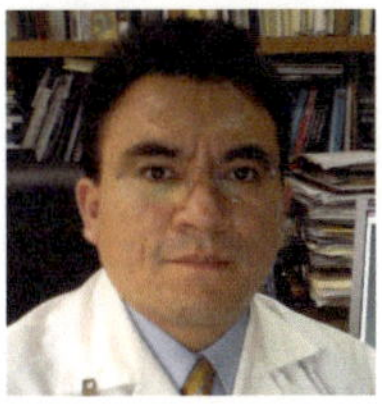

Dr. Juan Manuel Mejia-Arangure was born in Nayarit, Mexico. He received a Medical Doctor degree by the Universidad Nacional Autonoma de Mexico (UNAM). Afterwards he obtained MSc Sociomedical in the area of Epidemiology and in 2004 his PhD degree, with thesis: "Molecular epidemiology of childhood acute leukemias. An assessment of a causal model, interaction of three factors: susceptibility, exposition and vulnerable time", for which he obtained Acknowledgement of Merit. Dr. Mejia-Arangure is member of Mexican and international societies including: Sistema Nacional de Investigadores, Academia Mexicana de Pediatria, Agrupacion Mexicana para el Estudio de la Hematologia, American Society of Hematology, the Society of Epidemiologic Research and the International Society for Environmental Epidemiology. He wrote 71 scientific articles and 13 book chapters and the present is his second book as Editor.

Contents

Preface XI

Section 1 **Hypothesis on the Etiology of ALL 1**

Chapter 1 **Model for Identifying the Etiology of Acute Lymphoblastic Leukemia in Children 3**
Juan Manuel Mejía-Aranguré

Chapter 2 **Infectious Etiology of Childhood Acute Lymphoblastic Leukemia, Hypotheses and Evidence 19**
Abigail Morales-Sánchez and Ezequiel M. Fuentes-Pananá

Section 2 **Pathophysiology of ALL 41**

Chapter 3 **Pathophysiology of Acute Lymphoblastic Leukemia 43**
M. P. Gallegos-Arreola, C. Borjas-Gutiérrez, G. M. Zúñiga-González, L. E. Figuera, A. M. Puebla-Pérez and J. R. García-González

Chapter 4 **Multi-Role of Cancer Stem Cell in Children Acute Lymphoblastic Leukemia 75**
Dong-qing Wang, Hai-tao Zhu, Yan-fang Liu, Rui-gen Yin, Liang Zhao, Zhi-jian Zhang, Zhao-liang Su, Yan-Zhu, Hui-qun Lu, Juan Hong and Jie Zhang

Chapter 5 **Adult T-Cell Leukemia/Lymphoma (ATL): Pathogenesis, Treatment and Prognosis 87**
Shoko Kobayashi and Shigeki Iwasaki

Section 3 Epidemiology of ALL 113

Chapter 6 **Etiological Research of Childhood Acute Leukemia with Cluster and Clustering Analysis 115**
David Aldebarán Duarte-Rodríguez, Richard J.Q. McNally, Juan Carlos Núñez-Enríquez, Arturo Fajardo-Gutiérrez and Juan Manuel Mejía-Aranguré

Chapter 7 **Sociodemographic and Birth Characteristics in Infant Acute Leukemia: A Review 145**
ML Pérez-Saldivar, JM Mejía-Aranguré, A Rangel-López and A Fajardo Gutiérrez

Chapter 8 **Infection During the First Year of Life and Acute Leukemia: Epidemiological Evidence 171**
Janet Flores-Lujano, Juan Carlos Núñez-Enríquez, Angélica Rangel-López, David Aldebarán-Duarte, Arturo Fajardo-Gutiérrez and Juan Manuel Mejía-Aranguré

Section 4 Prognostic of ALL 191

Chapter 9 **Genetic Markers in the Prognosis of Childhood Acute Lymphoblastic Leukemia 193**
M.R. Juárez-Velázquez, C. Salas-Labadía, A. Reyes-León, M.P. Navarrete-Meneses, E.M. Fuentes-Pananá and P. Pérez-Vera

Chapter 10 **Survival of Patients with Acute Lymphoblastic Leukemia 237**
Jorge Organista-Nava, Yazmín Gómez-Gómez, Berenice Illades-Aguiar and Marco Antonio Leyva-Vázquez

Chapter 11 **Bone Marrow Transplantation (BMT) in Philadelphia-Positive Acute Lymphoblastic Leukemia (Ph+ ALL) 265**
Jorge Milone and Enrico Alicia

Chapter 12 **Alterations of Nutritional Status in Childhood Acute Leukemia 277**
Alejandra Maldonado-Alcázar, Juan Carlos Núñez-Enríquez, Carlos Alberto García-Ruiz, Arturo Fajardo-Gutierrez and Juan Manuel Mejía-Aranguré

Chapter 13 **Acute Lymphoblastic Leukemia (ALL) Philadelphia Positive (Ph1) (Incidence Classifications, Prognostic Factor in ALL Principles of ALL Therapy) 297**
Alicia Enrico and Jorge Milone

Chapter 14 **Invasive Fungal Infections in ALL Patients 317**
Roman Crazzolara, Adrian Kneer, Bernhard Meister and Gabriele Kropshofer

Preface

Clinical Epidemiology of Acute Lymphoblastic Leukemia: From the Molecules to the Clinic, is a book which has the goal of introducing the reader into the principal advances in the molecular biology of acute lymphoblastic leukemia (ALL) with application to the clinic.

There are four sections in the book. The first section is about the hypothesis on the etiology of ALL; two chapters were selected at this point. The model for identifying the etiology of ALL is my personnel viewpoint about the etiology of All, mainly in children. I believe that all cancer in children would have a similar behavior in its etiology, however my principal work as researcher during the last twenty years lies on the etiology of ALL in children, therefore the hypothesis centers specially on this group of disease.

In the second section the pathophysiology of ALL is described in three interesting articles. Epidemiology of ALL is mentioned in the third section where the review of different topics we want to work with in the future is showed to detail.

Finally where reference is specially made to the participation of molecular rearrangements in the prognostic of ALL, in different countries like Mexico, the molecular diagnostic is not done in all the hospitals that attend children with ALL. It is important that the entire policy marker understands the importance that all patients would be diagnosed with the tools that increased the possibility of a better answer to the treatment. I decided to include malnutrition in this section because in undeveloped countries like Mexico malnutrition would explain the high mortality of ALL, specially in children; however in other parts of the world malnutrition is not an important prognostic factor in the survival of children with ALL.

In the last year the development of the molecular biology has contributed in the advance of the survival of patients with ALL. However, current epidemiological findings have not been able to fully explain the etiology of the ALL. If this is a mystery we need to claim God for an answer, after all "He revealeth the deep and secret things: he knoweth what is in the darkness, and the light dwelleth with him" (Daniel 2:22).

Today the patients with ALL are treated better than in the past however, today we cannot prevent the development of the disease. The cure of ALL increases the family's and patients' hope, which is great. However if we can prevent the disease we will reduce the parents' and patient's broken heart when children are diagnosed with ALL.

I thank all the contributors, many of whom are long-time friends and co-workers. Others are colleagues with whom I have collaborated, or learned from in the literature. Particular thanks go to Arturo Fajardo who has provide me with invaluable guidance over my years in the IMSS.

I dedicate this book to my wife (Norma Luque) and my son (Yurian Mejia) who are my inspiration and the principal motif of my life.

Dr. Juan Manuel Mejia-Arangure
Pediatric Hospital, Centro Médico Nacional "Siglo XXI",
Mexico

Section 1

Hypothesis on the Etiology of ALL

Chapter 1

Model for Identifying the Etiology of Acute Lymphoblastic Leukemia in Children

Juan Manuel Mejía-Aranguré

Additional information is available at the end of the chapter

http://dx.doi.org/10.5772/52716

1. Introduction

The incidence of ALL varies throughout the world; however, there is a greater frequency of the disease in those countries with a higher socio-economic level [1], with the exception that a higher frequency of ALL has been reported for some Hispanic cities [2]—cities that generally are considered to have a lower standard of living. The highest incidence of ALL has been reported for Costa Rica and for Mexico City [3].

It is accepted that ALL is the result of the interaction, which occurs at a specific moment of life, between environmental factors and susceptibility to the disease [4]. The theories concerning the origin of this illness have been focussed fundamentally on the B-cell precursors of ALL [1]. The most important of these theories was proposed by Greaves and Kinlen; several more recent variations, such as the adrenal theory and infective lymphoid recovery hypothesis have attempted to include these theories [5-8].

The theory of Greaves and that of Kinlen have been discussed in one of the chapters in this book. One of the limitations of the theory of Greaves is that it has not been possible to demonstrate it empirically. In his theory, Greaves argues that some cases of the pre-B ALL observed in the peak age of 2 to 5 years could be associated with an aberrant immune response displayed by an immature immune system. The early exposition to common infectious agents are required for the proper maturation of the immune system, lack of these expositions results in aberrant responses when children are finally in contact with the agent When follow-up studies were carried out in order to evaluate whether children who suffered infections during the first months of life had a greater risk of leukemia, it was not possible to demonstrate any such correlation. When kindergarten registries were used as information source, it was also not possible to demonstrate that there was an association with B-cell precursors of ALL, or in a specific manner in which ALL appears between two and five years of age [9,10]. In addition, data are emerging from epidemiological databases that the idea of early infection being a protective factor for ALL originated due to a bias (non-differential misclassification) [11] and that, in reality, no such association exists. At any rate, determination of whether a child suffered from different infections during the first year of life is extremely difficult; for this reason, the empirical reference will need to be improved in order to lend greater support to this hypothesis.

Nevertheless, the principal importance of the hypothesis of Greaves cannot be questioned, because it does not exclude what epidemiological methods have been able to demonstrate concerning late infection [12]. These data are conclusive in showing that, in the majority of cases, ALL originates during intrauterine life [13] and that proliferation of the B cells, in fact, the time in which the highest peak of proliferation occurs, is during the first year of life [12]. All these findings permit the deduction that ALL requires a first "hit" in the intrauterine stage and another hit during a later stage of life and that some infections may play a very important role in the causality of B-cell precursors of ALL.

2. Exposure

ALL has been associated with different environmental risk factors [14,15]; however, the only environmental factor that is universally accepted as being associated with ALL is exposure to X-rays *in utero*[14]. The identification of environmental factors has had various problems, one of which is the effect of the sample size on statistical power [15-18]. ALL is an infirmity with a very low frequency, which makes it difficult for studies to attain a sample size appropriate for identifying an association with an environmental risk factor [16,17]. Another problem is that most of the environmental factors that are associated with leukemia, such as exposure to X-rays or exposure to very low frequency magnetic fields, have a very low frequency of occurrence [16,19,20]. The study design that has been used the most to search for associations with ALL is the case-control study; this type of study has the limitation that it has low efficiency for identifying associations when the frequency of exposure is very low [16,17]. Another limitation in determining environmental exposure is that the greater part of the instruments used to evaluate such exposures either have not been validated for this purpose or are not sufficiently sensitive to detect the presence of such exposure, as is the case for exposure to infections during the first year of life [11] or for exposure to extremely low frequency magnetic fields [19].

Most experimental designs have the limitation that they cannot evaluate various independent variables at the same time [21]. Multivariate analysis that is used to evaluate the effect of an independent variable, adjusted for the effect of various control variables or potential confounders, implies a modeling with only one or two predictor variables for the disease [21]. ALL is potentially the result of the presence not of one or two independent variables, but of many risk factors that act at the same time to provoke the development of the illness [1]. According to the multicausal theory, illnesses must have at least two risk factors that lead to the development of the illness; the majority of multivariate models, such as logistic regression, do not permit this type of simultaneous evaluations.

One of the limitations in trying to identify the association between environmental factors and the development of ALL is that not taken into account is the idea that, in order for a child to develop leukemia, it is not enough that the child be exposed to leukemiogenic factor, but that it is necessary that the child be susceptible to the infirmity [22-24]. If we start with the premise, postulated by Greaves, that ALL is the result of two hits, one that occurred in the intrauterine stage or in a stage very early in life and another hit that was necessary afterward [25,26], then this would predict that each child that develops ALL must have had a prior susceptibility for developing the infirmity; otherwise, the children that are exposed to the "second hit", given that they do not have the first, will not be able to develop the disease [13,27,28].

Consequently, an error that has been committed in many epidemiological studies is that these studies have been carried out without taking into account the susceptibility of the child for the infirmity [29]. Our group was the first to demonstrate that environmental factors have an important weight in the development of ALL in children with a high susceptibility for the illness, such as those with Down syndrome (DS) [7,29]. By including children with DS, not only as cases but also as controls, it has been possible to improve the precision of the sampling size, because even with relatively small sample sizes, it was possible to identify a number of important environmental factors associated with ALL [7,30].

3. Susceptibility

Susceptibility to ALL has been studied from two perspectives: one that deals with genes or syndromes that increase the risk of developing ALL; the other, with the genes or alterations that increase the effect of the environmental exposure for a child to develop ALL.

There are genetic rearrangements, such as MLL/AF4, the involvement of which in the development of ALL in children is indisputable [13]. In fact, Greaves postulated that the MLL/AF4 is a necessary and sufficient cause for the development of ALL in children, especially in infants [13,26]. However, some researchers have demonstrated that this rearrangement may appear with an important frequency in older children and that even the twin of the children that develop ALL could lose the MLL/AF4 rearrangement in later years of life [31,32]. In a chapter of this book, it is shown how exposure during pregnancy to inhibitors of topoisomerase II is a risk factor for the offspring of the pregnancy to develop ALL with the presence of genetic rearrangements MLL. There are no studies that demonstrate that children that are born with genetic rearrangements in MLL, upon exposure to determined environmental factors, have a greater risk of developing ALL. Such studies are difficult to perform, because the frequency of genetic rearrangements in MLL in children without ALL is estimated to be less that 1 in 10000 live births [13].

Among the syndromes that predispose to ALL are SD, ataxia, telangiectasia, and Fanconi anemia [24]. Although these children present an elevated risk for developing ALL, not all develop the disease [33]. It is possible that these children would have to be exposed to some environmental factor in order to develop ALL, as has been demonstrated for children with SD [4,15,29,33,34].

There also exists susceptibility determined by polymorphisms that increase the effect of luekemiogenic factors, through which children develop ALL. Examples are those related to the polymorphisms of methyl-n-transferase and cytochrome p-450. Some polymorphisms of these genes have been associated to a greater toxic effect for benzene and other factors that are potentially leukemiogenic [35-39].

Some nutritional alterations also have been seen to increase the effect of some potentially leukemiogenic factors, a possible examples is reduction in the consumption of vitamin A, as it is known that vitamin A reduces the effect of exposure to carcinogens in tobacco smoke [40]. Tobacco smoke contains substances, such as benzene, which are known to have a leukemiogenic effect [41,42].

4. Vulnerable period

The frequency of ALL has a characteristic peak at 2–5 years of age [23,24]. In the Mexican population, there appears another age peak at 6–9 years of age [43]. This peak primarily results from B-cell precursor ALL and that has the genetic rearrangement ETV6/RUNX1 [13,23].

In an attempt to explain the cause of this peak, a series of hypotheses have been generated [23], among which that proposed by Greaves stands out. Greaves commented that this age peak reflects the start of a greater immunological response and, in particular, it is in direct relation to the capacity to produce immunoglobulins [12]. Greaves assumes that, after the first year of life, the possibility is increased that a previously mutated cell may undergo a second mutation and this brings with it the development of ALL [12].

In the case of ALL, it has been established that, for children who are born with a greater susceptibility to ALL, such as those children born with the genetic rearrangement that involves MLL, the age at onset of ALL is earlier, generally during the first year of life. It is estimated that those children have a 100% probability of developing ALL [13]. In contrast, children who are born with the genetic rearrangement ETV6/RUNX1 have a 25% probability of developing ALL and their peak age at onset (2–5 years of age) is later than that for the children born with the genetic rearrangement that involves MLL [13]. This leads one to think that the peak age of onset of ALL reflects the degree of susceptibility with which a child is born and, on the other hand, the degree of proliferation of the cells involved in the development of the disease [1,43]. A similar situation exists for retinoblastoma, in which the age at onset of ALL reflects the degree of proliferation of the cells in the retina and for osteosarcoma which appears earlier in females than in males, starting at the growth spurt in adolescence [1,28,44].

Another aspect that, despite its great importance in epidemiological research, is on occasions overlooked is the stage of life at which the exposure to a carcinogenic agent occurs. Greaves has pointed out the importance of the infection occurring at a particular period, 2–3

http://dx.doi.org/10.5772/52716

years of age [25], for development of ALL. Exposure of a child to radiation (x ray for example) in the earlier stages of life has been associated with a greater risk of ALL [45] and, in addition, the leukemia has a shorter latency period. Hertz-Picciotto et al. underscored the importance of evaluating the time of life or stage of development of the tissues at which the exposure occurs [46], because for two individuals who may have been exposed to the same factor, the effect of said exposure will vary according to the stage of development of the individual or of the particular organ [47-52]. Some of the factors that can influence the toxicity of a substance in an organism may vary according to the individual's age. Such is the case for the absorption, metabolism, detoxification, and excretion of xenobiotic compounds. Similarly, for children, there can exist an immaturity in the biochemical and physiological functions of the majority of the systems of the body, as well as variation in the bodily composition (content of water, fat, protein, and minerals) [48,52-54]. These factors may make the neonate, for example, very sensitive to chemical substances [52,53,55].

Considering the importance of the time at which the exposure occurs separately from the stage of development of the organism that may be affected, it is important to evaluate whether the exposure occurred in the prenatal stage, during the pregnancy, or in the postnatal period [28,50]. For example, exposures that affect a maternal ovum may have occurred peri-conceptionally or even a long time before conception, given that the ova are present, already formed, in the woman [47]. Among the exposures that affect the sperm or the substances that can concentrate in the semen, said exposures can only cause damage periconceptionally, because sperm and seminal fluid involved in the fertilization were formed hours, or a few days, prior to the conception [47]. It has also been observed that some substances that are stored in the fat or in the bones of the mother may be removed during the pregnancy and cause injury to the fetus [47]. Some significant exposure during pregnancy may be more related to the presence of the rearrangement MLL/AF4 [13,56], because the cases of leukemia that occur in infants generally belong to this type of leukemia, whereas exposures that occur at 2–4 years of age may be more related to the B-cell precursor ALL with ETV6/RUNX1, because this is the peak age of onset for this disease [13,43,57].

Infections may have another action: an increase in the proliferation of B cells may increase the risk that the cells being exposed to leukemiogenic agent would lead to ALL [7,12].

On the other hand, it is not only necessary that the cells have proliferated, but also it is necessary that, in that moment, there be a niche in the bone marrow which would permit the growth and the expansion of that leukemia clone [28]. In a book in the series In Tech, Pelayo has described the function of the microenvironment of the bone marrow in the development of ALL [58,59]. Today, it is known that the alterations not only must occur in the cancerous cells, what confers upon them the capacity for mutations and genomic instability, that changes the cycles of cell regulation and energy consumption, evades or destroys the immune system and generates mechanisms of inflammation that lead to tumor propagation [60]. In addition to all this, cancerous cells are capable of causing changes in their microenvironment to generate an environment in which a cancerous cell can form a "nest", a microenvironment that generates tumor invasion, and a microenvironment that favors the development of metastasis [58-61]. Such changes in the cells make them even more vulnerable to exposure to carcinogenic substances [62-64].

5. Down syndrome model: Advantage of a design with cases and controls selected for susceptibility

Robinson was one of the first to propose that if a child with DS is studied, identification of the effect of the major portion of environmental factors in the development of ALL in children could be achieved [33]. Children with DS have a higher risk for developing leukemias, not only myeloid leukemias, but also lymphoblastic leukemias. In the lymphoblastic leukemias, the participation of the genes, *JAK 1* and *JAK2*, have a definite affect in these children developing the disease [65].

The study of children with a high susceptibility to ALL has permitted, even with a smaller sample size, the identification of the role that some environmental factors play in the development of ALL. The risks (odds ratios) encountered when comparing the population of children with ALL with DS and a population of healthy children with DS have been relatively higher than those reported when comparing healthy children without high susceptibility to the disease as controls. We have called this approach "studies of cases and controls selected by susceptibility". The advantages that we have reported about this design is that it improves the sampling power and the precision of the estimators [66].

6. Theory as a model of prediction

Theories are considered as a tool or instrument that can be used to predict [67].

The epidemiological theory that attempts to predict the origin of diseases in human populations is the Sufficient-Component Cause model [68]. This theory underscores the idea that diseases are multicausal and that it is necessary that at least two component causes must be present or have occurred for an individual to develop said disease. Upon completing the component causes of the disease, then a sufficient cause has been completed and, in such case, the person will develop the disease [68].

The criteria of demarcation to determine if a hypothesis is scientific or not are that the refutationism proposes that the hypothesis be deducible, that there exists a way to test the hypothesis empirically, and that the hypothesis be be falsifiable [67,68].

With respect to the multicausal theory and the Sufficient-Component Causes model, the empirical referent that the sufficient cause has been completed is only the disease itself; its origin is deducible because this theory assumes that all illnesses arises from the action of at least two component causes. However, there is no manner in which this hypothesis can be falsified, because whatever model proposed to show that the sufficient cause has been completed at the time of the attempt at falsification and consequently to demostrate that with

http://dx.doi.org/10.5772/52716

the "sufficent cause completed" the diseases was not developed. An argument that could emerge is that, as the sufficient cause was not reality completed, it is for this reason that the individual did not develop the disease. At this point, we are left without possibilities of demonstrating that said hypothesis may be falsifiable. In one sense, the illness itself is the sufficient cause and therefore stops being two separate variables and no longer fulfills its function of prediction, given that one cannot say that an individual completed the sufficient cause and consequently goes on to develop the disease; we know that the sufficient cause has been completed only when the individual becomes ill.

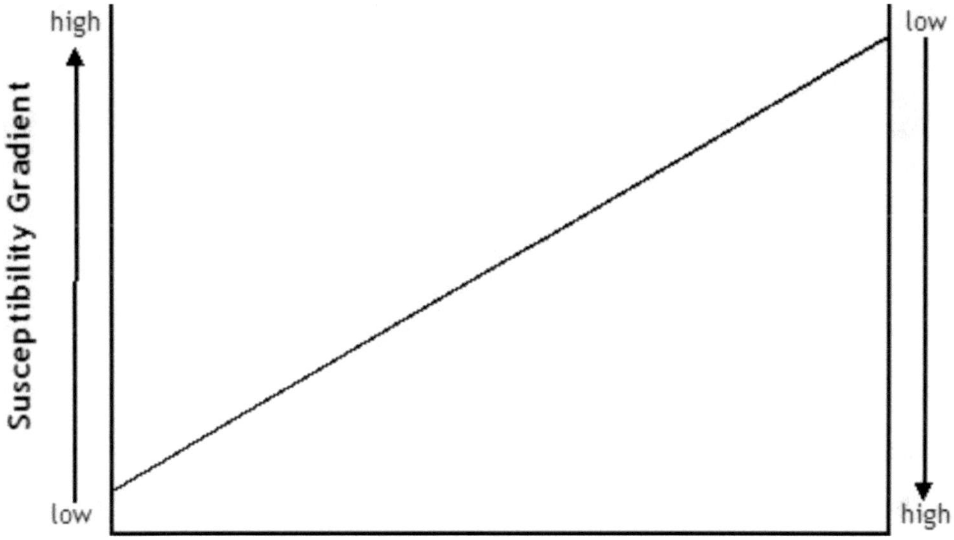

Figure 1. Interaction between a gradient of susceptibility to a disease and a gradient of exposure to environmental risk factors. To develop ALL, an individual with a higher susceptibility, as determined by the interplay of genetic factors, would need only a lower exposure, as determined by the unknown, possibly synergistic, interplay of the characteristics of the exposure. Conversely, the higher the exposure, the lower the susceptibility that would be needed to result in development of the disease.

The hypothesis that is set forth here is bounded by three phenomena, the "exposure", the "susceptibility", and the "vulnerable period" (Fig. 2). This model includes only these three component causes that are necessary for a child to develop the illness. As was described in the initial part of this chapter, these three phenomena are interrelated and there exists a gradient which indicates that, when there is an excess of one of these components, less is needed of the other two components in order to develop the illness (Fig. 1).

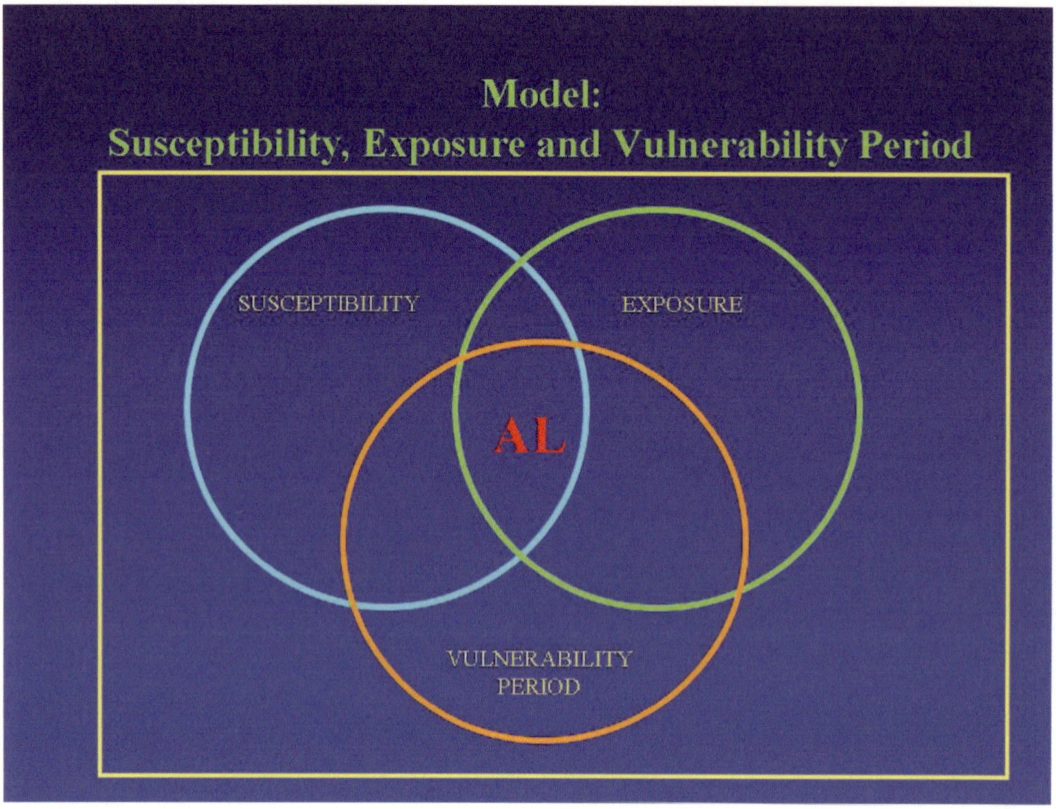

Figure 2. Interaction among the three phenomena. Acute lymphoblastic leukemia (AL) in childhood is the result of the interactions among three phenomena: the gradient of susceptibility, the gradient of exposure to carcinogenic environmental factors, and the tissue vulnerability period.

7. Conclusions

Current models to identify the environmental causes of ALL have limitations that could lead to years of studies and the investment enormous sums of money, yet still continue without successfully determining the factors associated with ALL.

This proposed model of susceptibility, exposure, and vulnerable period permits boundaries to be drawn around the factors that could potentially influence the development of the disease and, in addition, permits the development of new methods for the study of the environmental causes of ALL in children, such as the study of cases and controls selected by susceptibility.

Children that are born with a high susceptibility to ALL, such as children with SD, should be the first among those that should be protected from exposure to environmental factors that potentially provoke ALL, such as tobacco smoke [29], exposure to magnetic fields of extremely low frequency [69], etc. The approach of the precautionary principle should be followed, in that although the causal evidence is not absolute, the risk or the effect of the illness is so serious that putting oneself in contact the risk factor should be avoided [66,70]. Similarly, for children of parents who underwent elevated exposure to leukemiogenic factors during the pregnancy, it may happen that, although these children may have been born "normal", it is possible that they had been born with a high susceptibility to the ALL, which is not possible to identify simply by observation.

Susceptibility to ALL is a constitutive condition or one that is acquired in an early stage of life. Exposure to a leukemiogenic agent will have an affect to the extent of the intensity of the exposure and the degree of susceptibility to the disease or the intrinsic factors that modify the form in which the child's bodily tissues respond to this exposure. However, this must occur at a specific moment when a cell is proliferating and where the conditions around the cell are appropriate for the cell to be converted into a leukemic clone and finally develops the disease.

As the absolute truth described in the Bible says, "There is a time for everything…" [71]

Acknowledgments

This chapter contains results of studies that were funded by grants from the National Council of Science and Technology (CONACYT, Mexico; CB-2007-83949; 2007-C01-71223; and 2010-1-141026) and from the Mexican Institute of Social Security (IMSS, Mexico; FIS/PROT/56 and FIS/IMSS/PROT/G10/846). Translation of the original Spanish into English was financed by CONACYT and the Coordination of Research in Health through the Division of Development and Research. The author thanks Dr. Arturo Fajardo-Gutiérrez (Unit of Clinical Epidemiology, IMSS, Mexico) whose comments enriched the hypothesis presented here and Veronica Yakoleff for translating the text.

Author details

Juan Manuel Mejía-Aranguré

Address all correspondence to: juan.mejiaa@imss.gob.mx

Coordination of Research in Health, Mexican Institute of Social Security, Mexico City, Mexico

References

[1] Mejía-Aranguré JM, Pérez-Saldivar ML, Pelayo-Camacho R, Fuentes-Pananá E, Bekker-Mendez C, Morales-Sánchez A, Duarte-Rodríguez DA, Fajardo-Gutiérrez A.

Childhood Acute Leukemias in Hispanic Population: Differences by Age Peak and Immunophenotype. In: Faderl S. (ed.) Novel aspects in acute lymphoblastic leukemia. Rijeka: In Tech; 2011. P3-32.

[2] Mejía-Aranguré JM, Bonilla M, Lorenzana R, Juárez-Ocaña S, de Reyes G, Pérez-Saldivar ML, Guadalupe González-Miranda, Roberto Bernáldez-Ríos, Antonio Ortiz-Fernández, Manuel Ortega-Alvarez, María del Carmen Martínez-García, Arturo Fajardo-Gutiérrez. Incidence of leukemias in children from El Salvador and Mexico City between 1996 and 2000: Population-based data. BMC Cancer 2005; 5:33

[3] Pérez-Saldivar ML, Fajardo-Gutiérrez A, Bernáldez-Ríos R, Martínez-Avalos A, Medina-Sanson A, Espinosa-Hernández L, Flores-Chapa JD, Amador-Sánchez R, Peñaloza-González JG, Álvarez-Rodríguez FJ, Bolea-Murga V, Flores-Lujano J, Rodríguez-Zepeda MC, Rivera-Luna R, Dorantes-Acosta EM, Jiménez-Hernández E, Alvarado-Ibarra M, Velázquez-Aviña MM, Torres-Nava JR, Duarte-Rodríguez DA, Paredes-Aguilera R, Campo-Martínez MA, Cárdenas-Cardos R, Alamilla-Galicia PH, Bekker-Méndez VC, Ortega-Alvarez MC, Mejia-Arangure JM. Childhood acute leukemias are very frequent in Mexican population: descriptive epidemiology from all boroughs of Mexico City. BMC Cancer 2011; 11:355.

[4] Taylor GM. Immunogenetics and the aetiology of childhood leukemia. Archives of disease in childhood1994; 70(2):77-81.

[5] Schmiegelow K, Vestergaard T, Nielsen SM, Hjalgrim H. Etiology of common childhood acute lymphoblastic leukemia: the adrenal hypothesis. Leukemia 2008; 22(12): 2137-41

[6] Azevedo-Silva F, Camargo B, Pombo-de-Oliveira MS. Implications of infectious diseases and the adrenal hypothesis for the etiology of childhood acute lymphoblastic leukemia. Brazilian journal of medical and biological research2010; 43(3):226-9

[7] Mejia-Arangure JM, Perez-Saldivar ML, Flores-Lujano J, Bekker-Mendez C, Pinto-Cardoso S, Duarte-RodíguezDA, Fajardo-Gutierrez A. Infections and acute leukemia in children with Down Syndrome. In: Dey S (ed.) Prenatal diagnosis and screening for Down Syndrome. Rijeka: In Tech; 2011. p79-106.

[8] Richardson RB. Promotional etiology for common childhood acute lymphoblastic leukemia: The infective lymphoid recovery hypothesis. Leukemia research 2011; 35(11):1425-31.

[9] Roman E, Simpson J, Ansell P, Kinsey S, Mitchell CD, McKinney PA, Birch JM, Greaves M, Eden T. United Kingdom Childhood Cancer Study Investigators. Childhood acute lymphoblastic leukemia and infections in the first year of life: a report from the United Kingdom Childhood Cancer Study. Am J Epidemiol2007; 165: 496–504.

[10] Rosenbaum PF, Buck GM, Brecher ML. Early child-care and preschool experience and the risk of childhood acute lymphoblastic leukemia. American journal of epidemiology 2000; 152(5):1136-44.

http://dx.doi.org/10.5772/52716

[11] Roman E, Simpson J, Ansell P, Lightfoot T, Smith A. Infectious proxies and childhood leukaemia: findings from the United Kingdom Childhood Cancer Study (UKCCS).Blood cells, molecules & diseases2009; 42(2):126-8.

[12] Greaves M. Infection, immune responses and the aetiology of childhood leukaemia. Nature reviews. Cancer 2006; 6(3): 193-203.

[13] Greaves MF, Wiemels J. Origins of chromosome translocations in childhood leukaemia. Nature reviews. Cancer 2003;3(9):639-49.

[14] Mejía-Aranguré JM, Ortega-Alvarez MC, Fajardo-Gutiérrez A. Epidemiología de las leucemias agudas en niños (Parte I). Revistamédica del InstitutoMexicano del Seguro Social 2005; 43(4):323-33

[15] Mejía-Aranguré JM, Ortega-Alvarez MC, Fajardo-Gutiérrez A. Epidemiología de las leucemias agudas en niños (Parte II). RevistamédicadelInstitutoMexicano del Seguro Social 2005; 43(5):401-9.

[16] Gufferman S. Methodologic approaches to studying environmental factors in childhood cancer. Environmental health perspectives 1998; 106:(Suppl 3):881-6.

[17] Linet MS, Wacholder S, Zahm SH. Interpreting epidemiologic research: lessons from studies of childhood cancer. Pediatrics 2003; 112(1 Pt 2):218-32.

[18] Woodruff TJ, Axelrad DA, Kyle AD, Nweke O, Miller GG, Hurley BJ. Trends in Environmentally related childhood illnesses. Pediatrics 2004; 113(4 Suppl):1133-40.

[19] Greenland S, Kheifets L. Leukemia attributable to residential magnetic fields: Results from analyses allowing for study biases. Risk analysis: an official publication of the Society for Risk Analysis 2006; 26(2):471-82.

[20] Kheifets L, Afifi AA, Shimkhada R. Public health impact of extremely low-frequency electromagnetic fields. Environmental health perspectives 2006; 114(10):1532-7.

[21] Kleinbaum DG, Klein M. Important special cases of the logistic model. In Logistic Regression. Springer Science: New York 2010: 41-71.

[22] Stewart A. Aetiology of childhood malignancies. British medical journal 1961:1(5224): 452-60.

[23] Greaves MF. Aetiology of acute leukaemia. Lancet 1997; 349(9048):344-9.

[24] Eden T. Aetiology of childhood leukaemia. Cancer treatment reviews 2010; 36(4): 286-97.

[25] Greaves M. Molecular genetics, natural history and the demise of childhood leukaemia. European journal of cancer 1999; 35(14):1941-53.

[26] Greaves M. Biology of leukemia: An overview. In: Henderson ES, Lister TA, Greaves MF. Leukemia. 7hd ed. Philadelphia:Saunders 2002:8-18.

[27] Dickinson HO. The causes of childhood leukaemia. British medical journal 2005; 330(7503):1279-80.

[28] Huntly BJP, Gilliland G. Leukemia stem cells and the evolution of cancer-stem-cell research. Nature reviews. Cancer 2005; 5(4):311-21.

[29] Mejía-Aranguré JM, Fajardo-Gutiérrez A, Flores-Aguilar H, Martínez-García MC, Salamanca-Gómez F, Palma-Padilla V, Paredes-Aguilera R, Bernáldez-Ríos R, Ortiz-Fernández A, Martínez-Avalos A, Gorodezky C. Environmental factors contributing to the development of childhood leukemia in children with Down's syndrome. Leukemia 2003; 17(9):1905-07.

[30] Flores-Lujano, Perez-SaldivarML , Fuentes-PananaEM, GorodezkyC, Bernaldez-RiosR, Del Campo-MartinezMA, Martinez-AvalosA, Medina-Sanson A, Paredes-AguileraR, Flores-ChapaJ De Diego, Bolea-MurgaV, Rodriguez-ZepedaMC, Rivera-LunaR, Palomo-ColliMA, Romero-GuzmanL , Perez-VeraP , Alvarado-IbarraM, Salamanca-GómezF, Fajardo-Gutierrez A,Mejía-ArangnuréJM. Breastfeeding and early infection in the aetiology of childhood leukaemia in Down syndrome. British journal of cancer2009; 101(5):860-4.

[31] Alondra Daniel-Cravioto, Cesar R. Gonzalez-Bonilla, Juan Manuel Mejia-Arangure, Maria Luisa Perez-Saldivar, Arturo Fajardo-Gutierrez, Elva Jimenez-Hernandez, Milagros Hernandez-Serrano, Vilma Carolina Bekker-Mendez. Genetic rearrangement MLL/AF4 is most frequent in children with acute lymphoblastic leukemias in Mexico City. Leukemia & lymphoma 2009; 50(8): 1352–60.

[32] Chuk MK, McIntyre E, Small D, Brown P. Discordance of MLL-rearranged (MLL-R) infant acute lymphoblastic leukemia in monozygotic twins with spontaneous clearance of preleukemic clone in unaffected twin. Blood 2009; 113(26):6691-4.

[33] Ross JA, Spector LG, Robison LL, Olshan AF. Epidemiology of leukemia in children with Down syndrome. Pediatric blood & cancer 2005;44(1):8-12.

[34] Canfield KN, Spector LG, Robison LL, Lazovich D, Roesler M, Olshan AF, Smith FO, Heerema NA, Barnard DR, Blair CK, Ross JA. Childhood and maternal infections and risk of acute leukemia in children with Down syndrome: a report from the Children's Oncology Group. British journal of cancer 2004; 91(11):1866-72.

[35] Krajinovic M, Labuda D, Richer C, Karimi S, Sinnett D. Susceptibility to childhood acute lymphoblastic leukemia: influence of CYP1A1, CYP2D6, GSTM1, and GSTT1 genetic polymorphisms. Blood 1999; 93(5):1496-501.

[36] Krajinovic M, Richer C, Sinnet H, Labuda D, Sinnett D. Genetic polymorphisms of N-Acetyltransferases 1 and 2 and gene-gene interaction in the susceptibility to childhood acute lymphoblastic leukemia. Cancer epidemiology, biomarkers & prevention 2000; 9(6):557-62.

[37] Infante-Rivard C, Krajinovic M, Labuda D, Sinnett D. Childhood acute lymphoblastic leukemia associated with parental alcohol consumption and polymorphisms of carcinogen-metabolizing genes. Epidemiology 2002; 13(3):277-81.

[38] Krajinovic M, Sinnett H, Richer C, Labuda D, Sinnett D. Role of NQO1, MPO and CYP2E1 genetic polymorphisms in the susceptibility to childhood acute lymphoblastic leukemia. International journal of cancer 2002; 97(2):230-6.

[39] Gast A, Bermejo JL, Stanulla M, Burwinkel B, Schrappe M, Bartram CR, Hemminki K, Kumar R. Folate metabolic gene polymorphisms and childhood acute lymphoblastic leukemia: a case-control study. Leukemia 2007; 21(2):320-5.

[40] Bartsch H, Nair U, Risch A, Rojas M, Wikman H, Alexandrov K. Genetic polymorphism of CYP genes, alone or in combination, as a risk modifier of tobacco-related cancers. Cancer epidemiology, biomarkers & prevention 2000; 9(1):3-28.

[41] InfanteRivard C, Krajinovic M, Labuda D, Sinnett D. Parental smoking, CYP1A1 genetic polymorphisms and childhood leukemia (Quebec, Canada). Cancer causes & control 2000; 11(6):547-53.

[42] Pyatt D, Hays S. A review of the potential association between childhood leukemia and benzene. Chemico-biological interactions 2010; 184(1-2):151-64

[43] Bernaldez-Rios R, Ortega-Alvarez M, Perez-Saldivar ML,Alatoma-Medina NE, Del Campo-Martinez MA, Rodriguez-Zepeda MC, Montero-Ponce I, Franco-Ornelas S, Fernandez-Castillo G, Nuñez-Villegas N, Taboada-Flores MA, Flores-Lujano J, Argüelles-Sanchez ME, Juarez-Ocaña S, Fajardo-Gutierrez A, Mejia-Arangure JM. The age incidence of childhood B-cell precursor acute lymphoblastic leukemia in Mexico City. Journal of pediatric hematology/oncology 2008; 30 (3):199-203.

[44] Mejía-Aranguré JM, Flores-Aguilar H, Juárez-Muñoz I, Vázquez-Langle J, Games-Eternod J, Pérez-Saldivar ML, Ortega-Alvarez MC, Rendón-Macías ME, Fajardo-Gutiérrez A. Edad de aparición de los diferentestumoresmalignos en la infancia. RevistaMédica delInstitutoMexicano delSeguro Social 2005;43 (1):25-37.

[45] Miller RW. Special Susceptibility of the child to certain radiation-induced cancers. Environmental health perspectives 1995; 103(Suppl 6):41-44.

[46] Hertz-Picciotto I, Pastore LM, Beaumont JJ. Timing and patterns of exposures during pregnancy and their implications for study methods. American journal of epidemiology1996; 143:597-607.

[47] Bearer CF. How are children different from adults? Environmental health perspectives 1995; 103(Suppl 6):7-12.

[48] Losan AF, Anderson L, Roman E, Fear N, Wolf M, Whyatt R y cols. Workshop to identify critical windows of exposure for children's health: cancer work group summary. Environmental health perspectives 2000; 108(Suppl 3):595-597.

[49] Selevan SG, Kimmel CA, Mendola P. Indentify critical windows of exposure for children's health. Environmental health perspectives 2000; 108(Suppl 3):451-455.

[50] Anderson LM, Diwan BA, Fear NT, Roman E. Critical windows of exposure for children's health: cancer in human epidemiological studies and neoplasms in experimental animal models. Environmental health perspectives 2000; 108(Suppl 3):573-594.

[51] Charnley G, Putzrath RM. Children's health, susceptibility, and regulatory approaches to reducing risk from chemical carcinogens. Environmental health perspectives 2001; 109(2): 187-192.

[52] Perera FP, Illman SM, Kinney PL, Whyatt RM, Kelvin EA, Shepard P y cols. The challenge of preventing environmentally related disease in young children: community-based research in New York City. Environmental health perspectives 2002; 110(2): 197-204.

[53] Thomas RD. Age-specific carcinogenesis: Environmental exposure and susceptibility. Environmental health perspectives1995; 103(Suppl 6):45-48.

[54] Smith A, Lightfoot T, Simpson J, Roman E. Birth weight, sex and childhood cancer: A report from the United Kingdom Childhood Cancer Study. Cancer Epidemiology 2009; 33(5):363-7.

[55] Anderson LM, Jones AB, Rice JM. Perinatal carcinogenesis: current directions. British journal of cancer 1991; 63:1025-8.

[56] Ross JA. Environmental and Genetic Susceptibility to MLL-Defined Infant Leukemia. Journal of the National Cancer Institute Monographs 2008;2008(39):83–86.

[57] Kang H, Wilson CS, Harvey RC, Chen IM, Murphy MH, Atlas SR, Bedrick EJ, Devidas M, Carroll AJ, Robinson BW, Stam RW, Valsecchi MG, Pieters R, Heerema NA, Hilden JM, Felix CA, Reaman GH, Camitta B, Winick N, Carroll WL, Dreyer ZE, Hunger SP, Willman CL. Gene expression profiles predictive of outcome and age in infant acute lymphoblastic leukemia: a Children's Oncology Group study. Blood 2012;119(8):1872-81.

[58] Pelayo R, Dorantes-Acosta E, Vadillo E, Fuentes-Panana E. From HSC to B-Lymphoid cells in normal and malignant hematopoiesis. In: Pelayo R. (ed.) Advances in hematopoietic stem cell research. Rijeka: In Tech; 2011. p277-98.

[59] Purizaca J, Meza I, Pelayo R.Early lymphoid development and microenvironmental cues in B-cell acute lymphoblastic leukemia.Archives of medical research 2012; 43(2): 89-101

[60] Hanahan D, Weinberg RA. Hallmarks of cancer: the next generation. Cell 2011; 144(5):646-74.

[61] Stratton MR. Exploring the genomes of cancer cells: Progress and promise. Science 2011; 331(6024):1553-8.

[62] Lander ES. Initial impact of the sequencing of the human genome. Nature 2011; 470(7333):187-97.

[63] Willyard C. Breaking the cancer habit. Nature 2011; 471(7339):S16-S17.

[64] Brower V. Portents of malignancy. Nature 2001; 471(7339):S19-S21.

[65] Pui CH, Mullighan CG, Evans WE, Relling MV. Pediatric acute lymphoblastic leukemia: where are we going and how do we get there? Blood 2012; 120(6):1165-74.

[66] Mejia-Arangure JM,Fajardo-Gutierrez A. Selection by Susceptibility as a Design to Identify Environmental Risk Factors in Children's Acute Leukemia. Epidemiology 2006; 17(16):S505-S506

[67] Popper K. The logic of scientific discovery. London: Routledge 2002

[68] Rothman KJ. What is causation. In: Epidemiology. An introduction. New York: Oxford University Press 2012. p23-37

[69] Mejia-Arangure JM, Fajardo-Gutierrez A, Perez-Saldivar ML, Gorodezky C, Martinez-Avalos A, Romero-Guzman L, Campo-Martinez MA, Flores-Lujano J, Salamanca-Gomez F, Velasquez-Perez L. Magnetic Fields and Acute Leukemia in Children With Down Syndrome. Epidemiology 2007; 18(1):158-61.

[70] Ebi K, von Ehrenstein OS, Radon K. Electromagnetic fields. In: Tamburlini G, Ehrenstein OV, Bertollini R. Children's health and environment: a review of evidence. Environmental issue report No. 29. Regional Office for Europe, Germany: World Health Organization 2002. p172-87.

[71] Ecclesiastes 3:1. Holy Bible, New International Version® Anglicized, NIV® Copyright © 1979, 1984, 2011 by Biblica, Inc.®

Infectious Etiology of Childhood Acute Lymphoblastic Leukemia, Hypotheses and Evidence

Abigail Morales-Sánchez and
Ezequiel M. Fuentes-Pananá

Additional information is available at the end of the chapter

http://dx.doi.org/10.5772/54455

1. Introduction

Research on the role of infectious agents in the etiology of cancer has grown remarkably in recent decades. A causal association between infection events and the development of different types of cancer has been strongly suggested in epidemiologic studies, while the direct oncogenic capacity of a set of pathogens has been demonstrated in the laboratory.

It is now recognized that between 15 and 20% of all tumors are associated with infection by direct tumorigenic agents [1]. However, the transforming mechanisms of carcinogenic infectious agents are not restricted to the expression of oncogenes and their ability to modulate the expression and function of oncogenes and anti-oncogenes in target cells. Other routes of transformation have been described, in which, an agent participates through more indirect mechanisms, such as promoting immune suppression or chronic inflammation. Although, in indirect mechanisms of transformation the infectious agent usually does not reside in the cell that will form the tumor mass, it contributes to cancer development making favorable conditions for tumor initiation or growth.

One of the malignancies proposed to be etiologically related to infection is childhood acute lymphoblastic leukemia (ALL). ALL is a heterogeneous group of hematologic malignancies in which the process of differentiation and limited proliferation that characterizes normal lymphopoiesis is altered and replaced by a malignant clonal expansion of immature lymphocytes. ALL is the most common type of childhood malignancy worldwide, unfortunately, little is known about the origin of ALL, some cases are associated with genetic predisposition conferred by Down syndrome, Bloom syndrome, ataxia-telangiectasia, Nijmegen breakage syndrome or exposure to environmental agents such as ionizing radiation or mutagenic chemicals, however these events account for less than 5% of ALL cases [2], therefore, discernible causal factors involved in cancer initiation or promotion are unknown for the bulk of primary leukemia.

Several etiologic factors have been proposed to cause ALL. One of the most reported in the literature and the subject of this chapter is related to infections. Independently, Greaves, Kinlen and Smith have suggested different mechanisms by which certain events related to infection may explain at least some cases of childhood leukemia [3-5]. Interestingly, the suggested role of infectious agents in leukemogenesis varies from one hypothesis to another, favoring either direct or indirect mechanisms of transformation. It is our main goal to describe these hypotheses highlighting the type of evidence in favor and against them and providing a biological frame in which to discuss possible mechanisms of leukemogenesis by the infectious agents. Due to the large number of publications in the field, this is not intended as an in-deep and complete review of all published literature but a summary in which to set the basis for discussion.

2. 'Delayed infection' hypothesis and 'two-hits' minimal model by Greaves

One of the most cited proposals on the infectious etiology of ALL is the *delayed infection* hypothesis, in which Greaves argues that some cases of the common B-ALL ($CD10^+$ $CD19^+$ preB cALL) observed in the peak age of 2 to 5 years could be associated with an aberrant immune response displayed by an immature immune system [3]. This hypothesis is based in the theory that early exposures to common infectious agents are required for the proper maturation of the immune system, lack of these exposures results in aberrant responses when children are finally in contact with the agent(s). In Greaves view, ALL develops in the biological context of an aberrant immune response due to delayed infections, and thus, the infectious agents are only an indirect trigger of the leukemogenic process.

More recently, Greaves has added to his proposal the most frequent chromosomal aberrations in pre-B cALL, hyperdiplody and the translocation TEL-AML1 (also known as ETV6-RUNX1), as susceptibility factors. Molecular analysis has shown shared clonotypic TEL and AML1 breakpoints in leukemic blasts from monochorionic monozygotic identical twins [6]. The same result has been observed when comparing the patients' blood at diagnosis and their blood archived at birth (Guthrie cards) [7]. These results have supported that these genetic insults are often generated *in utero*, based on such findings, Greaves has proposed a minimal 'two-hits' model to explain the development of pre-B cALL [8]. According to this model, hyperdiploidy or the TEL-AML1 translocation originate *in utero* and provide the first oncogenic hit, which is not sufficient for the occurrence of the disease but generates a preleukemic clone. In the presence of additional postnatal oncogenic hits, this susceptible clone then evolves into a malignant leukemic clone. Such additional hits could be promoted indirectly by the aberrant immune response to infection of children growing in microbiological isolated environments.

Greaves' hypothesis is based on the observation of the steady increase of childhood leukemia parallel to the increase of upscale living conditions in developed countries. Since its publication, a series of epidemiological studies have been designed to test the *delayed infection* hypothesis. Evaluation of parity, breastfeeding, improved hygiene conditions, neonatal or infant infections, vaccination against some viruses, day care attendance [9-13] among others, have been used as markers of exposure to infectious agents during the first years of life. As we will see next, these studies have found heterogeneous and even contradictory results.

The United Kingdom Childhood Cancer Study (UKCCS), a nationwide, population based case-control study, was designed to investigate different hypotheses about risk factors in childhood cancer, one of them referred to the association between day care attendance during the first year of life and the risk of developing leukemia [11]. Day care attendance was used as a surrogate marker for exposure to infectious agents, assuming that as more contacts a child has, there is a larger chance for exposure to infections. Data were obtained through interviews with parents of 1286 children with ALL between 2 and 14 years of age and 3605 controls from 10 different regions of the UK. The results showed an inverse relationship between 'social activity' and the risk of leukemia, OR=0.73 (95% confidence interval (CI): 0.62-0.87), showing also a dose-response trend. The interpretation of these findings was that early exposure to infections, indicated by day care attendance, is a protective factor against childhood leukemia, thus supporting Greaves' *delayed infection* proposal [11].

Another study from the same UKCCS data set was published two years later. In this report, it was analyzed the relationship between neonatal infections and risk of leukemia; the data were extracted from primary-care records compiled before diagnosis and interviews with parents. According to this study, children with ALL (ages 2-5 years) had more clinically diagnosed neonatal infections than their counterpart control: episodes number=3.6 (95% CI: 3.3-3.9) *vs* 3.1 (95% CI:2.9-3.2) [14]. These results contrast with the ones from the previous UKCCS study and argue that early infections are a risk factor for ALL, and therefore, give no support to the *delayed infection* hypothesis.

The study by Cardwell and colleagues using hospital records of clinically diagnosed infections in the first year of life from the UK General Practice Research Database (GPRD), compared 162 ALL cases with 2215 matched controls, no differences were found between cases and controls OR=1.05 (95%CI:0.64-1.74), then this study provided no support to Greaves' hypothesis [15]. Another large group, the Northern California study group analyzed day care attendance and parental recall of children ear infections between 294 ALL cases (ages 1-14) and 376 matched controls. Both markers were found protective, OR=0.42 (95% CI:0.18-0.99) and OR=0.32 (95% CI:0.14-0.74), respectively, but only for non-Hispanic white children, supporting Greaves' hypothesis but suggesting ethnic differences in the etiology of ALL [16].

The number of children born in a family has also been used as a marker for microbiological exposure. Dockerty and colleagues investigated the association between parity and risk of ALL in children aged 0-14 from England and Wales. They found a statistically significant protective effect for ALL in children of houses with increasing parity, OR=0.5 (95% CI: 0.3-0.8) [9]. Infante-Rivard et al also evaluated parity and day care attendance in a population based study (491 leukemia cases of children under 10 years old and 491 matched controls) in Quebéc Canada. This group found a protective association with day care attendance, OR=0.49 (95% IC:0.31-0.77) and breast-feeding OR=0.68 (95% IC:0.49-0.95), while having older siblings was associated with increased risk of leukemia, OR=2.12 (95% IC: 1.57-2.85) [12].

The study by Flores-Lujano evaluated the frequency of severe infections that required hospitalization in the first year of life in children with Down's syndrome (DS) with or without ALL (57 cases and 218 controls aged 19 years or younger). In this study, DS children were chosen because it is known that they have an around 10 to 30 fold higher incidence of B cell ALL. They also found an association between infection an increased risk of leukemia, OR=3.45 (95% CI:1.37–8.66), which is against the Greaves' hypothesis [17].

In summary, many studies have explored the *delayed infection* hypotheses with heterogeneous results, with some studies actually showing an increased risk given by infections in the first years of life. The lack of consistency among investigations deserves further analysis and it is beyond the aim of this chapter. Some of the variables among studies are concerned with the methodological approach, study design, statistical tests and the representativeness of the studied population, among many others that could explain the heterogeneity of the results. Many other considerations are more related to the biological aspects of the hypothesis as it is discussed in the integrated discussion with the other hypotheses concerning an infectious origin of childhood leukemia.

3. 'Population mixing' hypothesis by Kinlen

In early 1980, an unusual increase in the incidence of childhood leukemia was observed in young people living in the vicinity of nuclear reprocessing plants in Cumbria, England and Dounreay, Scotland. It was thought that such increase in leukemias was the result of radioactive contamination, which might have caused somatic or germinal line mutations in the population [18-20]. However, in deep tests showed no evidence of radioactive leaks (Committee on Medical Aspects of Radiation in the Environment) or many other types of population occupational exposures [20].

In 1988 Kinlen proposed that the observed leukemia clusters could result from the unusual population mixing occurring in regions receiving the influx of workers and their families who were attracted by new jobs in nuclear plants. Disease outbreaks associated with population growth and migration had been previously documented, and Kinlen hypothesized that this was also the case for the leukemia clusters. During populations mixing, resident people would be naive to infection by different agents carried by the newcomers and vice versa, exposure to such agents would cause an abnormal response leading to the outbreak [4].

Kinlen first proved his *population mixing* hypothesis in Thurso, Scotland, an isolated rural area that received large influxes of people who had migrated to work at a nuclear plant. The results showed that during the period when the population doubled (1951-1967) there was

http://dx.doi.org/10.5772/54455

an increased incidence of childhood leukemia, returning to normal numbers in subsequent years [4]. Other relevant studies of Kinlen's group are concerned with new military settlements; for instance, in post-war Britain between 1949 and 1950, when national military service was mandatory for all men reaching 18 years of age and the period of service was increased from 1 to 2 years. During the following years there was a significant increase of leukemia in areas with the highest proportion of military servicemen. A similar phenomenon was observed in Fallon, Nevada US when there was a considerable increase in the number of trainee recruits in the nearby naval base [21].

Virtually every study that has been led by Kinlen's working group has shown similar results, *i.e.* they have observed a significant increase in childhood leukemia matching large-scale mixing between rural and urban populations. [22-27]. In favor of Kinlen proposal, childhood leukemia clusters were more evident when people from urban regions were mixed with people from isolated areas with low population density, and those who develop leukemia were mostly children from the most immunologically isolated. Also, the leukemia peaks were transitory coinciding with the largest flow of people, arguing against a common source of a persistent chemical/radiation contaminant.

Other researchers have addressed the same question. For example, Koushik and colleagues conducted an ecologic study of childhood leukemia and population mixing in Ontario, Canada. The percent of population change was employed as indicator of mixing population. In this study, 1394 leukemia cases recorded between 1978 and 1992 were included. The results showed that population growth was also associated with a high incidence of leukemia, but only in rural and not in urban areas [28]. Other studies have shown no support for the Kinlen's hypothesis, among them is Laplanche & de Vathaire's [29]. This study included all French communities and covered the period between 1968 and 1990 during which occurred a rapid population increase. According to the results during the mentioned period, deaths from leukemia in children or young adults under 25 years of age were slightly lower than the expected estimate and no differences in risk according to the size of population increase or region were found. Another French study carried around the nuclear reprocessing plant of La Hague found no evidence of increase in childhood leukemia cases [30].

Although, not all the studies carried out around areas of population mixing have correlated with clusters of childhood leukemia, it is relevant that most do. It is also important that, although the original observation was done around nuclear plants, there is evidence of a similar phenomenon occurring in many other regions around non-nuclear sites, including military settlements. From his observations, Kinlen proposed that a common infectious agent could be responsible and adults are the main transmitters, thus population mixing could be responsible for the leukemia cases seen even in the first year of life.

If Kinlen proposal is true, it is possible that the data against his hypothesis had different explanations: 1) the effect may be dose dependent, so, high levels of contact might be necessary; 2) the hypothesis has been proposed for large-scale rural-urban population mixing and many studies might not reach the required population threshold, and 3) other genetic and/or environmental differences might be affecting the outcome [4, 22].

Similar to the Greaves' hypothesis, the identity of the infectious agent(s) involved in Kinlen model is still not known. In fact, most of the population mixing studies had failed to find an increase in a symptomatic infection in adults or children, paralleling the increase in leukemia incidence. Considering that there are viruses of recognized leukemia causality in animals and one human's leukemia caused by a virus, Kinlen has proposed that the agent involved could be a prevalent virus causing an uncommon infection [31]. Kinlen also considers that the putative causative virus is not transmitted as a typical acute infection virus, a characteristic common of tumorigenic viruses. However, the viral family known to be involved in animal leukemia is the retroviridae, and specifically for adult humans the causative agent is the human T cell leukemia/lymphoma virus type 1 (HTLV-1), which is endemic of areas with no recognized picks of childhood leukemia. Because both Kinlen and Greaves models fail to identify the causative agent, both hypotheses seem similar pointing out to a common mechanism of response rather than a possible direct mechanism of infection.

4. Direct viral leukemogenesis hypothesis by Smith

A third hypothesis regarding the infectious etiology of childhood leukemia was proposed by Smith and colleagues. According to the *delayed infection* hypothesis, children exposed to infectious agents during the first months of life (e.g. in developing countries) should have almost no leukemogenic potential, whereas children that become infected later (e.g. in affluent societies), exposure to the same agent would be potentially leukemogenic. Smith disagrees with this scenario, especially for children aged 2 and 3, which represent the larger proportion of children within the peak incidence of 2 to 5 years old, and suggested that there should be an alternative mechanism by which the infection leads to leukemia and that could explain all age-related picks of disease, including infant leukemias [5].

In his publication *Considerations on a possible viral etiology for B-precursor acute lymphoblastic leukemia of childhood* Smith proposed that the infectious process leading to leukemia occurs during intrauterine life by mother to fetus transmission [5]. *De novo* infected seronegative women or those in which the agent reactivation occurred during pregnancy were especially vulnerable to infect their fetus. This hypothesis also considers possible infections during the first year of life of children from seronegative mothers unable to passively immunize their offspring. According to Smith's hypothesis, the pathogen acts through a direct mechanism of B cell infection, initiating or complementing the process of cellular transformation together with additional oncogenic hits either intrauterine or postnatal.

Considering that more than 60% of cases of ALL-B are associated with chromosomal abnormalities, Smith hypothesized that the agent involved should be a virus, since many viral agents present a variety of mechanisms that promote genetic instability. According to Smith's hypothesis the putative virus should have the ability to cross the placenta, to infect B lymphocytes and to have oncogenic potential. However, such agent should not have the ability to induce severe abnormalities, since ALL is not associated with other cancers or birth defects. Thus, an important difference of Smith's hypothesis is that the infection *per se*

http://dx.doi.org/10.5772/54455

carries the power to trigger the chromosomal abnormalities often present in childhood leukemia, while for Greaves, the genetic insult is already present and the infection indirectly promotes the acquisition of additional hits.

Several viral families fulfill Smith's criteria for a causative agent. Members of the adenovirus, herpesvirus and polyomavirus are transmitted very early pre- or post-natally, have tropism for bone marrow cells and have oncogenic potential; we know that most of the population carries all these viruses asymptomatically, with only a few of them developing a related-neoplasia. On the other hand, the retroviruses are also good candidates, as they already have been implicated in leukemias. Several transforming mechanisms have been described for all of these viruses, including expression of constitutively active viral signaling proteins, transcriptional activation of cellular oncogenes and/or disruption of tumor suppressor genes, and importantly, induction of genetic instability; for instance Epstein Barr Virus (EBV or human herpesvirus-4) is associated with Burkitt's lymphoma, in which it also correlates with translocation of the cellular oncogene c-Myc [32].

Studies showing that maternal infections are associated with an increased risk of ALL supported Smith's model. Lehtinen et al analyzed sera of the first trimester from 342 Finnish and Icelandic mothers of children with ALL, searching for antibodies against herpesvirus EBV, cytomegalovirus and HHV-6 (human herpesvirus-6). Only an increase of anti-EBV antibodies was found correlating with leukemia cases, OR=2.9 (95% CI:1.5-5.8) [33]. Because of the nature of the antibodies found, this data suggested EBV reactivation as a potential event leading development of ALL. This same group confirmed the above observation with an additional 304 mothers: anti-EBV reactivation antibodies, OR=1.9 (95% CI:1.2-3.0) [34]. The possible role of EBV reactivation during pregnancy is still awaiting confirmation from other groups. Naumberg's group also found a similar positive association when the mother had lower genital tract infections, OR=1.78 (95% CI:1.2-2.7), especially in children older than 4 years of age at diagnosis, OR=2.01 (95% CI:1.1-3.8) [35].

Many other studies have shown conflicting results between viral infection during pregnancy and subsequent childhood leukemia in offspring, either by influenza virus or by other unspecified common infections [10, 12, 36]. On the other hand, several small studies have found an association between maternal varicella-zoster virus (causing chicken-pox) reactivation and childhood leukemia [37, 38]. Note, however, that none of these approaches have addressed viruses with recognized oncogenic potential and that they are epidemiological studies based on the mother recalled history of infection during pregnancy.

A distinct approach to explore direct transformation occurring *in utero* has been conducted through retrospective analyses of children who developed leukemia; in these studies, viral genomes have been searched in archived blood spots collected at birth with very heterogeneous results. For instance, an early study found blood spots positive to adenovirus-C in two children that developed leukemia, but other groups have not reproduced such result [39]. Bogdanovic et al searched for viral genomes from herpesvirus EBV and HHV-6, polyomavirus JCV and BKV (from the patients' initials from whom the viruses were isolated) and parvovirus 19 in Guthrie cards from 54 Swedish patients, finding no association [40-42]. Parvovirus B19 was another good candidate for causality since it has been associated with several childhood hematological diseases. One should consider that, although the search for viral genomes in Guthrie cards is more stringent, the negative result does not mean that there is not increased viral infection/reactivation during pregnancy and the titer and type of antibodies are probably more reliable markers for this.

Based on Smith's original proposal, the notion of a direct oncogenic mechanism in the etiology of childhood leukemia was widened to include infections with a transforming agent occurring postnatally but prior to the onset of the disease. In this possible leukemogenic mechanism, infection is not necessarily the first oncogenic hit. To test this proposal derived from Smith's hypothesis, different viral agents have been screened directly in the leukemia blast (Table 1). One study evaluated the presence of the viral genome of polyomavirus JCV and BKV in 15 samples at diagnosis of pre-B ALL and a second study included 25 samples in which the viral genome of JCV, BKV and SV40 (simian virus 40) were searched. In both studies, the screening was performed by PCR without finding any of these viruses present in the leukemia samples [43, 44].

Virus	Leukemia subtype	Age (years)	Sample	Screening method	N	Ref.
Polyomaviruses JVC and BKV	B-precursor ALL	1-12	BM or PB	Endpoint PCR	15	[43]
Polyomaviruses JVC, BKV and SV40	B-precursor ALL	2-5	BM	Real-time PCR	25	[44]
Polyomaviruses JVC and BKV	B-precursor ALL T-ALL	0.75-17	Archived neonatal blood spots	Nested PCR	50 4	[40]
Herpesviruses EBV y HHV-6	B-precursor ALL T-ALL	0.75-17	Archived neonatal blood spots	Nested PCR	50 4	[41]
Herpesviruses EBV, HHV-6, -7 and -8	B-precursor ALL	1.5-13	BM or PB	Southern blot (only for EBV) and Real-time PCR	47	[45]
Parvovirus B19	B-precursor ALL T-ALL	0.75-17	Archived neonatal blood spots	Nested PCR	50 4	[42]
Retrovirus BLV	ALL	≤16	BM and PB	Southern blot	131	[46]
Annelovirus TT	ALL	us	BM, PB and CFS	Nested PCR, dot blot and Southern blot	28	[47]

* In this study, the samples were obtained at diagnosis or during treatment. BM: bone marrow, PB: peripheral blood, CSF: cerebrospinal fluid, us: unspecified.

Table 1. Screening for viral sequences in ALL.

Mackenzie et al searched for human herpesvirus-4 (EBV), -6, -7 and -8 (KSHV); 20 peripheral blood or bone marrow samples were tested by Southern blot (EBV) or conventional PCR (HHV -6, -7 and -8). The authors found that seven samples were positive for some of these viruses; however, the low viral load found indicated that the viral genome was not present in every leukemia blast and therefore the result did not support that infection was part of the initial insult that preceded the malignant clonal expansion [45].

Bender et al screened for Bovine leukemia virus (BLV) years before the publication of Smith's proposal. BLV is an exogenous retrovirus whose direct role in the genesis of bovine leukemia has been well documented. 131 samples of ALL (the article did not address a specific subtype of leukemia) and 136 controls were screened by Southern blot for the BLV genome. Cases and controls were negative to the virus arguing against a positive role of BLV in childhood leukemia [46]. Screening for transfusion-transmitted virus (TTV) have also been negative [47].

In summary, different studies have failed to identify viral agents within the leukemia cells indicative of a a viral direct leukemogenic mechanism. However, it is important to consider that these studies included only a small number of samples, 50 or less. These studies at the most suggest that if an infectious agent is involved in leukemogenesis, this would occur in a limited number of cases. A larger number of samples from more geographical regions and different social strata should be included for a more definitive conclusion.

The list of candidate viruses is not exhausted yet and the pathogen involved in the genesis of leukemia (if any) could still be unknown, Kaposi sarcoma associated herpesvirus (KSHV) and Merkel cell polyomavirus (MCPV) were discovered a few years ago and have already been associated with several neoplasias including the ones from which the virus were isolated, Kaposi's sarcoma and Merkel cell carcinoma, respectively [48]. Under this idea, the study of MacKenzie et al was designed to identify undescribed members of the Herpesviridae family by a degenerate PCR, but no new herpesviruses were found in any of the 18 samples analyzed [45]. As the individual virus "hunt" is a limited method, next generation sequencing technologies are an attractive approach to ask for the presence of known and unknown infectious agents in leukemic cells.

5. Space-time clustering of childhood leukemia by Alexander

As we learn in the previous section, childhood leukemia has been shown to be a disease often presented in space and time clusters correlating with communities with large influx of people. Population based morbility/mortality maps are used in public health to inform us of points of an excess of cases (the cluster) relative to the expected incidence, which are then unlikely to have happened by chance and points out to possible etiological factors and the population at risk. Leukemia aggregates have been studied for decades and to date, a number of studies have reported an unusual increase in the number of cases associated with space-time patterns, some of them have been anecdotal reports but others have been discovered through employment of formal statistical analysis. We describe next some cluster studies that have been specifically designed to test the hypothesis of the involvement of infectious agents in the development of childhood leukemia.

Alexander's work is one of the pioneering reports using rigorous statistical methods to determine the existence of spatial temporal clusters as indirect evidence of an infectious etiology for childhood leukemia. The analysis was performed using data obtained from the censuses of 1971 and 1981 in England, Wales and Scotland and was restricted to wards whose contribution to spatial clustering test exceeded an expected, arbitrarily established threshold, from a Poisson distribution on uniform risk of the disease. The report included 487 cases of ALL and other unspecified leukemias. The location at birth was extrapolated from the location data at diagnosis (assuming no changes in residence). The association infection-leukemia was tested from 3 hypothesis envisioned from three different scenarios based on the period of exposure and age of disease presentation:

Period of exposure	Age at presentation
I In utero or around the time of birth	5 years or older
II Post-natal	Under 5 years
III Recent first exposure previous to the onset	'Childhood peak' (ages 2-4 years)

Table 2.

To test these hypotheses, the cases were divided into series A and B, the 'susceptibles' (not exposed) and the 'infectives'. To evaluate spatial and temporal associations, the data were analyzed as pairs of cases; spatial linkage was defined based in location within the same electoral ward. Temporal linkage was an overlap of at least 3 months between the time of presumed susceptibility of the child in series A and infectivity of the child in series B.

The results of this study showed support for the hypothesis I: exposure around the time of birth leads to an increased risk of leukemia whose onset takes place at 5 years or older. At the biological level, the authors interpreted the silent and persistent infection of an agent acquired *in utero* as potentially contributing to the development of the malignancy at any time prior to its presentation. The authors exemplified the process similar to an infection by pestivirus, which however, has not been associated with carcinogenic processes in animals and they are known to induce death even *in utero*. According to this paper, infections did not explain the cases in the 2-5 years old peak, which is the most common in developed countries such as those included in this study [49].

The report of Birch et al, included 798 cases of acute leukemia diagnosed between 1954 and 1985 taken from the Manchester Children's Tumour Registry (MCTR) and aimed to evaluate various scenarios for the infectious etiology of leukemia (cluster criteria were established *a priori* as less than 5 km and less than 1 year apart). To support Greaves', Kinlen's and Smith's proposals, two working hypotheses were established: H1 is true (Greaves and Kinlen hypotheses) and H2 is false (Smith hypothesis). This study also considered 4 possible space-time interactions in which the potentially leukemogenic infection would occur. The different hypothetical scenarios and their associated proposals depending on the type of interaction were as follows:

Interactions	Hypothetical Scenery	Support to
I Between times and places of birth	The infection occurred *in utero* or in early infancy	Smith's hypothesis
II Between times and places of diagnosis	The infection occurred before diagnosis	Greaves' and Kinlen's hypothesis
III Between time of diagnosis and place of birth	The infection occurred before diagnosis	Greaves' and Kinlen's hypothesis
IV Between time of birth and place of diagnosis	No plausible according to previous results	---

Table 3.

To analyze the data, different statistical tests were used and the authors considered mobilization of children from the records of changes of residence. The results showed evidence of space-time clustering based on place of birth and time of diagnosis for the sub-groups aged 0-4 years, but no evidence based on place and time of birth, thus the results lent support to Greaves and Kinlen hypotheses but they did not support Smith's [50].

Methodologies used to search time clusters have also been used to address seasonal variation for childhood leukemia. According to this idea, if an infection is associated with disease, then a seasonal pattern would be expected, either at birth or diagnostic. Perhaps the largest study of this type is the one conducted by Higgins et al, using the population based data from the UK National Registry of Childhood Tumors that included 15,835 leukemia cases from children born and diagnosed between 1953-1995. No seasonality was found in this study after leukemia classification by age, gender or immunophenotype [51]. Similar studies have been conducted in the USA, Singapore and Sweden, founding the same negative result. In all of these studies only some temporal peaks (but no evidence of seasonality) have been observed [52].

Many other studies have provided evidence for space-time clustering of childhood leukemia [53-56]. Some have not addressed a possible infectious explanation but correlated with population mixing. An extreme example was Greece, which experienced one of the largest influx of people from rural to urban settings and presented one of the highest incidences of childhood leukemia around that time [57]. Although, these studies based on the observation of space-time clusters are considered an indirect evidence of the involvement of infectious agents in the etiology of leukemia, the identity of such agent(s) is unknown and therefore the participation of other environmental factors cannot be presently ruled out.

6. Integrative discussion

Indirect evidence supports an association between infections in childhood leukemia, and three hypotheses have been proposed to explain and/or address this question with variable and even opposite results. From these hypotheses, the *delayed infection* by Greaves argues for an indirect role for infection, Smith's hypothesis for a direct causative role and Kinlen's seems to sit in the middle, favoring a direct infection of the cell that will become the leukemic blast but also an indirect mechanism of response still unexplained. In other words, for Greaves, infections in early life are protective and for Kinlen and Smith are a risk factor; for Greaves and Kinlen almost any type of infectious agents (for Kinlen mostly viral) able to trigger aberrant immune or cellular responses could be the causative agent, for Smith it would be viruses with direct oncogenic capacities.

Based mainly in adult cancers, we now know that pathogens contribute to neoplasia through different mechanisms. The classical ones are those in which the agents infect cells and promote oncogenic transformation 'from within', through altering signaling pathways and gene expression programs (supports Smith). Indirect roles (supports Kinlen) include promotion of an inflammatory microenvironment, loss of cancer immune surveillance and a cofactor role helping the tumor through secretion of growth and angiogenic factors. The latter one is the mechanism proposed to explain cytomegalovirus oncomodulatory role in high-grade gliomas and it is thought to be a tumor maintenance rather that an initiating mechanism [58]. From these mechanisms, a direct role would be very possible but so far multiple studies have failed to find evidence of infection by oncogenic agents in the leukemic blast. On the other hand, an inflammatory role is very unlikely because it is generally associated with chronic diseases lasting decades (e.g. *Helicobacter pylori* and hepatitis B and C virus infections). A cofactor or immune suppressive roles are possible, especially for preleukemic clones (e.g. the ones with an early chromosomal abnormality).

Considering all these mechanisms, it is important to acknowledge that the term childhood leukemia harbors many different biological entities, and it is very likely that they involve different mechanisms of origin. Examples of important known differences are the lineage origin of the leukemic blast, myeloid *vs* lymphoid or T cell *vs* B cell. Also, there are at least three recognized B cell immature developmental stages where the leukemia is originated: early proB, preB-I and large preB-II, which are recognized for the differential expression of lineage- and stage- specific antigens and are dependent on the activity of different signaling pathways and transcriptional programs [59].

As mentioned before, childhood leukemia is also associated to chromosomal abnormalities: hyperdiploidy, hypodiploidy and translocations t(12;21)(p13;q22) (TEL-AML1), t(1;19)(q23;p13) (E2A-PBX1), t(9;22)(q34;q11) (BCR-ABL) and t(4;11)(q21;q23) (MLL-AF4) are among the most common in B-ALL. These genetic abnormalities affect specific signaling pathways and favor transcriptional expression profiles related to the developmental stage of the B cell leukemic blast. Therefore, the risk and protection factors driven these known and still many unknown different childhood leukemia entities are probably different and models of the origin of the disease should be restrained to specific subtypes. Because most reports

http://dx.doi.org/10.5772/54455

group together several subtypes of leukemia, ethnic, stage, age and genetic insult, it is difficult to interpret whether they support or reject the different hypothesis of the infectious origin of the disease.

It should be noted that Greaves' hypothesis concerns the common form of B-cell ALL ($CD19^+$, $CD10^+$). This form comprises most of the ALL cases that peak at 2–5 years of age observed in developed countries or in affluent communities that have improved their living standards and have become 'more hygienic' [60]. Through comparison of international reports, variations in the peaks of childhood ALL have been identified. The aforementioned peak at 2–5 years of age is reduced, or even absent, for Black Africans and for other developing communities [61-63]. In Mexico, for example, two incidence peaks have been reported; the first occurring at 2–3 years of age and the second at 6–9 [64]. There is also the infant leukemia (of children under one year old) that is of very bad prognostic and is at least 80% positive to MLL translocations, supporting different etiologies between age groups.

Although, the *delayed infection* and *mixing population* hypotheses exhibit several points in common, they exhibit important differences too, for instance, Greaves' hypothesis is concerned to common childhood leukemia seen in age group of 2 to 5 years, while, Kinlen has not associated the leukemia clusters with a particular subtype of disease and has interpreted his results as all types of childhood leukemia might have a common cause. This argument could weak his hypothesis since a common etiologic mechanism for the different subtypes of the disease is difficult to envision. Also, the largest increase in leukemia cases has been reported for developed countries and Kinlen has not provided an explanation of how his model of large mixing of urban and rural populations can be extrapolated to or represent an affluent or aseptic setting.

Given the multifactorial nature of cancer, the role of other environmental and genetic factor in Kinlen's proposal is also missing. Kinlen's studies often seem to be based in the sole action of an infectious agent, but there are not known examples of infectious agents or oncogenic insults with full penetrance.

Some studies supporting the population mixing proposal have observed a specific increase of infant leukemia, which is mostly associated with MLL translocations. It has been reported that topoisomerase II inhibitors, consumed in some foods during pregnancy or present in drugs commonly used to treat cancer, are a risk factor for this type of translocation [65, 66]. There are not infectious agents known to promote MLL translocation or to inhibit topoisomerase II enzyme. Therefore, how other environmental insults take part in events of population mixing should also be considered. In this scenario, Greaves model seems more complete, since it includes the genetic lesions that characterize childhood leukemia. Greaves usees these genetic lesions to frame a biologically plausible mechanism in which children are more vulnerable to a leukemogenic process after an untimely infection episode. Still, in Greaves model, the first and perhaps more important oncogenic hit happens by chance and therefore his model does not provide an easy target for controlled intervention.

The rise of several types of diseases in recent years, mainly in developed countries, has been proposed to be associated with increasing hygienic conditions. This hygiene hypothesis states that lack of early childhood exposure to microorganisms triggers the appearance of disease [67]. Although Greaves has modeled his *delayed infection* proposal in the *hygiene hypothesis,* there might be subtle differences between both hypotheses. While the *hygiene hypothesis* is highly concerned with acquisition of the human normal flora, Greaves is also concerned with pathogens that are not life threatening when acquired early. There are many examples of the latter and several diseases have been associated to delayed infection, examples of them are EBV or cytomegalovirus-related infectious mononucleosis, measles and chickenpox. In these cases, infection in the first years of life leads to mild to no symptoms, but when acquired late leads to serious and even life threatening diseases and in the case of EBV, it has been proposed that it predisposes to lymphoma. However, the window in which these infections become dangerous are usually beyond the years of the higher incidence pick of childhood leukemia and could only explain leukemia of the teenager or young adult.

Studies in mice are strongly indicative that animals grown in germ free conditions are often immunologically unsuited to fight infections and that perhaps one of the most important components of the immune instruction program is the normal flora [68]. Inoculation of probiotics in germ free mice is associated with development of a regulatory immune response in mucosa (based mainly in frequencies of regulatory T cells and levels of cytokines IL-10 and TGF-β) and equilibrated Th1/Th2/Th17 environments. Same results have been obtained after inoculation with several members of *Bifidobacterium,* which are normal residents of infant feces [69]. Animals without a normal microbiota often develop fatal responses when they are challenged with low doses of otherwise controllable pathogens. These results have supported a model in which humans have co-evolved with their flora and this flora is more than a passive passenger providing multiple benefits to the host. Several lines of evidence support that a normal microbiota is necessary for a healthy host metabolism, and also for what is now known as the microbial immunotraining.

The example of germ free animals, although extreme, points out that looking for infection markers of childhood common pathogens might not be indicative of the normal development and equilibrium of the human microbiota and the immune system, and if it is true that leukemia is the result of an aberrant immune response, then markers of infections are not representative of homeostatic acquisition of the normal human flora. In a similar scenario, infections that may confer risk or protection for leukemia are not necessarily symptomatic, thus, data collection of infections with clinical symptoms would exclude relevant infections to normal immune system development. Also, studies that finding that early symptomatic infections are a risk factor for leukemia might only be reflecting on the antibiotics used to treat those infections and the effects that they had on the establishment of the children normal microbiota.

There are many diseases with increased incidence in affluent societies. Among the most studied are asthma, allergies and type 1 diabetes; several studies have tried to link some of these diseases to childhood leukemia. Linabery et al published a meta-analysis of the different studies searching for association between childhood leukemia and allergy, asthma, eczema and hay fever. Although, this meta-analysis shows a protective effect of these diseases, OR=0.69 (95% CI:0.54-0.89), OR=0.79 (95% CI:0.61-1.02), OR=0.74 (95% CI:0.58-0.96), OR=0.55 (95% CI: 0.46-0.66), respectively, the authors observed high heterogeneity of the data with several studies failing to find an effect [70]. Moreover, the overall protection observed argues that the same hygienic conditions driving allergies are protecting from childhood leukemia. An alternative explanation is that the molecular pathway leading to allergy and the leukemogenesis pathway are mutually exclusive.

A similar approach has been proposed for parasitic infections, since the fall of this type of infection has been parallel to the increase in allergies and childhood leukemia in most developed countries. Furthermore, many parasites drive Th1 immune responses while allergies are associated with Th2 responses providing a feasible biological frame for protection to allergies and perhaps childhood leukemia. A few studies have found a correlation between lack of infection of intestinal parasites and childhood leukemia [71]. However, many autoimmune diseases also explained by the hygiene hypothesis are triggered by Th1 responses, such as type 1 diabetes, confusing a mechanistic explanation for this phenomenon and arguing against a common origin for all these diseases.

7. Conclusion

Different hypotheses have tried to relate the origin of childhood acute lymphoblastic leukemia to infections and epidemiological, clinical and molecular evidence have been searched to support them with highly variable results. ALL is a common term that harbors several diseases varying in their age of presentation, associated genetic lesions, cellular origin and prognosis, probably reflecting different biological origins and thus suggesting different causative factors. Hence, although some of the accumulated evidence favors one or other of the hypotheses there is not a consensus whether infections participate and this participation is through direct or indirect mechanisms of transformation. Although, the postulated mechanisms differ from each other, they are not mutually exclusive. The causal factors of leukemia most probably are influenced by complex environmental and genetic interaction with some of them having greater or lesser roles in different individuals or subtypes of the disease. New approaches and methodologies should be used to provide further data supporting the role of infections. In that scenario, more direct markers of aberrant immune responses should be analyzed to support Greaves proposal. Th1/Th2/Th17 and/or regulatory immune environments should be tested as early as during pregnancy, lactation or in stored newborn blood. Next generation technologies should be used to identify novel infectious agents in ALL samples and to study the microbiota of patients. All these efforts together will result in a better understanding of the role of infectious agents in childhood ALL, their mechanisms of leukemogenesis and will provide better points for disease control.

Acknowledgements

This work was funded by CONSEJO NACIONAL DE CIENCIA Y TECNOLOGIA (CONACYT), Grant 2010-1-141026, IMSS/FIS/PROT 895; CB-2007-1-83949; 2007-1-18-71223, IMSS/FIS/PROT 056.

This chapter constitutes a partial fulfillment of the Graduate Program of Doctor Degree in Biomedical Sciences, Medicine Faculty, National Autonomous University of Mexico, Mexico City, Mexico. A Morales-Sánchez acknowledges the scholarship and financial support provided by the National Council of Science and Technology (CONACyT) and National Autonomous University of Mexico.

Author details

Abigail Morales-Sánchez and Ezequiel M. Fuentes-Pananá*

*Address all correspondence to: empanana@yahoo.com

Unit of Medical Research in Clinical Epidemiology, High Specialty Medical Care Unit of the Pediatric Hospital, National Medical Center XXI Century, Mexican Institute of Social Security, Mexico City, Mexico

References

[1] Parkin DM. The global health burden of infection-associated cancers in the year 2002. International journal of cancer Journal international du cancer 2006;118(12) 3030-3044.

[2] Pui CH, Robison LL, Look AT. Acute lymphoblastic leukaemia. Lancet 2008;371(9617) 1030-1043.

[3] Greaves MF. Speculations on the cause of childhood acute lymphoblastic leukemia. Leukemia 1988;2(2) 120-125.

[4] Kinlen L. Evidence for an infective cause of childhood leukaemia: comparison of a Scottish new town with nuclear reprocessing sites in Britain. Lancet 1988;2(8624) 1323-1327.

[5] Smith M. Considerations on a possible viral etiology for B-precursor acute lymphoblastic leukemia of childhood. Journal of immunotherapy 1997;20(2) 89-100.

[6] Wiemels JL, Cazzaniga G, Daniotti M, Eden OB, Addison GM, Masera G, et al. Prenatal origin of acute lymphoblastic leukaemia in children. Lancet 1999;354(9189) 1499-1503.

[7] Gale KB, Ford AM, Repp R, Borkhardt A, Keller C, Eden OB, et al. Backtracking leukemia to birth: identification of clonotypic gene fusion sequences in neonatal blood spots. Proceedings of the National Academy of Sciences of the United States of America 1997;94(25) 13950-13954.

[8] Greaves M. Childhood leukaemia. British Medical Journal. 2002;324(7332) 283-287.

[9] Dockerty JD, Draper G, Vincent T, Rowan SD, Bunch KJ. Case-control study of parental age, parity and socioeconomic level in relation to childhood cancers. International journal of epidemiology 2001;30(6) 1428-1437.

[10] McKinney PA, Juszczak E, Findlay E, Smith K, Thomson CS. Pre- and perinatal risk factors for childhood leukaemia and other malignancies: a Scottish case control study. British journal of cancer 1999;80(11) 1844-1851.

[11] Gilham C, Peto J, Simpson J, Roman E, Eden TO, Greaves MF, et al. Day care in infancy and risk of childhood acute lymphoblastic leukaemia: findings from UK case-control study. British Medical Journal 2005;330(7503) 1-6.

[12] Infante-Rivard C, Fortier I, Olson E. Markers of infection, breast-feeding and childhood acute lymphoblastic leukaemia. British journal of cancer 2000;83(11) 1559-1564.

[13] Groves FD, Gridley G, Wacholder S, Shu XO, Robison LL, Neglia JP, et al. Infant vaccinations and risk of childhood acute lymphoblastic leukaemia in the USA. British journal of cancer 1999;81(1) 175-178.

[14] Roman E, Simpson J, Ansell P, Kinsey S, Mitchell CD, McKinney PA, et al. Childhood acute lymphoblastic leukemia and infections in the first year of life: a report from the United Kingdom Childhood Cancer Study. American journal of epidemiology 2007;165(5) 496-504.

[15] Cardwell CR, McKinney PA, Patterson CC, Murray LJ. Infections in early life and childhood leukaemia risk: a UK case-control study of general practitioner records. British journal of cancer 2008;99(9) 1529-1533.

[16] Ma X, Buffler PA, Wiemels JL, Selvin S, Metayer C, Loh M, et al. Ethnic difference in daycare attendance, early infections, and risk of childhood acute lymphoblastic leukemia. Cancer epidemiology, biomarkers & prevention: a publication of the American Association for Cancer Research, cosponsored by the American Society of Preventive Oncology 2005;14(8) 1928-1934.

[17] Flores-Lujano J, Perez-Saldivar ML, Fuentes-Panana EM, Gorodezky C, Bernaldez-Rios R, Del Campo-Martinez MA, et al. Breastfeeding and early infection in the aetiology of childhood leukaemia in Down syndrome. British journal of cancer 2009;101(5) 860-864.

[18] Black D, editor. Investigation of the Possible Increased Incidence of Cancer in West Cumbria. Proceedeings of Report of the Independent Advisory Group HMSO. 1984; London.

[19] Heasman MA, Kemp IW, Urquhart JD, Black R. Childhood leukaemia in northern Scotland. Lancet 1986;1(8475) 266.

[20] Gardner MJ, Snee MP, Hall AJ, Powell CA, Downes S, Terrell JD. Results of case-control study of leukaemia and lymphoma among young people near Sellafield nuclear plant in West Cumbria. British Medical Journal 1990;300(6722) 423-429.

[21] Francis SS, Selvin S, Yang W, Buffler PA, Wiemels JL. Unusual space-time patterning of the Fallon, Nevada leukemia cluster: Evidence of an infectious etiology. Chemico-Biological Interaction 2012;196(3) 102-109.

[22] Kinlen LJ. Epidemiological evidence for an infective basis in childhood leukaemia. British journal of cancer 1995;71(1) 1-5.

[23] Kinlen LJ, Balkwill A. Infective cause of childhood leukaemia and wartime population mixing in Orkney and Shetland, UK. Lancet 2001;357(9259) 858.

[24] Kinlen LJ, Clarke K, Hudson C. Evidence from population mixing in British New Towns 1946-85 of an infective basis for childhood leukaemia. Lancet 1990;336(8715) 577-582.

[25] Kinlen LJ, Hudson C. Childhood leukaemia and poliomyelitis in relation to military encampments in England and Wales in the period of national military service, 1950-63. British Medical Journal 1991;303(6814) 1357-1362.

[26] Kinlen LJ, John SM. Wartime evacuation and mortality from childhood leukaemia in England and Wales in 1945-9. British Medical Journal 1994;309(6963) 1197-1202.

[27] Kinlen LJ, Dickson M, Stiller CA. Childhood leukaemia and non-Hodgkin's lymphoma near large rural construction sites, with a comparison with Sellafield nuclear site. British Medical Journal 1995;310(6982) 763-768.

[28] Koushik A, King WD, McLaughlin JR. An ecologic study of childhood leukemia and population mixing in Ontario, Canada. Cancer causes & control : CCC 2001;12(6) 483-490.

[29] Laplanche A, de Vathaire F. Leukaemia mortality in French communes (administrative units) with a large and rapid population increase. British journal of cancer 1994;69(1) 110-113.

[30] Guizard AV, Boutou O, Pottier D, Troussard X, Pheby D, Launoy G, et al. The incidence of childhood leukaemia around the La Hague nuclear waste reprocessing plant (France): a survey for the years 1978-1998. Journal of Epidemiology and Community Health 2001;55(7) 469-474.

[31] Kinlen L. Childhood leukaemia, nuclear sites, and population mixing. British journal of cancer 2011;104(1) 12-18.

[32] Sompallae R, Callegari S, Kamranvar SA, Masucci MG. Transcription profiling of Epstein-Barr virus nuclear antigen (EBNA)-1 expressing cells suggests targeting of chromatin remodeling complexes. PLoS One 2010;5(8) e12052.

[33] Lehtinen M, Koskela P, Ogmundsdottir HM, Bloigu A, Dillner J, Gudnadottir M, et al. Maternal herpesvirus infections and risk of acute lymphoblastic leukemia in the offspring. American journal of epidemiology 2003;158(3) 207-213.

[34] Tedeschi R, Bloigu A, Ogmundsdottir HM, Marus A, Dillner J, dePaoli P, et al. Activation of maternal Epstein-Barr virus infection and risk of acute leukemia in the offspring. American Journal of Epidemiology 2007;165(2) 134-137.

[35] Naumburg E, Bellocco R, Cnattingius S, Jonzon A, Ekbom A. Perinatal exposure to infection and risk of childhood leukemia. Medical and pediatric oncology 2002;38(6) 391-397.

[36] Little J. Epidemiology of Childhood Cancer. 1st edition. 1999.

[37] Blot WJ, Draper G, Kinlen L, Wilson MK. Childhood cancer in relation to prenatal exposure to chickenpox. British Journal of Cancer 1980;42(2) 342-344.

[38] Adelstein AM, Donovan JW. Malignant disease in children whose mothers had chickenpox, mumps, or rubella in pregnancy. British Medical Journal 1972;164(5841) 629-631.

[39] Vasconcelos GM, Kang M, Pombo-de-Oliveira MS, Schiffman JD, Lorey F, Buffler P, et al. Adenovirus detection in Guthrie cards from paediatric leukaemia cases and controls. British Journal of Cancer 2008;99(10) 1668-1672.

[40] Priftakis P, Dalianis T, Carstensen J, Samuelsson U, Lewensohn-Fuchs I, Bogdanovic G, et al. Human polyomavirus DNA is not detected in Guthrie cards (dried blood spots) from children who developed acute lymphoblastic leukemia. Medical and Pediatric Oncology 2003;40(4) 219-223.

[41] Bogdanovic G, Jernberg AG, Priftakis P, Grillner L, Gustafsson B. Human herpes virus 6 or Epstein-Barr virus were not detected in Guthrie cards from children who later developed leukaemia. British Journal of Cancer 2004;91(5) 913-915.

[42] Isa A, Priftakis P, Broliden K, Gustafsson B. Human parvovirus B19 DNA is not detected in Guthrie cards from children who have developed acute lymphoblastic leukemia. Pediatric Blood Cancer 2004;42(4) 357-360.

[43] MacKenzie J, Perry J, Ford AM, Jarrett RF, Greaves M. JC and BK virus sequences are not detectable in leukaemic samples from children with common acute lymphoblastic leukaemia. British journal of cancer 1999;81(5) 898-899.

[44] Smith MA, Strickler HD, Granovsky M, Reaman G, Linet M, Daniel R, et al. Investigation of leukemia cells from children with common acute lymphoblastic leukemia for genomic sequences of the primate polyomaviruses JC virus, BK virus, and simian virus 40. Medical and pediatric oncology 1999;33(5) 441-443.

[45] MacKenzie J, Gallagher A, Clayton RA, Perry J, Eden OB, Ford AM, et al. Screening for herpesvirus genomes in common acute lymphoblastic leukemia. Leukemia 2001;15(3) 415-421.

[46] Bender AP, Robison LL, Kashmiri SV, McClain KL, Woods WG, Smithson WA, et al. No involvement of bovine leukemia virus in childhood acute lymphoblastic leukemia and non-Hodgkin's lymphoma. Cancer Research 1988;48(10) 2919-2922.

[47] Shiramizu B, Yu Q, Hu N, Yanagihara R, Nerurkar VR. Investigation of TT virus in the etiology of pediatric acute lymphoblastic leukemia. Pediatric Hematology and Oncology 2002;19(8) 543-551.

[48] Feng H, Shuda M, Chang Y, Moore PS. Clonal integration of a polyomavirus in human Merkel cell carcinoma. Science 2008;319(5866) 1096-1100.

[49] Alexander FE. Space-time clustering of childhood acute lymphoblastic leukaemia: indirect evidence for a transmissible agent. British Journal of Cancer 1992;654 589-592.

[50] Birch JM, Alexander FE, Blair V, Eden OB, Taylor GM, McNally RJ. Space-time clustering patterns in childhood leukaemia support a role for infection. British Journal of Cancer 2000;82(9) 1571-1576.

[51] Higgins CD, dos-Santos-Silva I, Stiller CA, Swerdlow AJ. Season of birth and diagnosis of children with leukaemia: an analysis of over 15 000 UK cases occurring from 1953-95. British Journal of Cancer 2001;84(3) 406-412.

[52] Gao F, Nordin P, Krantz I, Chia KS, Machin D. Variation in the seasonal diagnosis of acute lymphoblastic leukemia: evidence from Singapore, the United States, and Sweden. American Journal of Epidemiology 2005;162(8) 753-763.

[53] Alexander FE, Boyle P, Carli PM, Coebergh JW, Draper GJ, Ekbom A, et al. Spatial temporal patterns in childhood leukaemia: further evidence for an infectious origin. EUROCLUS project. British Journal of Cancer 1998;77(5) 812-817.

[54] Alexander FE, Boyle P, Carli PM, Coebergh JW, Draper GJ, Ekbom A, et al. Spatial clustering of childhood leukaemia: summary results from the EUROCLUS project. British Journal of Cancer 1998;77(5) 818-824.

[55] Alexander FE, Chan LC, Lam TH, Yuen P, Leung NK, Ha SY, et al. Clustering of childhood leukaemia in Hong Kong: association with the childhood peak and common acute lymphoblastic leukaemia and with population mixing. British Journal of Cancer 1997;75(3) 457-463.

[56] McNally RJ, Alexander FE, Birch JM. Space-time clustering analyses of childhood acute lymphoblastic leukaemia by immunophenotype. British Journal of Cancer 2002;87(5) 513-515.

[57] Kinlen LJ, Petridou E. Childhood leukemia and rural population movements: Greece, Italy, and other countries. Cancer Causes Control 1995;6(5) 445-450.

[58] Michaelis M, Doerr HW, Cinatl J. The story of human cytomegalovirus and cancer: increasing evidence and open questions. Neoplasia 2009:11(1) 1-9.

[59] Perez-Vera P, Reyes-Leon A, Fuentes-Panana EM. Signaling proteins and transcription factors in normal and malignant early B cell development. Bone Marrow Research 2011:502751.

[60] Greaves M. Childhood leukaemia. British Medical Journal 2002;324(7332) 283-287.

[61] Brown WM, Doll R. Leukaemia in Childhood and Young Adult Life. British Medical Journal 1961;1(5231) 981-988.

[62] Hewitt D. Some features of leukaemia mortality. British Journal of Preventive & Social Medicine 1955;9(2) 81-88.

[63] Ramot B, Magrath I. Hypothesis: the environment is a major determinant of the immunological sub-type of lymphoma and acute lymphoblastic leukaemia in children. British Journal Haematology 1982;50(2) 183-189.

[64] Bernaldez-Rios R, Ortega-Alvarez MC, Perez-Saldivar ML, Alatoma-Medina NE, Del Campo-Martinez Mde L, Rodriguez-Zepeda Mdel C, et al. The age incidence of childhood B-cell precursor acute lymphoblastic leukemia in Mexico City. Journal of Pediatric Hematology/Oncology 2008;30(3) 199-203.

[65] Felix CA. Secondary leukemias induced by topoisomerase-targeted drugs. Biochimica et Biophysica Acta 1998;1400 233–255.

[66] Spector LG, Xie Y, Robison LL, Heerema NA, Hilden JM, Lange B, Felix CA, Davies SM, Slavin J, Potter JD, Blair CK, Reaman GH, Ross JA. Maternal diet and infant leukemia: the DNA topoisomerase II inhibitor hypothesis: a report from the children's oncology group. Cancer Epidemiology, Biomarkers and Prevention 2005;14(3) 651-655.

[67] Yazdanbakhsh M, Kremsner PG, van Ree R. Allergy, parasites and the hygiene hypothesis. Science 2002;296(5567) 490-494.

[68] Tlaskalova-Hogenova H, Stepankova R, Kozakova H, Hudcovic T, Vannucci L, Tuckova L, et al. The role of gut microbiota (commensal bacteria) and the mucosal barrier in the pathogenesis of inflammatory and autoimmune diseases and cancer: contribution of germ-free and gnotobiotic animal models of human diseases. Cellular and Molecular Immunology 2011;8(2) 110-120.

[69] Qiurong L. Reciprocal Interaction between commensal microbiota and mucosal immune system. Journal of Immunodeficiency and Disorders 2012;1(1) 1-2.

[70] Linabery AM, Jurek AM, Duval S, Ross JA. The association between atopy and childhood/adolescent leukemia: a meta-analysis. American Journal of Epidemiology 2010;171(7) 749-764.

[71] Rivera-Luna R, Cardenas-Cardos R, Martinez-Guerra G, Ayon A, Leal C, Rivera-Ortegon F. Childhood acute leukemia and intestinal parasitosis. Leukemia 1989;3(11) 825-826.

Section 2

Pathophysiology of ALL

Chapter 3

Pathophysiology of Acute Lymphoblastic Leukemia

M. P. Gallegos-Arreola, C. Borjas-Gutiérrez,
G. M. Zúñiga-González, L. E. Figuera,
A. M. Puebla-Pérez and J. R. García-González

Additional information is available at the end of the chapter

http://dx.doi.org/10.5772/54652

1. Introduction

The Acute lymphoblastic leukemia (ALL), it produced as a result of a process of malignant transformation of a progenitor lymphocytic cell in the B and T lineages. In ALL, the majority of the cases, the transformation affects the B lineage cells. Leukemia and other cancers share biological characteristics, as clonality. The molecular alterations that are required for the development of a malignant disease is a rare phenomenon when one considers the large number of target cells susceptible to this condition, in other words, a single genetic change rarely be sufficient for developing a malignant tumor. This means that a small percentage of people (1%) who develop malignant hematological disease, probably only 1 cell mutated in a critical gene for the proliferation, differentiation and survival of progenitor cells. There is evidence supporting a sequential multistep process, of alterations in several oncogenes in tumor suppressor genes or microRNA genes in cancerigen cells.

Genes Involved in leukemia

Most of what is known of the influence of some mutant genes of the origin of leukemia, derived from studies in molecular virology, in the gene transfection, and in the generation of leukemia in-vivo in transgenic mice. These studies are based on bacterial DNA recombinant methods. Most of the mutations in leukemia are acquired and occur in the lymphoid cell progenitor, less frequently (1% to 5% of leukemia) the mutated genes are inherited, this involved a numerical chromosome abnormality, for example: constitutive trisomy 21.

Genetic factors of acute leukemia have been extensively studied. The results of studies of gene expression analysis of high resolution whole genome, copy number alterations of DNA, loss of heterozygosity epigenetic changes and whole genome sequencing, have allowed the recognition of new genetic alterations, so that virtually all patients with ALL can be classified according to the specific genetic abnormality. This information has increased our knowledge of leukemogenesis, the prognosis and has served as the basis for the development of the target therapy. However, the understanding of how genetic alterations collaborate to induce leukemic transformation remains unclear.

The altered genes in the leukemia can be result in loss or gain of the function through several mechanisms, for example: abnormal recombination (chromosomal, translocation, inversion, insertion) loss of genetic material (deletion) gain of genetic material (duplication) point mutation and the presence additional copies of certain chromosomes as in the case of hyperdiploidy; previous alterations favoring the activation of oncogenes, this encode proteins that control cells proliferation, apoptosis or both.

The advances in the conventional cytogenetic techniques, as the fluorescence *in situ* hybridization, have shown the chromosomal rearrangements. In this sense, recently has been reported that the incidence of chromosomal change is related with the age, so the translocation t(9;22)(q34;q11) increases in each successive decade, up to 24% between the 40-to 49 years old, the t(4;11) (q21;q23) and t(1;19) (q23;q13) are rare in patients older than 60 years old, but t (8;14)(q24;q32) and t(14;18)(q32;q21) increased with age. The hiperdipoidia occurs in 13% of patients under 20 years old and only 5% of elderly patients. The hypodiploidy and complex karyotype (presence of more than 2 chromosomal abnormalities) also increase with age of 4% in the range of 15 to 19 years old to 16% older than 60 years old.

When an oncogen is activated by mutation, encoded protein is structurally modified so that enhances its transforming activity, thus remains on active status, continuously transmitting signals through the binding of tyrosine and treonina cinasa. These signals induce cell growth continued incessant. This mechanism of activation of ocogenes is more evident in others forms of leukemia, for example: severe myeloblastic leukemia and other myelodysplastic syndromes where the genes NRAS are mutated. There are mutations that suppress the function and are observe in tumor suppressor genes such as TP53, however, less than 3% of patients with ALL are TP53 mutations, although all cells have a resistance abnormal apoptosis induced by lack of significant proportion of p53, which is explained in large part by epigenetic medications.

By other hand, some authors have found alterations in the number of copies (ANCs) to 50 recurrent regions in ALL, some are really small and they have less than 1 Mb, however occur in genes encoding regulatory proteins of normal lymphoid development in 40% of cases of ALL progenitors B. The target most common are lymphoid transcription factor PAX5 that have deletions or amplifications until 30% of cases with ALL-B, also found in genes ANCs of transcription factor IKZF1 the IKZF3, EBF1, LEF1 and TCF3, RAG1 and RAG2.

Another important point, is the dihydrofolate reductase (DHFR) gene amplification has been considered as the most relevant in the ALL, this amplification produce cytogenetic abnormalities evident as the amplified of high DNA segment that included some hundreds of kilobases.

The ALL of T-cell type represents about 10% to 15% of the ALL in adults and the 25% in children and their clinical behavior is the most aggressive, the patients have a higher percentage of failure of remission induction, relapse rate is also higher, and had infiltration at central nervous system compared with B-cell ALL. In this sense, is known that the oncogenes and tumor suppressor genes are implicated in ALL-T are: c-MYC, NOTCH, LMO1 / 2, LYL1, TAL1 / 2, Hox11 and HOX11L2. It is clear that NOTCH activated is able to induce leukemogenesis of T cell and this is critical for the progression to ALL-T. Family members of NOTCH are transmembrane receptors that are involved in controlling the differentiation, proliferation and apoptosis in several cell types including T cells. The binding of its ligand to the extracellular domain, resulting in cleavage of the intracellular domain of NOTCH, this reaction is catalyzed by γ-secretase complex, and the intracellular domain free of translocase to the nucleus, that regulates transcription of genes regulated by NOTCH.

The NOTCH target genes are mainly cyclina D1 and c-Myc. Both NOTCH as c-MYC regulate cell cycle progression by inducing expression of cyclins and reduced expression of p27. An important aspect is that NOTCH is able to inhibit apoptosis induced by p53 allowing the tumor regression. In the development of ALL-T there is strong evidence of pro-oncogenic function of signals transduced by NOTCH, and that modulates the activity of downstream signaling pathways, through transcriptional regulation of their target genes. Is possible regulators of signaling downstream of NOTCH especially in murine models are some intermediate signaling routes as: phosphatidylinositol 3-kinase (PI3K), Akt / protein kinase B, extracellular signal-regulated kinase-1/2, and nuclear factor kB. In general, the products of oncogenes can be classified into six categories: transcription factors, chromatin remodeling, growth factors, growth factor receptors, signal transducers, and finally regulators of apoptosis. Transcription factors generally require interacting with other proteins to act, for example: Fos transcription protein dimerizes with the transcription factor Jun to form the AP1 transcription factor is really a complex, and this increases the expression of several genes control cell division, all they have been involved in the development of leukemia.

Aberrant methylation of CpG sites in promoter regions of genes has been identified in ALL cell lines, to respect it is important to note that methylation of CpG dinucleotides in position near the site of transcription initiation can silence gene expression, hypermethylation of tumor suppressor genes and hypomethylation of oncogenes can lead to various forms of cancer.

Other mechanism important in the development of the ALL is the angiogenesis and signal transducers on the binding of tyrosine kinase receptors, finally the molecules regulators of the apoptosis, where the BCL2 gene encodes for a cytoplasmic protein that is localized in the mitochondria and increases the survival of the cell by inhibiting apoptosis.

Secondary leukemias

Secondary hematological malignancies are a serious complication of cancer treatment. They usually manifest as acute leukemias and myelodysplastic syndromes. This also touch the item on secondary leukemias and its frequency is high and has increased possibly due to increasingly frequent use of genotoxic agents and by increased survival to other types of cancer. So, learn more about these could eventually help reduce its appearance. It is known that this type of leukemia may arise as a result to exposure to cytotoxic treatments (side effects of genotoxicity) and / or radiation therapy and as a result of other blood disorders; probably as a result of environmental or genetic causes. In particular in this we will focus more on the former. In most cases it is suggested that the mechanism of leukemogenesis is associated with DNA damage of hematopoietic cells from bone marrow by agents such as those used in chemotherapy. Although the majority of secondary leukemias are acute myeloid leukemia (AML) has been reported cases of lymphoid leukemia and chronic myeloid leukemia (CML) associated with chemotherapy treatments. Finally, we intend to touch points as the classification of secondary leukemias, its relationship to chemotherapeutic agents and ionizing radiation, etiology, individual susceptibility, pathogenesis, and treatment as well as their behavior in infants and adults.

In this way one can conclude that the pathophysiology of ALL involved mechanisms genetic and environmental complex at different levels, and also have a close and complex relationship. The key features in the pathophysiology of the ALL is its monoclonal origin, uncontrolled cell proliferation by sustained self-stimulation of their receptors for growth, no response to inhibitory signals, and cellular longevity conditioned by decreased apoptosis.

Acute lymphoblastic leukemia (ALL) is the result of a process of malignant transformation of progenitor cell lineage of the B and T lymphocytes. (Pui et al, 2011) In most cases of ALL, this transformation affects B lineage cells. (Heltemes et al, 2011)

In the last 3 decades, there has been a significantly improvement in treatment outcome of ALL in children, 70% to 80% of children can get cured of their disease, a situation that is different in adults with ALL, since only 30% -35% of them may heal. (Sotk et al, 2000; Mullighan and Downing, 2009)

The required molecular alterations, for the development of malignant disease, are a rare phenomenon, when it is considered the large number of target susceptible cells to such alteration (Greaves, 2002) ie, a single genetic change is unlikely to be sufficient for the development of a malignant tumor (Croce, 2008), this means that in a very low percentage of people (1%) is developed a hematologic malignancy, only 1 cell will likely experience a mutation in a critical gene for proliferation, differentiation and survival of progenitor cells (Greaves, 2002), that`s what we mean when we mention the monoclonal origin of cancer.

It is important to mention that when we refer to the origin of cancer, in this cases ALL, reference is made to the terms: Cell Origin and Stem Cell Cancer. Actually, the concept implies that normal cells of distinct origin acquire the first mutation(s) to promote cancer, ie, that is the cell that will initiate the cancer, while the cancer stem cell will disseminate it (figure 1). (Visvader, 2011)

Malignant diseases, including acute leukemias, show a marked heterogeneity in cellular morphology, rate of proliferation, genetic lesions and, as a result, the response to treatment. The molecular mechanisms, underlying the heterogeneity of malignant neoplasia, are important points in the study of the cancer's biology. (Visvader, 2011) Above mentioned alterations may be due to somatic mutations, although alterations in the germline may predispose to familial (or hereditary) cancers. (Croce, 2008)

http://dx.doi.org/10.5772/54652

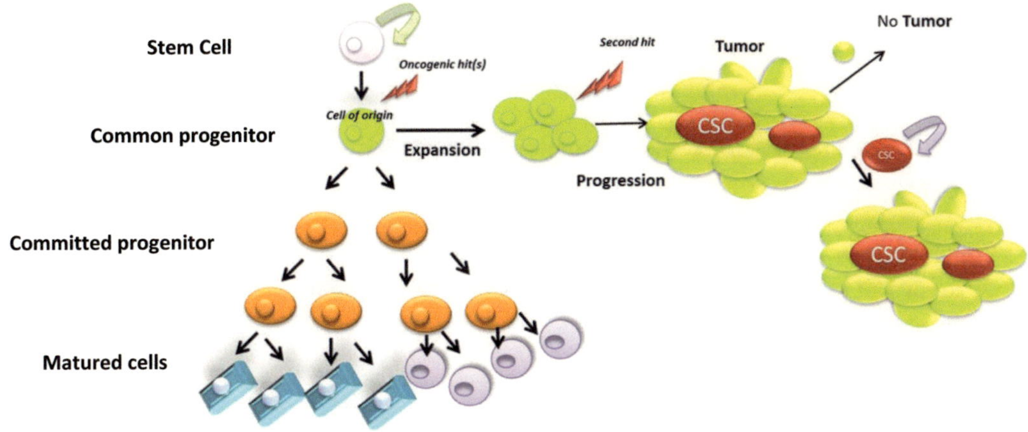

Figure 1. Cell origin and evolution of a cancer stem cell (modified of Visvader, 2011)

There is growing evidence that supports a multi-step process in leukemogenesis, ie, sequential steps and serial number of alterations in oncogenes, tumor suppressor genes, or microRNA genes in cancer cells. (Greaves, 2002; Croce, 2008) Oncogenes are dominant genes that once mutated, from a normal cellular gene (proto), encode abnormal proteins that cannot control cell proliferation, apoptosis, or both, thereby contributing to cancer development. (Pierce, 2009)

A suppressor gene normally inhibits cell division, and favors the growth of cancer when both alleles are mutated, i.e., they are recessive mutations, where the lack of function of both alleles is promoting the development of malignancy. (Pierce, 2009)

Unlike the genes involved in cancer development, microRNA genes do not encode proteins, their products are small RNA molecules (single strands of 21 to 23 nucleotides) that recognize and bind a nucleotide sequence of messenger RNA (mRNA), to the complementary microRNA sequence, and thus blocking the translation of protein from mRNA; then, their function is to regulate gene expression. (Calin et al., 2002; Croce, 2008)

2. Genes involved in the leukemias

Much of what we know about the great influence of certain mutant genes, in the origin of leukemia, is derived from mouse transgenesis studies in molecular virology, with gene transfection and the generation of leukemia *in vivo*. These studies are based on bacterial recombinant DNA methods. (Pui et al, 2011)

This knowledge has increased our understanding of leukemogenesis and prognosis, and additionally has served as foundation for the development of targeted therapy. However, the comprehension of how genetic alterations that collaborate to induce leukemic transformation is not clear yet.(Pui et al, 2011)

Most mutations in leukemia are acquired, and occur *de novo* in the lymphoid progenitor cells, less frequently (1% to 5% of leukemias) the mutated genes are inherited (vgr, p53, DNA ligase), or a numeric chromosomal abnormality is involved, for example constitutive trisomy 21. (Greaves, 2002)

Acute leukemias are the most studied malignant disorders from a genetic standpoint, the results of whole-genome studies, e.g.: gene expression analysis of high-resolution, genome-wide alterations in DNA copy number variation (CNA), loss of heterozygosity, epigenetic changes, and complete genome sequencing have favored the recognition of new genetic alterations, then virtually all patients with LLA can be classified according to the specific genetic abnormality, as shown in Figure 2, which is evident in children with ALL the high frequency of genetic abnormalities. (Mullighan et al, 2007; Pui et al, 2011)

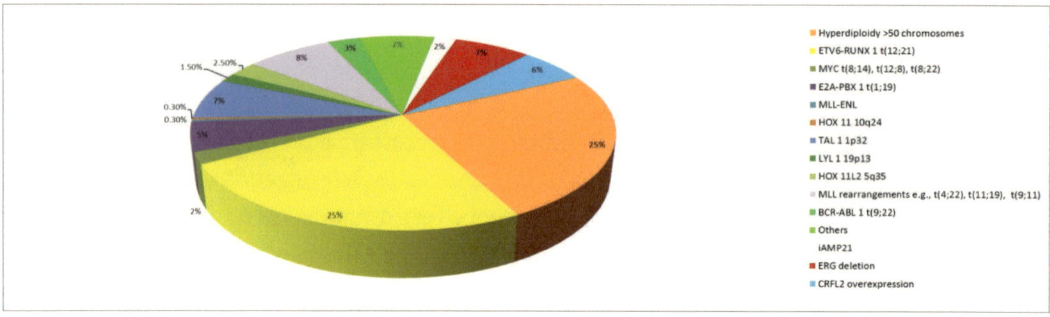

Figure 2. Frequency of genetic abnormalities in childrenwith ALL. (modified of Puiet al, 2011.)

As discussed previously, the altered genes in leukemia can result in loss or gain of function, and this is achieved through various mechanisms, for example, abnormal recombination (chromosomal translocation, inversion, or insertion), loss of genetic material (deletion), gain of genetic material (duplication), or mutation. Also can be present additional copies of certain chromosomes, as in the case of hyperdiploidy. With these chromosomal alterations, the activation of oncogenes is favored. Oncogenes can be activated by: chromosomal rearrangements, gene mutation and gene amplification. (Croce, 2008)

i. The demonstration of chromosomal rearrangements have been evidenced by improved conventional of cytogenetic study. The standard analysis can detect primary chromosomal abnormalities in more than 75% of all cases. (Liang et al, 2010)

Recently, it was reported that the incidence of chromosomal alterations is associated with age. (Moorman et al, 2010) In fact, age is a determining factor in the prognosis and treatment outcome for patients with ALL. In long term survival, the rates are close to 80% in children under 5 years of age, but will decrease to 50% or 60% in adolescents and young adults, and approximately 30% in adults of 45 to 54 years, but rarely exceed 15% in older adults. The Philadelphia chromosome (Ph) is the most common cytogenetic abnormality associated with ALL in adults. (Zuo et al, 2010; Lee et al, 2011)

http://dx.doi.org/10.5772/54652

The Philadelphia chromosome positive (Ph+) ALL is a product of reciprocal translocation between the long arm of chromosome 9(q34), where the oncogene *ABL1* is located, and the long arm of chromosome 22(q11), where the *BCR* gene lies, leading to the formation of the BCR-ABL1 chimeric protein (Figure 3), and as a result of this fusion the Bcr-Abl tyrosine kinase, constitutively active, is produced, which is responsible for the acute and chronic leukemia forms. (Martinelli et al, 2009)

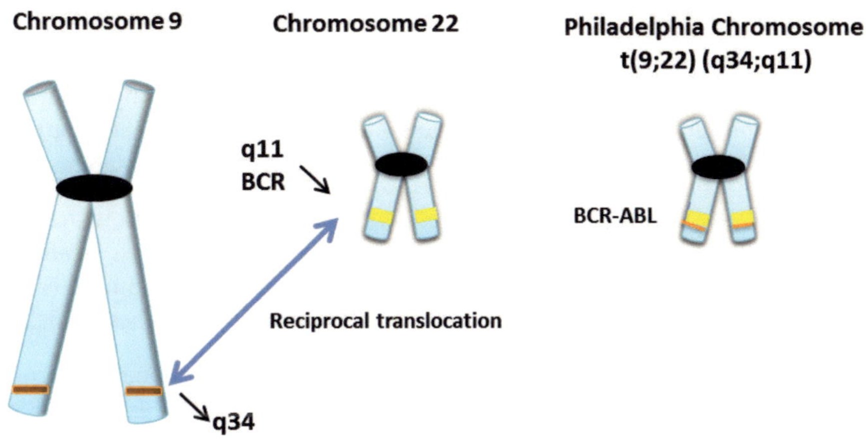

Figure 3. Philadelphia chromosome translocation (translocation between 9 and 22 chromosomes). (modified of Satter-and James, 2003)

This alteration is relatively rare (approximately 5%) in infants with ALL, but not in adults where its frequency range between 20% and 30%, it was the first known cytogenetic abnormality associated with chronic myeloid leukemia (CML) and Ph+ALL.

Despite the Ph+ ALL occurs in only about 5% of patients under 20 years of age, the incidence increases to 33% in patients over 40 years and it reaches 49% in patients over 40 years, to decrease the incidence to 35% in patients over 60 years. (Lee et al, 2011)

A significant proportion of patients with ALL Ph+ (approximately 85%), and high-risk ALL without BCR-ABL1 fusion (~28%), have *IKZF1* gene deletion, and both situations are associated with adverse prognosis. (Martinelli et al, 2009; Cazzaniga et al, 2011)

The gene *IKZF1* is located on 7p12, and encodes the transcription factor Ikaros, which is a member of the family of transcription factors containing zinc fingers (Martinelli et al, 2009). Deletion of *IKZF1* is not observed in the chronic phase of CML, but is detected in two out of three samples analyzed during the lymphoid blast crisis. (Mullighan et al, 2009) *IKZF1* genomic alterations, causing loss expression or expression of dominant negative isoforms, are critical in the pathogenesis of BCR-ABL1 ALL Ph+. (Mullighan et al, 2009)

Almost half of patients with BCR-ABL1 ALL and lymphoid blast crisis CML also harbor deletion of *CDKN2A/B and PAX5* genes; approximately 20% of these cases have deletion of the three genes. These data support the concept that it is required the alteration of several cellular pathways to induce the development of **ALL**. It has been correlated the *ALL IKZF1* focal deletion with clinical response to treatment, overall response rate of relapse and disease-free survival; and it has also been shown that deletion of Ikaros gene represents the most important prognostic factor so far described, in ALL Ph+.(Mullighanh et al, 2009; Martinelli et al, 2009)

Other chromosomal abnormalities associated with age are the t(4;11)(q21;q23) and t(1;19)(q23;p13), that are rare in patients older than 60 years of age, but on the other way t(8;14)(q24;q32) and t(14;18)(q32;q21) increases with age. (Moorman et al, 2010)

The translocation t(4;11)(q21;q23) leads to the formation of the *MLL-AF4* fusion gene, and is responsible for more than 50% of ALL cases in children younger than 6 months in 10-20% of older infants, in approximately 2% of children and only 10% of adults with *de novo* ALL. Chromosomal abnormality in adults with ALL is considered to be of high risk. (Marchesi et al, 2011)

The gene Mixed Lineage Leukemia (*MLL*) is frequently involved in hematological malignancies, particularly acute leukemia, both lymphoblastic and myeloblastic, it is located at 11q23, and plays an important role in the positive regulation of gene expression during early embryonic development (ie it is a HOX gene) and also in hematopoiesis. (Marchesi et al, 2011)

MLL gene encodes a 500 kD protein containing several conserved functional domains, a target of proteolytic activity of Caspasa 1, a cleaving protein specialized in N-terminal fragments of 320 kD and C-terminal of 180 kD. This latter is responsible for methyltransferase activity in lysine 4 of histone H3 (H3K4), which mediates changes in chromatin associated with epigenetic transcriptional activation. (Milne et al, 2002; Hsieh et al, 2003)

The main chromosomal alterations that may occur with the *MLL* gene are mainly reciprocal translocations, causing fusion with other different genes, and partial tandem duplication of genes. (Schnittger et al, 2000)

Translocations in which *MLL* gene is involved can result in a chimeric protein, that fuses the MLL N-terminal with the C-terminal portion of the associated genes; the methyltransferase domain (SET domain) is invariably lost in the MLL fusion protein. This fusion of genes can alter normal cellular proliferation and differentiation processes, which favors leukemogenesis. (Ayton et al, 2001)

MLL gene is a target of about 104 different rearrangements, of which 64 are translocations with other genes. The proteic products of the fusions are nuclear localization signals, and play an important function as potent transcription factors. (Meyer et al, 2009)

Genes that most commonly fuses with *MLL* gene are, in order of frequency: *AF4, AF9, ENL, AF10, AF6, ELL,* and *AF1P*. The leukemias that express the fusion gene *MLL-AF4* are diagnosed primarily as pro-B, in pediatric and adult patients, while the fusion with genes *AF9, AF6,* or *AF10* are common in AML subtypes myelomonocytic or monoblastic variety. (Kohlmann et al, 2005; Moriya et al, 2012)

The t(1;19)(q23;p13) is recurrent in children and adults, and results from the fusion of gene TCF3 transcription factor 3 (E2A immunoglobulin enhancer binding factors E12/E47) locat-

http://dx.doi.org/10.5772/54652

ed at 19p13.3, with gene pre-B-cell leukemia homeobox 1 (*PBX1*), located at 1q23.3, the fusion gene *TCF3 (E2A)-PBX1* encodes a chimeric protein with transforming properties. (Garg et al, 2009)

The gene encoding E2A transcription factors E12 and E47 binds enhancer elements of the gene of κ light chains of immunoglobulins, as well as some other gene regulatory elements. (Garg et al, 2009)

The transcriptional activator domain of the chimeric protein encoded by the fusion gene *E2A-PBX1* is provided by *E12/E47*, and the DNA binding domain is provided by the (HOX) Homebox *PBX1*, this protein promotes leukemogenesis by activation of several genes that are not normally expressed in lymphoid tissues. (Garg et al, 2009)

The t(12; 21)(p13, q22) is a consequence of gene fusion *ETV6/RUNX1* (also known as *TEL/AML1*) and is the hallmark of one of the most common genetic subtypes of ALL of precursor of B cells in children, in whom is the most common molecular genetic alteration occurring in 20% to 25% of pediatric cases; while in adults this translocation is rare. (Pui et al, 2011)

The current model involves several steps, the fusion of these genes can occur already during fetal development and is the initial event, but is not sufficient for the neoplastic transformation (Fuka et al, 2011). Indeed, the development of ALL of infancy B cell lineage involves (at least) 2 genetic events (hits), the first of which often arises in prenatal stage. (Thomsen et al, 2011)

The fusion gene that encodes a chimeric transcription factor, involves the N-terminus of the protein ETV6 and the most of the RUNX1 protein, it is believed that normally RUNX1 acts as a modulator of transcription; transcriptional repressor becomes the target genes *RUNX1*. (Fuka et al, 2011)

Hyperdiploidy is detected in approximately 25-30% of children with ALL precursor B cells. In these patients the clinical phenotype is usually associated with low risk and good prognosis. (Grumayer et al, 2002; Pui et al, 2011) It is interesting to mention that a hyperdiploid karyotype refers to a higher number of chromosomes than the normal diploid number (e.i., greater than 46 chromosomes), but having a *chromosome* number that is not a *multiple of the haploid number* (23 chromosomes), the modal number can be located between 47-57 chromosomes (Shaffer et al, 2009). This karyotype arises through a simultaneous gain of multiple chromosomes, from a diploid karyotype, during a single abnormal cell division. (Grumayer et al, 2002)

The hyperdiploidy occurs in 13% of young adults, and only 5% of elderly patients. The hypodiploidy and complex karyotype (presence of more than 2 chromosomal abnormalities) also increase with age, from 4% in the range of 15 to 29 years of age and 16% older than 60 years. (Moorman et al, 2010)

ii. When an oncogene is activated by mutation, the encoded protein is structurally modified in such a way that increases their transforming activity, ie, remains in the active state, continuously transmitting signals by binding of tyrosine and threonine kinase. These signals induce cell growth continued incessant. This mechanism of activation of oncogenes is more evident in other forms of leukemia, for example, AML and myelodysplastic syndromes (MDS) where the *NRAS* gene is mutated. There are mutations that suppress the function, and it is observed in tumor suppressor genes such as *TP53*, however, less than 3% of patients with ALL have *TP53* mutations, although all the cells have abnormal resistance to apoptosis induced by lack of a significant proportion of p53, which is explained in large part by epigenetic. (Zornoza et al, 2011)

On the other hand, some authors have found change in the number of copies (CNVs) to 50 regions in ALL recurring, some are very small and have less than 1 Mb, however, occur in genes encoding regulatory proteins of normal lymphoid development up to 40% of cases of ALL stem B. The most common targets are lymphoid transcription factor PAX5, that can hold deletions or amplifications in up to 30% of cases of ALL-B, also found CNVs in transcription factor genes IKZF1, the IKZF3, EBF1 (factor Cell B early), LEF1 and TCF3, and RAG1 and RAG2 genes. (Mullighan et al, 2009)

iii. The most relevant gene amplification in LLA is the dihydrofolatereductase (*DHFR*). The amplification of this gene causes evident cytogenetic alterations because the amplified DNA segment may involve several hundred kilobases. (Croce, 2008)

A variety of acute leukemia to consider is the T-cell ALL (ALL-T), it represents about 10% to 15% of ALL in adults and 25% of children. The clinical behavior is more aggressive, patients have a higher percentage of failure of remission, relapse rate is also higher as well, and the central nervous system infiltration compared with B-cell ALL type. (Demarest et al, 2011)

Oncogenes and tumor suppressor genes that have been implicated in T-ALL are: *c-MYC, NOTCH, LMO1 / 2, LYL1, TAL1 / 2, Hox11* and *HOX11L2*. It is clear that activated Notch is able to induce T cell leukemogenesis and is critical for the progression to T-ALL. (Demarest et al, 2008)

Members of the NOTCH family are transmembrane receptors that are critically involved in controlling the differentiation, proliferation and apoptosis in several cell types including T cells. The Notch receptor binding to its ligand exhibits a cleavage site for extracellular ADAM metalloproteinase, and a cleavage site in the transmembrane region for the γ-secretase, thus releasing the intracellular domain of Notch, which transmits this signaling to the cell nucleus, where it is associated with a DNA-binding complex. (Palomero et al, 2006; Chan et al, 2007; Sanda et al, 2010; Gomez et al, 2012)

Notch signaling cooperates with the signaling of T cell receptors (TCR) to expand the number of thymocytes undergoing β-selection. Over 50% of T-cell ALL have activating mutations in Notch1. (Gomez et al, 2012)

NOTCH target genes are mainly cyclin D1 and c-Myc. Both Notch and c-Myc regulates cell cycle progression by inducing expression of cyclins and reduced expression of *p27*. An important aspect to point out is that Notch is able to inhibit apoptosis induced by p53. When Notch expression is suppressed, the p53 pathway is activated and leads to tumor regression. (Demarest et al, 2008; Sanda et al, 2010)

An important aspect of Notch, is that depending on the type of cells, the extracellular environment, and the intensity of the signal, Notch can transmit signals as pro-oncogenic or

http://dx.doi.org/10.5772/54652

tumor suppressor (Leong and Karsan, 2006). In the development of T-ALL there is strong evidence of pro-oncogenic function of signals transduced by Notch, and that modulates the activity of downstream signaling pathways, through transcriptional regulation of its target genes. (Chan et al, 2007)

Possible regulators of signaling downstream of Notch, especially in murine models, are some intermediate signaling pathways, such as phosphatidylinositol 3-kinase (PI3K), Akt /protein kinase B, extracellular signal-regulated kinase-1/2, and nuclear factor kB. (Chan et al, 2007)

In general, the products of oncogenes can be classified as described below:

1. **Transcription factors:** They generally require interacting with other proteins to act, for example: Fos transcription protein dimerizes with the transcription factor Jun to form the AP1 transcription factor which is a complex, and this increases the expression of several genes control cell division.

2. **Chromatin remodeling:** It plays an important role in the degree of compaction of chromatin and therefore in the control of gene expression, replication and chromosome segregation, by the action of two types of enzymes: the ATP-dependent enzymes, which have important role in changing the position of histones, and enzymes that modify N-terminal tails of histones. (Peterson and Workman, 2000)

   Indeed, the epigenetic code is made by the pattern of histone modification, and determines in this way the interaction between nucleosomes and chromatin-associated proteins, thereby determining its transcriptional capacity. (Croce, 2008)

   On this basis it is important to note that methylation of CpG-dinucleotides in position near the site of transcription initiation can silence gene expression, hypermethylation of tumor suppressor genes and hypomethylation of oncogenes can lead to various forms of cancer. Aberrant methylation of CpG sites in promoter regions of genes has been identified in ALL cell lines. (Milani et al, 2009)

   In this way it has been found some improperly methylated genes that are involved in the p53 pathway suggesting that despite not having an activating mutation of this gene in ALL, there is an abnormal function of p53 mediated by epigenetic mechanisms. In fact, hypermethylation of genes involved in the TP53 pathway is an independent poor prognostic factor in patients with ALL. (Zornoza et al, 2011)

3. **Growth factor receptors:** They are altered in many cancers. A deletion of the ligand binding domain causes constitutive receptor activation in the absence of ligand binding sites of interaction by providing cytoplasmic proteins containing the SRC homology domain binding and other domains, this way deregulates multiple signaling pathways. Vascular endothelial growth factor (VEGF) regulates hypoxia-dependent control of gene transcription. VEGF activity is mediated by three tyrosine kinase receptors: VEGFR1 (FLT1), VEGFR2 (Flk1-KDR) and VEGFR3 (FLT4).

   The importance of angiogenesis and signaling pathways related to angiogenesis in the growth and expansion of cells in acute leukemia has been well established. *In vitro* in the leukemic cell, activation of VEGFR1 (FLT1) promotes cell migration and proliferation, whereas in vivo cells overexpressing FLT-1It accumulate in the bone marrow.

At the same time, the FLT-1 neutralization affects leukemia cell location (now in the bone marrow of the diaphysis), increased apoptosis, and prevents their departure to other tissues, which prolongs survival of mice inoculated. (Fragoso et al, 2006)

4. **Signal transducers:** They on the binding of receptor tyrosine kinases, to appropriate ligand receptor, lead to reorganization and autophosphorylation of tyrosine in the intracellular portion of the molecules, this increases the activity of the receptor or receptor interaction promotes intracytoplasmic domain with other proteins such as with the SRC homology domains. (Croce, 2008)

5. **Regulators of apoptosis:**Regulators that finally lead to apoptosis, where the *BCL2* gene encodes for a cytoplasmic protein that is localized in the mitochondria and increases the survival of the cell by inhibiting apoptosis.

Cytogenetics in acute lymphoblastic leukemia

The cytogenetic studies of human neoplasia began in 1960 with the discovery by Nowell and Hungerford of the Philadelphia chromosome in individuals with chronic myelogenous leukemia. Thirteen years after, Rowley performed chromosomal banding techniques and defined the origin of the Philadelphia chromosome as the result of the chromosomal translocation t(9;22)(q34;q11). (Mitelman et al, 2007; Croce, 2008; Pui et al, 2011; Dowing et al, 2012) These findings established the beginning for the cytogenetic studies of many solid and hematologic tumors. Currently, it has been consolidated a public database (Mitelman Database of Chromosome Aberrations and Gene Fusions in Cancer) containing 61,846 reported cases of cytogenetic studies and 975 different gene fusions in diverse human tumors. (Mitelman et al, 2012)

The ALL is the most common malignancy in pediatric population with a frequency of 19.7%. It is markedly different from the frequency observed in adults (1.2%). In both groups, the commitment of B-cell lineage is most frequent than the T-cell lineage. The variety of chromosomal abnormalities observed during the malignant development is also different between pediatric and adult ALL. The chromosomal abnormalities most frequent in pediatric ALL are the t(12;21)(p13;q22) with the *ETV6-RUNX1* gene fusion (21%) and hiperdiploidy of >50 chromosomes (19%). In adult ALL the most recurrent chromosomal abnormalities are the t(9;22)(q34;q11) with the *BCR-ABL1* gene fusion (25%) and *MLL* (11q23) gene fusions (10%). (Dowing et al, 2012)

The chromosomal translocation t(9;22) fuses the tyrosine kinase *ABL1* (*v-abl Abelson murine leukemia viral oncogene homolog 1*) gene located on 9q34 band with the *BCR* (*Breakpoint Cluster Region*) gene situated on 22q11 band raising the *5'-BCR/ABL1-3'* gene fusion. Various forms of this hybrid gene are generated depending on the breakpoint at BCR gene occurred. The e13a2 and e14a2 BCR/ABL1 transcripts code for a 210 KD protein and the e19a2 produces a 230 KD protein. These isoforms are related mainly to CML. The e1a2 transcript codes for a 190 KD protein which is mostly related to ALL and a trend towards poor-

http://dx.doi.org/10.5772/54652

er therapy outcome. Currently, BCR/ABL1 expressing cells can be selectively killed with the Imatinib (or STI571, imatinib mesylate, Gleevec or Glivec; Novartis) which inhibits the excessive tyrosine kinase activity of the hybrid protein. Most of the patients achieve complete remission with this approach; however, sometimes relapse occurs mainly by mutations in the *ABL1* segment that render resistance to the Imatinib. (Mitelman et al, 2007; Croce, 2008; Pui et al, 2011; Dowing et al, 2012)

During the progression of the disease multiple genetic alterations accumulate over time being selected by their potential to give fitness advantage to the new clones. Irrespective which is the primary change, the most frequent secondary numerical chromosomal changes in ALL are +X, +6, -7, +8, and +21; whereas, the most recurrent secondary structural aberrations are dup(1q), i(7q)(q10), and der(22)t(9;22). (Johansson et al, 1994)

Leukemia and immunity

Although little is known about the etiology of leukemia, this has a multifactorial behavior with risk factors that may contribute to its development such as ionizing radiation, chemotherapy and chromosomal abnormalities. (Han et al, 2010) By other hand, there are three hypotheses one called delayed infection, the second population mixing and the third hygiene hypothesis, (Strachan, 1989; Kinlen, 1995; Greaves, 2006) the first two suggest that the immune system deficiency in an early stage of development can cause an abnormal immune response to infections which may arise in the development of human beings. Both hypotheses are similar to third called hygiene hypothesis, which explains an increase in allergies in Western populations. (Chang et al, 2010) Although most studies support to infections and immune system factors in the etiology of ALL, little is known about the role of genes in this etiology. The relation of immune system in the ALL is a complex process that involves the interaction of many cells that including leukocytes, epithelial barriers, complement proteins, colexinas, pentraxins, cytokines (TNF, IL-1, chemokines, IL-2, IFN type I, IFN etc.), Th1, Th2, Treg and Th17 cells, CD28, FCGR2, GATA3, STAT4, STAT6 and may other. (Chang et al, 2010) Variations in the genes of these cells can affect their development and function in the immune response and therefore it may increase susceptibility to developing ALL. (Han et al, 2010; Chang et al, 2010) Moreover it was found that the CD47 molecule protects the macrophage leukemic clones to bind to a molecule on the surface of these cells. The interaction between macrophages and leukemic cells inhibits macrophage specific action which allows the cancer cell to proliferate. So that although the macrophage plays an important role in the destruction of cancer cells, leukemic cells with greater metabolic potential, and the potential escapes annihilating the macrophage. (Tesniere et al, 2008; Jaiswal et al, 2009) In the innate immune system, macrophages and other immune cells involved in immune surveillance protect the body permanently cell rate unexpectedly mutates. In contrast, the adaptive immune system through T and B cells upon activation attempt to destroy leukemic cells; however these also evade cellular immunity. It has been shown that the human genome sequencing is useful to identify oncogenic mutations useful in predicting the diagnosis, prognosis and therapeutic choice. What has provided important insights into the pathogenesis of leukemias. (Kalender et al, 2012)

Polymorphisms environmental in leukemia

Although the clinical and biological aspects of the ALL are well documented, little is known about individual susceptibility. Polymorphic variants of several genes, diet, environmental exposure to carcinogens and individualities of immune system are potential factors that could be increase predisposition to leukemia. (Buffleret al., 2005) However some speculation exist about the mechanism of the potential agents carcinogenic that could cause such alterations to ALL origin.(Smith, 1996; Kamdar et al., 2011)

Polymorphisms in the via of folate metabolism

The genetic regulation of folate metabolism have been the focus of many investigations that may influence in the preleukemic clone origin, by the via DNA hypomethylation of key regulatory genes, as well as uracil misincorporation into DNA leading to double-strand breaks and chromosomal aberrations.(Kamdar et al., 2011) The presence of some polymorphisms in genes involved in folate metabolism (*MTHFR, MTR, CBS, SHMT1* and *TYMS*) may cause deficiency in the enzyme activity and lead to inadequate folate metabolism and hypomethylation of DNA, which may lead to a neoplastic process. (Sharp and Little, 2004; Kamdar et al., 2011) The insufficient input of folate produces elevated plasma concentration of Homocysteine (Hcy) and adenosylmethionine (SAM) elevation, so that SAM is inhibitor methyltransferase enzyme. (Sharp et al., 2004) This inhibition may alter both, the DNA methylation process, and the regulation of gene expression. (Sharpand Little, 2004; Lightfoot et al., 2010) The hypomethylation is associated with activation of oncogenes and neoplastic processes, whereas the hypermethylation of CpG islands in promoter regions, of some tumor suppressor genes, prevents the transcription and promotes the development of tumors. (Das and Singal, 2004) (figure 4) Associations studies have been developed to identify genetic variants associated with ALL susceptibility, among them are: methylenetetrahydrofolatereductase (MTHFR), an enzyme that participates in Hcy and folate metabolism, plays an important role in DNA methylation and provision of nucleotides for DNA synthesis. (Robien and Ulrich, 2003)

Variations in the MTHFR gene sequence may result in enzymatic deficiency, low plasma folate levels and hyperhomocysteinemia, a risk factor for many diseases as: coronary diseases, neural tube defects, cancer, and leukemia, among others. (Lordelo et al, 2011) Association studies have been described between C677T and A1298C MTHFR polymorphisms and risk of leukemia (Skibola et al, 1999; Franco et al., 2001; Robien and Ulrich, 2003; Gallegos et al, 2008), which produces an decreased catalytic activity of MTHFR and subsequent availability of 5,10-MeTHF and SAM, have been extensively studied in relation to childhood leukemia, these findings have been inconsistent and their frequency vary among ethnic groups.(Robien and Ulrich, 2003)

Methionine synthase (MTR): Other studied polymorphisms, in association with ALL, are the missense polymorphism MTR c.2756A>G (D919G), that has been reported that alter the susceptibility to various cancers, (Linnebank et al, 2004; Yu et al, 2010) however the results have been contradictories. MTR is a vitamin B12-dependent enzyme, which catalyzes the remethylation of Hcy to methionine and the demethylation of 5-meTHF to THF, and has influence on DNA methylation, as well as on nucleic acid synthesis (Greene, 2010) (figure 4). A meta-analysis including 24896 cancer patients and 33862 controls, from 52 published papers, for MTR

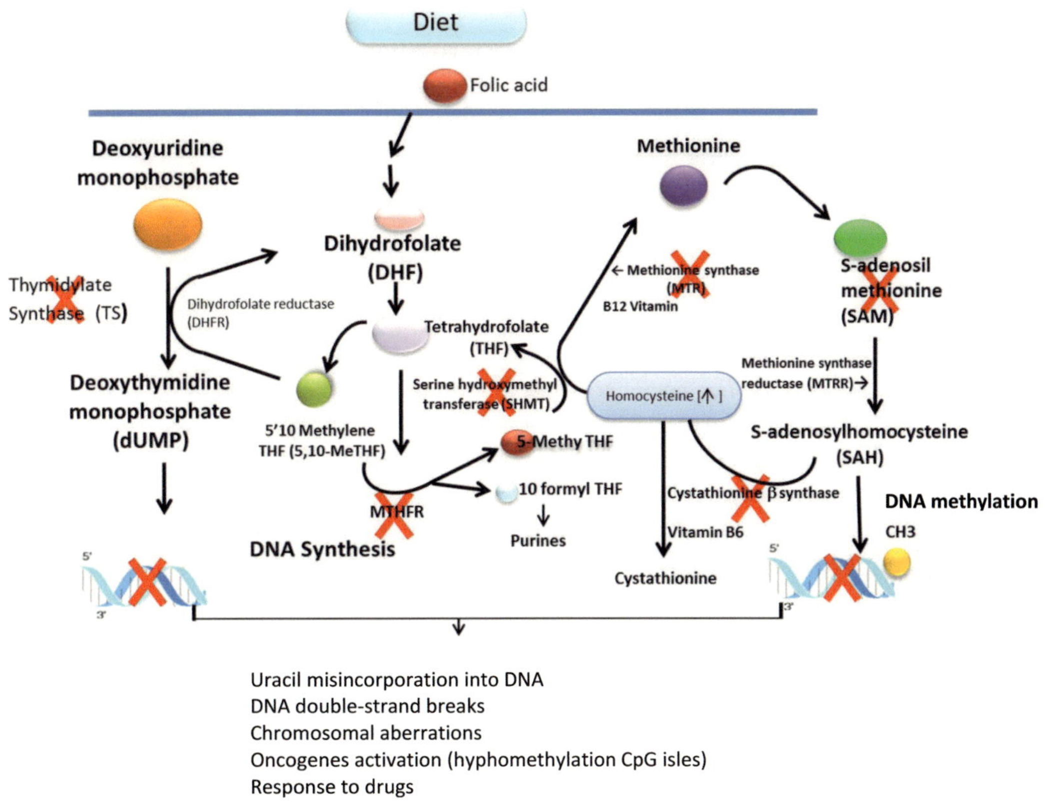

Figure 4. Polymorphisms (MTHFR, CBS and TS) of the via of folate in the development of ALL

A2756G was reviewed. Overall, individuals carrying MTR 2756GG genotype had a reduced cancer risk, under a recessive genetic model, in European populations. However, in Asian populations, it has a significantly high association. In stratified studies by tumor site, there was a *statistically significant* reduced risk with ALL. (Yu et al, 2010)

Cystathionine-β-synthase (CBS; gene localized to 21q22.3), the polymorphism most studied with leukemia are T833C, that co-segregates with 844ins68, and the G919A. (Ge et al, 2011) The frequencies of these polymorphisms are variable depending of the studied populations. The CBS participate in the trans-sulfuration pathway, catalyzes the condensation of serine and Hcy to form cystathionine, an intermediate step in the synthesis of cysteine. (figure 4) The 844ins68 polymorphism was associated in Down Syndrome (DS) with leukemia myeloblasts, detecting a 4.6-fold higher rate ($P < 0.001$) when compared to non-DS individuals. (Ge et al, 2011) The biological function of this polymorphism is even contradictory, it has been demonstrated that carriers of 844ins68 have significantly lower total plasma Hcy levels, after a methionine load, and concluded that this polymorphism was associated with higher CBS enzyme activities. (Ge et al, 2011)

Serine Hydroxymethyltransferase 1 (SHMT1)

Cytosolic SHMT1 regulates 5,10-MeTHF,that acts as substrate for MTHFR. The 1420C>T polymorphism of this gene reduces circulating folate levels, and may mimic folate deficiency, consequently shunting 5,10-MeTHF towards DNA synthesis, and have been shown that moderate the risk of hematological malignancies. (Lightfoot et al, 2005) Folate is a component important in the development of the embryogenesis and early fetal development, via its effects on DNA methylation and synthesis. Then, the well-documented in utero origin of ALL has led to hypothesize that deficient folate intake may be important in its etiology. (Lightfoot et al, 2005; de Jonge et al, 2009)

Thymidylate Synthase (TYMS)

Thymidylate synthase (TS) has been shown to moderate the risk of hematological malignancies. (Valiket al, 2004; Lightfoot et al, 2005) Although, it has been proposed that arise by genetics and environmental factors. (Krajinovic et al, 2004) Consistent with this paradigm, variants of genes involved in xenobiotic metabolism, DNA repair pathway and cell cycle checkpoint functions, have been shown to influence the susceptibility to ALL. (Pui, 2009) Many enzymes are involved in the folate metabolism, among which, thymidylate synthase (TS) is a crucial enzyme and hence a good candidate for studying the effect of polymorphisms in the folate metabolism gene, on the development of malignancies. TS, encoded by the *TS,* gene located on chromosome 18p11.32, plays a vital role in maintaining a balanced supply of deoxynucleotides, required for DNA synthesis and repair, by catalyzing the conversion of dUMP to dTMP. (Nazki et al, 2012)

The polymorphisms in *TYMS* gene include a 6-bp deletion (1494del6), in the 3′-untranslated region of *TS* that influences RNA levels; and a polymorphic tandem 28-bp repeat sequence within the promoter enhancer region of *TS*, where the triple repeat increases gene expression levels and reduces DNA damage. In fact, it is thought that the input of deoxynucleotides for DNA synthesis is controlled by TYMS, which has a polymorphic tandem repeat sequence within the promoter enhancer region containing a double (2R)or triple (3R) 28–bp repeat. The presence of the triple repeat leads to increased levels of gene expression and a reduction in DNA damage. (Skibola et al, 2004; Lightfoot et al, 2010) Methotrexate, an antifolic acid agent, has demonstrated to be an effective chemotherapeutic drug for the treatment of lymphoid malignancies, indicating an association between the folate metabolism and the development of such malignancies. (Hishidaet al, 2003) This increased expression may, in turn, increase the conversion of dUMP to dTMP, thereby; decreasing uracil levels and the consequent erroneous incorporation of uracil into DNA of rapidly dividing hematopoietic stem cells, and could work protectively against the development of ALL. (Skibola et al, 2004) The TS 28-bp repeat polymorphism has been shown to modulate the risk of ALL in various populations, but the obtained results are controversial and require further investigation to be confirmed and clarified. (Skibola et al, 2004; deJonge et al, 2009)

Polymorphisms in the xenobiotics metabolism

An ability that man has acquired in the course of evolution is the way to metabolize foreign compounds for the body to facilitate disposal. These compounds are called xenobiotics, in food and the environment are mostly lipophilic, so it tends to accumulate in lipophilic environments the body and are difficult to remove so they tend to trigger toxicity phenomena. (Gonzalez and Gelboin, 1994) The liver removes lipophilic xenobiotics, through a set of known reactions of biotransformation. The end result is the formation of metabolites less lipophilic and more soluble, which are easily eliminated in the urine or bile compounds. That is why these reactions are known as detoxification or deactivation. (DeAnn, 1998) In this sense, drugs are a class of compounds that are absorbed xenobiotics on the body and distributed in body fluids, tissue and organ. Where exert their pharmacological action and pharmacodynamics specified; only a small part reaches the tissue-receptor-target enzyme, while most are metabolized and eliminated. (Sheweita, 2000) Moreover, the processes of biotransformation of xenobiotics are subdivided into two phases: phase I metabolism, carried out by two families of enzymes oxygenases: those dependent on cytochrome P450 (CYP450) monooxygenases and the flavin (FMO). Their metabolism is characterized by the action of chemical processes of different nature mainly oxidation, oxygenation, reduction and hydrolysis, so as dealquilations and dehalogenations. These chemical reactions produce metabolites capable of binding covalently to endogenous molecules such as glucuronic acids, glutathione, sulfate and amino acids that generate conjugates, which are metabolized by Phase II which is characterized by solubility in generating molecules and decreased toxicity, generated by the modification of new functional groups, which transform the more polar metabolite, which facilitates their removal. In this regard, when a drug enters the body usually is modified by conjugation reactions to be easily removed. However, when there modifications in the concentrations concentration (high or low) of enzymes that perform the conjugation process and if the xenobiotic is lipophilic nature, tends to accumulate in the cell, which will lead to different processes: 1) accumulation of reactive metabolites adduct forming with DNA, 2) formation of a toxic compound 3) a nontoxic compound becomes a toxic derivative. This generates secondary metabolic pathways may have a carcinogenic action, toxicological, genotoxic or mutagenic in the body. (Marmiroli and Maestri, 2008) Different studies in the literature have suggested the association of polymorphisms in genes involved in xenobiotic metabolism phase I and II in patients with leukemia. (Aydin et al, 2006; Gallegos et al,2008, Lordelo et al, 2011)

Secondary leukemias

Secondary hematological malignancies represent a serious complication of cancer treatment. Usually manifiest as acute leukemia and MDS, and known more about these could eventually help reduce its appearance (Levine and Blomifield, 1992). It is known that this type of leukemias may arise as a result of exposure to cytotoxic treatments (with genotoxicity secondary effects) and/or radiotherapy (RT) and as a result of other hematological disorders (Harris et al, 1999; Brunning et al, 2001), and possibly also, product of environment or genetic causes. (Levine and Blomifield, 1992) In most cases it is proposed that the mechanism of leukemogenesis is associated with DNA damage in hematopoietic cells of the bone marrow by agents such as those used in chemotherapy (CT). (Levine and Blomifield, 1992) Although most secondary leukemias are acute AML, there have been reports of lymphoid leukemia and CML is associated with CT. (Andersen et al, 2000; Krishnan et al, 2000; Pedersen-Bjergaard et al, 2002)

The AML are hematologic malignancies characterized by the uncontrolled myeloid blast proliferation in the bone marrow and in peripheral tissues. (Sevilla et al, 2002) Differ according to the cytological, immunophenotypic and cytogenetic characteristics. (Paietta, 1995; Head, 1996) On the other hand the MDS are dis-hematopoietics processes of bone marrow, characterized by alteration in the maturation and differentiation of hematopoietic cell lines (with involvement of one, two or all three blood cell lineages) and in some cases, by the presence of bone marrow blasts, without showing acute leukemia criteria. (Bennet et al, 1982; Cheson, 1997)

The term secondary leukemia has referred to the development of AML as result of CT treatment, particularly alkylating agents (Levine and Blomifield, 1992) or topoisomerase II inhibitors, RT, or by exposure to environmental carcinogens (Harris et al, 1999; Brunning et al, 2001). Within the term of secondary acute leukemias (SAL) different entities are grouped by etiopathogenesis, prognosis and response to therapy. In general can be distinguished two groups: those that are a result of exposure to cytotoxic treatments such as CT and/or RT and those that are a result of the final evolution of other hematological disorders, such as, myeloproliferative syndromes, MDS, paroxysmal nocturnal hemoglobinuria. (Harris et al, 1999; Brunning et al, 2001)

In close relationship with these two groups of SAL also found leukemias result from environmental or occupational exposure to carcinogens, (Levine and Blomifield, 1992) or those that develop in patients with genetic disorders as chromosomal fragility syndromes such as Fanconi anemia and Bloom syndrome (Popp and Bohlander, 2010)

The increase is due to the increased number of survivors of other forms of cancer, (Ng et al, 2000) is important to know more about SAL, especially AML or MDS relating to previous therapies (AML-PT, MDS-PT). The cumulative risk of developing AML-PT/MDS-PT after ten years of receiving CT for breast cancer, non-Hodgkin´s lymphoma, ovarian cancer or Hodgkin ´s disease, has been estimated at 1.5, 7.9, 8.5, and 3.8% respectively. (Bolufer et al, 2006) Moreover, generally the cases of AML-PT/MDS-PT, the primary disease may be a solid tumor, other haematological malignancy or non-malignant disorder.

Today it is clear that AML-PT/MDS-PT can develop after exposure to cytotoxic CT with alkylating agents, topoisomerase II inhibitors, and/or RT, for the treatment of other neoplasias or in treating non-malignant disorders. In this sense, has been described after the use of immunosuppressants such as azathioprine (Harris et al, 1999; Brunning et al, 2001). While the study of these entities has been important, the maximum latency between exposure to leukemogenic agent and the development of AML-PT/MDS-PT has not been established with certainty.

Due to history of exposure to certain agents and the association with some cytogenetic abnormalities characteristic, two groups are recognized in AML-PT/MDS-PT: (Harris et al, 1999; Brunning et al, 2001)

Which appears as a result of the mutagenic effect of alkylating agents treatment, ionizing radiation or both, that occur after a long latency period between 5 to 7 years of exposure to cytotoxic agents and often show a phase of myelodysplasia prior to the evolution to AL, and often show a phase of myelodysplasia prior to the evolution to AL, which often produce alterations of chromosomes 5 and 7, (-5/5q- and -7/7q-) frequently refractory to treatment. (Andersen and Pedersen, 2000)

Those in patients treated with drugs that inhibit DNA-topoisomerase II as epipodophyllotoxins and anthracyclines, with a short latency period of between 2 to 3 years, without prior myelodysplasia phase and in which observed balanced translocations as 11q23 (MLL) and 21q22 (AML1/RUNX1), although there are some discrepancies. The treatment response is not significantly different from those of patients with *de novo* AML. (Penderse, 2002)

Leukemias have been associated with exposure to various agents as benzene and its metabolites (phenol, hydroquinone), environmental carcinogens demonstrated relationship to increased risk of developing leukemia. (Lan et al, 2004) Other compounds studied with controversial relationship, are some agricultural pesticides, heavy metals, smoke snuff, alcohol intake and exposure to cosmic rays of airlines pilots. (Larson, 2007) Ionizing radiation is a known leukemogenic agent and the main action mechanism includes the breakage of the DNA strands which can cause the aforementioned chromosomal deletions and translocations. Breaks may result from a direct effect of high doses of radiation or indirectly by free radicals generation. Furthermore, ionizing radiation can induce changes of bases in the DNA sequences, crosslinking strands, multiple damages or epigenetic alterations (Finch, 2007). In the case of RT, induced leukemia seems to start in the first 5 years after exposure, peaks at 10 years and decreases significantly after 15 years. The relative incidence of leukemias by RT is dose dependent, duration of exposure, and area of exposed bone marrow. (Finch, 2007) Fractionated doses of radiation are less leukemogenic than higher single doses, because it allows greater efficiency of DNA repair mechanisms. The leukemogenic risk appears to be greater when low-dose exposure affects large areas of bone marrow, whereas high doses of radiation over limited areas appear to have less effect. This is attributed to increased apoptosis induced by high doses of radiation on cells exposed. (Inskip, 1999; Smith et al, 2002) Estimates show, that patients undergoing RT for the treatment of malignancies or other non-malignant diseases has a risk of two to three times more to develop AML-PT/MDS-PT. (Smith et al, 2002) On the other hand, a younger ages at the time of exposure, greater the leukemogenic risk. The increased risk for developing AML-PT/MDS-PT, after treatment of non Hodkin lymphomas, breast cancer, cervical cancer and uterine body and Ewing's sarcoma, is attributed to the use of RT, while associated with Hodgkin's disease, ovarian cancer and testicular cancer, has been associated with the use of CT. (Levine and Blomifield, 1992; van Leeuwen et al, 1994; Inskip, 1999; Smith et al, 2002)

Many drugs used as CT in the treatment of a primary cancer, have been linked to the subsequent development of AML-PT/MDS-PT, thus, alkylating agents were the first to be evidenced leukemogenic potential, (Pedersen, 2002) effect related to the cumulative dose of the drug, the effect being greater with increasing patient age (Pedersen, 2002). All alkylating agents have effect leukemogenic, such is the case of drugs such as mechlorethamine, procarbazine, chlorambucil, cyclophosphamide, melphalan, semustine, lomustine, carmustine, prednimustine, busulfan. However, although the relative risk leukemogenic of these drugs has not been definitively established, drugs such melphalan and busulfan seem to condition an increased riesk than others as cyclophosphamide for reason which are unknown. (Stott et al, 1977; Greene et al, 1986; Krishnan et al, 2000) Although, this seems to suggest that more genotoxic and cytotoxic drugs are chosen that have less leukemogenic potential. Alkylating agents besides the aforementioned chromosomal damage can cause point mutations in some oncogenes like RAS. (Pedersen et al, 1988) However, these effects are no restricted to certain genes or chromosomal regions and possibly the selection of cells with abnormalities of chromosomes 5 and 7 come conditioned by a proliferative advantage to cells carrying these alterations. (Johansson et al, 1991; de Greef and Hagemeiger, 1996; Andersen et al, 2000)

Meanwhile, drugs that act by inhibiting topoisomerase II, as the epipodophyllotoxins (etoposide and teniposide) (et al, 1999) and intercalating agents such as anthracyclines (doxorubicin, daunorubicin, idarubicin) o las anthracenediones (mitoxantrone), have been associated with balanced translocations that originates function genes. The most common affect 11q23, 21q22, inv(16) and t(15;17) (Andersen et al, 1998; Rowley and Olney, 2002). Recently high-dose CT followed by autologous hematopoietic transplantation, have been associated with the development of AML-PT/MDS-PT, with time of onset of 47-50 months after transplantation. (Nademanee et al, 1995; Traweek et al, 1996; Krishnan et al, 2000; Pedersen et al, 2000; Gilliland and Gribben, 2002)

An important point to consider is individual susceptibility, since only a minority of patients develop secondary leukemia after exposure to CT, therefore it is suggested that differences in drug metabolism may predispose to the development of AML-PT/MDS-PT of some patients. (Bolufer et al, 2006) In this way, polymorphisms of genes encoding enzymes involved in drug metabolism could contribute to the risk of developing these pathologies. These genes could explain differences in metabolizing of these agents and condition a lower detoxification capacity or repair of genetic damage induced by the drug. (Bolufer et al, 2006) Genes have been studied encoding cytochrome P450 (CYPs) related to phase I metabolism, glutathione S-methyltransferase (GSTT1, GSTM1, GSTP1) involved in phase II metabolism (conjugation/detoxification), the NAD(P)H: qinone oxo-reductase 1 (NQO1) which acts on the metabolism of free radicals and oxidative stress, genes related to folate metabolism (MTHFR, TYMS, SHMT1, MTRR), also involved in DNA synthesis and genes related to DNA repair (hMLH1, hMSH2, hMSH3, RAD51, XRCC1, XRCC3, XPD, XPG, CHEK2, and ATM) that can cause genomic instability. (Bolufer et al, 2006)

The AML-PT/MDS-PT pathogenesis includes clonal alterations in the some genes function due to single mutations, chromosomal abnormalities or epigenetic phenomena. Many of the altered genes are tumor suppressor that have a recessive character and therefore, requires the loss of both alleles. The loss of a single copy of the gene can result in reduction of gene products and predispose to malignancy. Current evidence indicates that AML results from at least two mutations classes. The class I, confers proliferative advantage and/or cell survival without affecting their differentiation capacity, while the class II, prevent the normal hematopoietic cell differentiation. (Deguchi and Gilliland, 2002)

The AML-PT represent 10 to 15% of total AML and its incidence is increasing substantially in recent years, (Ng et al, 2000) the AML-PT are often associated with clonal cytogenetic abnormalities similar to those found in newly diagnosed AML, but with higher incidence of poor prognosis karyotypes and have particular clinical and biological features that include a poor response to CT commonly used in the treatment of AML and therefore have a significantly adverse prognosis.

Different authors have been relationship to drugs and radiation with specific emphasis on the balanced rearrangements chromosomes. (Andersen et al, 1998) Increased frequency of dicentric chromosomes in therapy-related MDS and AML compared to de novo disease is significantly related to previous treatment with alkylating agents and suggests a specific susceptibility to chromosome breakage at the centromere. (Andersen and Pedersen, 2000)

3. Conclusion

In this way one can conclude that the pathophysiology of acute lymphoblastic leukemia is very complex and involves various factors (genetic, immunes, environmental, and drugs) at different levels, and also has a close and complex relationship. The key features in the pathophysiology of the ALL is its monoclonal origin, uncontrolled cell proliferation by sustained self-stimulation of their receptors for growth, no response to inhibitory signals, and cellular longevity conditioned by decreased apoptosis.

Author details

M. P. Gallegos-Arreola[1], C. Borjas-Gutiérrez[3], G. M. Zúñiga-González[2], L. E. Figuera[4], A. M. Puebla-Pérez[5] and J. R. García-González[4]

1 Laboratorio de Genética Molecular, División de Medicina Molecular, CIBO-IMSS, Guadalajara, Jal., México

2 Laboratorio de Mutagénesis, División de Medicina Molecular, CIBO-IMSS, Guadalajara, Jal., México

3 División de Genética, CIBO-IMSS, &UMAE-Hospital de Especialidades, Servicio de Hematología, CIBO-IMSS, Guadalajara, Jal., México

4 División de Genética, CIBO-IMSS, Guadalajara, Jal., México

5 Laboratorio de Inmunofarmacologia, CUCEI, UdeG, Guadalajara, Jal., México

References

[1] Andersen MK, Johansson B, Larsen SO, Pedersen-Bjergaard J, Chromosomal abnormalities in secondary MDS and AML. (1998) Relationship to drugs and radiation with specific emphasis on the balanced rearrangements. Haematologica. 83(6):483–488.

[2] Andersen MK, Pedersen-Bjergaard J. (2000) Increased frecuency of dicentric chromosomes in terapy-related MDS and AML compared to de novo disease is significantly related to previous treatment with alkylating agents and suggests a specific susceptibility to chromosome breakage at the centromere. Leukemia. 14(1):105–111.

[3] Aydin M, Hatirnaz O, Erensoy N, Ozbek U. (2006) Role of CYP2D6, CYP1A1, CYP2E1, GSTT1, and GSTM1 genes in the susceptibility to acute leukemias. Am J Hematol.81(3): 162-70.

[4] Ayton PM, Cleary ML. (2001) Molecular mechanism of leukemogenesis mediated by MLL fusion proteins. Oncogene. 20(40):5695–707.

[5] Bennett JM, Catovsky D, Daniel MT, Flandrin G, Galton DA, Gralnick HR, Sultan C. (1982) Proposals for the classification of myelodisplastic syndromes. Br J Haematol. 51(2):189–199.

[6] Bolufer P, Barragan E, Collado M, Cervera J, López JA, Sanz MA. (2006) Influence of genetic polimorphisms on the risk of developing leukemia and on disease progression. Leuk Res. 30(12):1471–1491.

[7] Brunning RD, Matutes E Harris NL, Stein H, Vardiman JW (eds). (2001) World Health Organization Classification of tumours: Pathology and Genetics of tumours of Haematopoieyic and Lymphoid Tissues. Lyon: IARC Press. pp. 88–89.

[8] Buffler PA, Kwan ML, Reynolds P, Urayama KY. (2005) Environmental and genetic risk factors for childhood leukemia: appraising the evidence. Cancer Invest. 23(1):60-75.

[9] Calin GA, Dumitru CD, Shimizu M, Bichi R, Zupo S, Noch E, Aldler H, Rattan S, Keating M, Rai K, Rassenti L, Kipps T, Negrini M, Bullrich F, Croce CM. (2002) Frequent deletions and down-regulation of micro- RNA genes miR15 and miR16 at 13q14 in chronic lymphocytic leukemia. ProcNatlAcadSci USA. 99(24):15524-9.

[10] Cazzaniga G, van Delft FW, Luca Lo Nigro, Ford AM, Score J, Iacobucci I, Mirabile E, Taj M, Colman SM, Biondi A, (2011) Greaves M. Developmental origins and impact of BCR-ABL1 fusion and IKZF1 deletions in monozygotic twins with Ph+ acute lymphoblastic leukemia. Blood.18(20):5559–64.

[11] Chan SM, Weng AP, Tibshirani R, Aster JC, Utz PJ. (2007) Notch signals positively regulate activity of the mTOR pathway in T-cell acute lymphoblastic leukemia. Blood. 110 (1):278-86.

[12] Chang JS, Wiemels JL, Chokkalingam AP, Metayer C, Barcellos LF, Hansen HM, Aldrich MC, Guha N, Urayama KY, Scélo G, Green J, May SL, Kiley VA, Wiencke JK, Buffler PA. (2010) Genetic polymorphisms in adaptive immunity genes and childhood acute lymphoblastic leukemia. Cancer Epidemiol Biomarkers Prev. 9(9):2152-63.

[13] Cheson BD. (1997) The Myelodisplastics Syndromes. Oncologist. 2(1):28–39.

[14] Croce CM. (2008) Oncogenes and cancer. N Engl J Med. 358(5):502-11

[15] Das PM, Singal R. (2004) DNA methylation and cancer. J ClinOncol. 15;22(22):4632-42.

[16] de Greef GE, Hagemeiger A. (1996) Molecular and cytogenetic abnormalities in acute myeloid leukemia and myelodisplastic syndromes. Ballieres Clin Hematol. 9(1):1–18.

[17] de Jonge R, Tissing WJ, Hooijberg JH, Jansen G, Kaspers GJ, Lindemans J, Peters GJ, Pieters R.(2009) Polymorphisms in folate-related genes and risk of pediatric acute lymphoblastic leukemia. Blood.113(10):2284–89.

[18] DeAnn J. (1998) The detoxification enzyme systems. Alternative Medicine Review. 3 (3):187–98

[19] Deguchi K, Gilliland DG. (2002) Cooperativity between mutations in tyrosine kinases and in hematopoietic transcription factors in AML. Leukemia. 16(4):740–744.

[20] Demarest RM, Dahmane N, Capobianco AJ. (2011) Notch is oncogenic dominant in T-cell acute lymphoblastic leukemia. Blood.117(24):2901-09.

[21] Demarest RM, Ratti F, Capobianco AJ. (2008) It's T-ALL about Notch. Oncogene. 27(38): 5082-91.

[22] Downing JR, Wilson RK, Zhang J, Mardis ER, Pui CH, Ding L, Ley TJ, Evans WE. (2012) The Pediatric Cancer Genome Project. Nat Genet. 44(6):619-22.

[23] Finch SC. (2007) Radiation-induced leukemia: Lessons from history. Best Pract Res Clin Haematol. 20(1):109–118.

[24] Fragoso R, Pereira T, Wu Y, Zhu Z, Cabeçadas J, Dias S. (2006) VEGFR-1 (FLT-1) activation modulates acute lymphoblastic leukemia localization and survival within the bone marrow, determining the onset of extramedullary disease. Blood. 107(4):1608-16.

[25] Franco RF, Simões BP, Tone LG, Gabellini SM, Zago MA, Falcão RP. (2001) Themethylenetetrahydrofolatereductase C677T gene polymorphism decreases the risk of childhood acute lymphocytic leukaemia. Br J Haematol. 115(3):616-8.

[26] Fuka G, Kauer M, Kofler R, Haas OA, Panzer-Grümayer R (2011) The leukemia-specific fusion gene ETV6/RUNX1 perturbs distinct key biological functions primarily by gene repression. PLoS One. 6(10):e26348.

[27] Gallegos MP, Figuera LE, Delgado JL, Puebla-Pérez AM, Zúñiga-González GM. (2008) The MTHFR polymorphism C677T in adult patients with acute lymphoblastic leukemia is associated with an increased prevalence of cytogenetic abnormalities. Blood Cells Mol Dis. 40(2):244-5.

[28] Gallegos MP, González-García JR, Figuera LE, Puebla-Pérez AM, Delgado-Lamas JL, Zúñiga-González GM. (2008) Distribution of CYP1A1*2A polymorphism in adult patients with acute lymphoblastic leukemia in a Mexican population. Blood Cells Mol Dis. 41(1):91-4.

[29] Garg R, Kantarjian H, Thomas D, Faderl S, Ravandi F, Lovshe D, Pierce S, O'Brien S. (2009) Adults with acute lymphoblastic leukemia and translocation (1;19) abnormality have a favorable outcome with hyperfractionated cyclophosphamide, vincristine, dox-

orubicin, and dexamethasone alternating with methotrexate and high-dose cytarabine chemotherapy. Cancer. 15;115 (10):2147-54.

[30] Ge Y, Jensen T, James SJ, Becton DL, Massey GV, Weinstein HJ, Ravindranath Y, Matherly LH, Taub JW.(2002) High frequency of the 844ins68 cystathionine-beta-synthase gene variant in Down syndrome children with acute myeloid leukemia.Leukemia. 16(11):2339-41.

[31] Gilliland DG, Gribben JG. (2002) Evaluation of the risk of theraphy-related MDS/AML after autologous stem cell transplantation. Biol Blood Marrow Transplant. 8(1):9–16.

[32] Gómez del Arco P, KashiwagiMariko,.Jackson AF, Naito T, Zhang J, Liu F, Kee B, Vooijs M, Radtke F, Redondo JM, Georgopoulos K. (2010) Alternative promoter usage at the Notch1locus supports ligand-independent signaling in T cell development and leucemogénesis. Immunity. 33(5):685–98.

[33] Gonzalez FJ, Gelboin HV.(1994) Role of human cytochromes P450 in the metabolic activation of chemical carcinogens and toxins.Drug Metab Rev.26(1-2):165–83.

[34] Greaves M. Childhood leukaemia.(2002) BMJ. 324(7332):283-7.

[35] Greaves M. Infection, immune responses and the aetiology of childhood leukaemia. Nat Rev Cancer 2006;6(3):193–203

[36] Greene MH, Harris EL, Gerhenson DM, Malkasian GD Jr, Melton LJ 3rd, DemboAJ, Bennett JM, Moloney WC, Boice JD Jr. (1986) Melphalan may be a more potent leukemogen than cyclophosphamide. Ann Inter Med. 105(3):360–367.

[37] Greene ND, Stanier P, Moore GE.(2011) The emerging role of epigenetic mechanisms in the etiology of neural tube defects. Epigenetics. 6(7):875-83.

[38] Grumayer ER, Fasching K, Panzer S, Hettinger K, Schmitt K, Ipsiroglu S, Haas O. (2012) Nondisjunction of chromosomes leading to hyperdiploid childhood B-cell precursor acute lymphoblastic leukemia is an early event during leukemogenesis. Blood. 100 (1): 347-49.

[39] Han S, Lan Q, Park AK, Lee KM, Park SK, Ahn HS, Shin HY, Kang HJ, Koo HH, Seo JJ, Choi JE, Ahn YO, Chanock SJ, Kim H, Rothman N, Kang D. (2010) Polymorphisms in innate immunity genes and risk of childhood leukemia. Hum Immunol. 71(7):727-30.

[40] Harris NL, Jafee ES, Diebold J, Flandrin G, Muller-Hermelink HK, Vardiman J, Lister TA, Bloomfield CD. (1999) World Health Organization classification of neoplastic diseases of the hematopoietic and lymphoid tissues: report of the Clinical Advisory Committee meeting- Airlie House, Virginia, November 1997. J Clin Oncol. 17(12):3835–3849.

[41] Head DR. (1996) Revised classification of acute myeloid leukemia. Leukemia. 10(11): 1826–1831.

[42] Heltemes-Harris LM, Willette MJ, Ramsey LB, Qiu YH, Neeley ES, Zhang N, Thomas DA, Koeuth T, Baechler EC, Kornblau SM, Farrar MA. (2011) Ebf1 or Pax5 haploinsuf-

ficiency synergizes with STAT5 activation to initiate acute lymphoblastic leukemia. J Exp Med. 208(6):1135-49.

[43] Hishida A, Matsuo K, Hamajima N, Ito H, Ogura M, Kagami Y, Taji H, Morishima Y, Emi N, Tajima K. (2003) Associations between polymorphisms in the thymidylate synthase and serine hydroxymethyltransferase genes and susceptibility to malignant lymphoma. Haematologica.88(2):159-66.

[44] Hsieh JJ, Ernst P, Erdjument-Bromage H, Tempst P, and Korsmeyer SJ. (2003) Proteolitic cleavage of MLL generates a complex of N and C terminal fragments that confers protein stability and subnuclear localization, Molecular and Cellular Biology. 23(1):186–94.

[45] Inskip PD. (1999) Second cancer following radiotherapy. In: Neugut AI, Meadows AT, Robinson E (eds). Multiple primary cancers. Philadelphia, USA: Lippincott Williams & Wilkins. pp. 91–135.

[46] Jaiswal S, Jamieson CH, Pang WW, Park CY, Chao MP, Majeti R, Traver D, van Rooijen N, Weissman IL. (2009) CD47 is upregulated on circulating hematopoietic stem cells and leukemia cells to avoid phagocytosis. Cell. 138(2):271-85.

[47] Johansson B, Mertens F, Heim S, Kristoffersson U, Mitelman F. (1991) Cytogenetics of secondary myelodisplasia (sMDS) and acute nonlymphocytic leukemia (sANLL). Eur J Haematol. 47(1):17–27.

[48] Johansson B, Mertens F, Mitelman F. (1994) Secondary chromosomal abnormalities in acute leukemias. Leukemia. 8(6):953-62.

[49] Kalender Atak Z, De Keersmaecker K, Gianfelici V, Geerdens E, Vandepoel R, Pauwels D, Porcu M, Lahortiga I, Brys V, Dirks WG, Quentmeier H, Cloos J, Cuppens H, Uyttebroeck A, Vandenberghe P, Cools J, Aerts S. (2012) High accuracy mutation detection in leukemia on a selected panel of cancer genes. PLoS One.7(6):e38463

[50] Kamdar KY, Krull KR, El-Zein RA, Brouwers P, Potter BS, Harris LL, Holm S, Dreyer Z, Scaglia F, Etzel CJ, Bondy M, Okcu MF. (2011) Folate pathway polymorphisms predict deficits in attention and processing speed after childhood leukemia therapy. Pediatr Blood Cancer.57(3):454-60.

[51] Kinlen LJ. Epidemiological evidence for an infective basis in childhood leukaemia. Br J Cancer 1995;71(1):1–5.

[52] Kohlmann A, Schoch C, Dugas M, Schnittger S, Hiddemann W, Kern W, Haferlach T. (2005) New insights into MLL gene rearranged acute leukemias using gene expression profiling: shared pathways, lineage commitment, and partner genes. Leukemia. 9(6): 953-64.

[53] Krajinovic M, Lemieux-Blanchard E, Chiasson S, Primeau M, Costea I, Moghrabi A. (2004) Role of polymorphisms in MTHFR and MTHFD1 genes in the outcome of childhood acute lymphoblastic leukemia. Pharmacogenomics J. 4(1):66-72

[54] Krishnan A, Bhatia S, Slovak ML, Arber DA, Niland JC, Nademanee A, Fung H, Bhatia R, Kashyap A, Molina A, O'Donnell MR, Parker PA, Sniecinski I, Snyder DS, Spielberger R, Stein A, Forman SJ. (2000) Predictors of therapy-related leukemia and myelodysplasia following autologous transplantation for lymphoma: an assessment of risk factors. Blood. 95(5):1588–1593.

[55] Lan Q, Zhang L, Li G, Vermeulen R, Weinberg RS, Dosemeci M, Rappaport SM, Shen M, Alter BP, Wu Y, Kopp W, Waidyanatha S, Rabkin C, Guo W, Chanock S, Hayes RB, Linet M, Kim S, Yin S, Rothman N, Smith MT. (2004) Hematotoxicity in workers exposed to low levels of benzene. Science. 306(5702):1774–1776.

[56] Larson RA. (2007) Is secondary leukemia an independent poor prognostic factor in acute myeloid leukemia? Best Pract Res Clin Haematol. 20(1):29–37.

[57] Lee HJ, Thompson JE, Wang ES, Wetzler M. (2011) Philadelphia Chromosome-Positive Acute Lymphoblastic Leukemia Current Treatment and Future Perspectives.Cancer. 117(8):1583-94

[58] Leong KG, Karsan A. Recent insights into the role of Notch signaling in tumorigenesis. (2000) Blood. 107(6):2223-33.

[59] Levine EG, Blomifield CD. (1992) Leukemias and myelodisplastic syndromes secondary to drug, radiation and environmental exposure. Semin Oncol. 19(1):47–84.

[60] Liang DC, Yang CP, Lin DT, Hung IJ, Lin KH, Chen JS, Hsiao CC, Chang TT, Peng CT, Lin MT, Chang TK, Jaing TH, Liu HC, Wang LY, Yeh TC, Jou ST, Lu MY, Cheng CN, Sheen JM, Chiou SS, Wu KH, Hung GY, Chen RL, Chen SH, Cheng SN, Chang YH, Chen BW, Ho WL, Wang JL, Lin ST, Hsieh YL, Wang SC, Chang HH, Yang YL, Huang FL, Chang CY, Chang WH, Lin KS. (2010) Long-term results of Taiwan Pediatric Oncology Group studies 1997 and 2002 for childhood acute lymphoblastic leukemia.Leukemia. 24(2):397-405.

[61] Lightfoot TJ, Johnston WT, Painter D, Simpson J, Roman E, Skibola CF, Smith MT, Allan JM, Taylor GM. (2010) United Kingdom Childhood Cancer Study. Genetic variation in the folate metabolic pathway and risk of childhood leukemia.Blood.115(19):3923-9.

[62] Lightfoot TJ, Skibola CF, Willett EV, Skibola DR, Allan JM, Coppede F, Adamson PJ, Morgan GJ, Roman E, Smith MT. (2005) Risk of non-Hodgkin lymphoma associated with polymorphisms in folate-metabolizing genes. Cancer Epidemiol Biomarkers Prev. 14(12):2999–3003.

[63] Linnebank M, Schmidt S, Kölsch H, Linnebank A, Heun R, Schmidt-Wolf IG, Glasmacher A, Fliessbach K, Klockgether T, Schlegel U, Pels H. (2004) The methionine synthase polymorphism D919G alters susceptibility to primary central nervous system lymphoma. Br J Cancer.90 (10):1969–71.

[64] Lordelo GS, Miranda-Vilela AL, Akimoto AK, Alves PC, Hiragi CO, Nonino A, Daldegan MB, Klautau-Guimarães MN, Grisolia CK. (2012) Association between methylene tetrahydrofolatereductase and glutathione S-transferase M1 gene polymorphisms

and chronic myeloid leukemia in a Brazilian population. Genet Mol Res. 19;11(2): 1013-26.

[65] Marchesi F, Girardi K, Avvisati G. (2011) Pathogenetic, Clinical, and Prognostic Features of Adult t(4;11)(q21;q23)/MLL-AF4Positive B-Cell Acute Lymphoblastic Leukemia. AdvHematol. 2011;2011:62162.

[66] Marmiroli N. Maestri E. (2008) Health Implications of trace elements in the environment and the Food Chain In: Trace Elements as Contaminants and Nutrients: Consequences in Ecosystems and Human Health, Ed. M.N.V Prasad, John Wiley & Sons, Inc., 23-54.

[67] Martinelli G, Iacobucci I, Storlazzi CT, Vignetti M, Paoloni F, Cilloni D, Soverini S, Vitale A, Chiaretti S, Cimino G, Papayannidis C, Paolini S, Elia L, Fazi P, Meloni G, Amadori S, Saglio G, Pane F, Baccarani M, Foa R. (2009) IKZF1 (Ikaros) Deletions in BCR-ABL1–Positive Acute Lymphoblastic Leukemia Are Associated With Short Disease-Free Survival and High Rate of Cumulative Incidence of Relapse: A GIMEMA AL WP Report. J ClinOncol. 27(31):5202-07.

[68] Meyer C, Kowarz E, Hofmann J, Renneville A, Zuna J, Trka J, Ben Abdelali R, Macintyre E, De Braekeleer E, De Braekeleer M, Delabesse E, de Oliveira MP, Cavé H, Clappier E, van Dongen JJ, Balgobind BV, van den Heuvel-Eibrink MM, Beverloo HB, Panzer-Grümayer R, Teigler-Schlegel A, Harbott J, Kjeldsen E, Schnittger S, Koehl U, Gruhn B, Heidenreich O, Chan LC, Yip SF, Krzywinski M, Eckert C, Möricke A, Schrappe M, Alonso CN, Schäfer BW, Krauter J, Lee DA, ZurStadt U, TeKronnie G, Sutton R, Izraeli S, Trakhtenbrot L, Lo Nigro L, Tsaur G, Fechina L, Szczepanski T, Strehl S, Ilencikova D, Molkentin M, Burmeister T, Dingermann T, Klingebiel T, Marschalek R. (2009) New insights to the MLL recombinome of acute leukemias. Leukemia. 23(8):1490-9.

[69] Milani L, Lundmark A, Nordlund J, Kiialainen A, Flaegstad T, Jonmundsson G, Kanerva J, Schmiegelow K, Gunderson KL, Lönnerholm G, Syvänen AC. (2009) Allele-specific gene expression patterns in primary leukemic cells reveal regulation of gene expression by CpG site methylation. Gen Research. 19 (1):1-11.

[70] Milne TA, Briggs SD, Brock HW. (2002) MLL targets SET domain methyltransferase activity to Hox gene promoters, Molecular Cell. 10(5):1107–17.

[71] Mitelman F, Johansson B and Mertens F (Eds.). (2012) Mitelman Database of Chromosome Aberrations and Gene Fusions in Cancer http://cgap.nci.nih.gov/Chromosomes/Mitelman. Last updated on August 15, 2012

[72] Mitelman F, Johansson B, Mertens F. (2007) The impact of translocations and gene fusions on cancer causation. Nat Rev Cancer. 7(4):233-45.

[73] Moorman AV, Chilton L, Wilkinson J, Ensor HM, Bown N, Proctor SJ. (2010) Apopulation-based cytogenetic study of adults with acute lymphoblastic leucemia. Blood. 115(6): 206-14.

[74] Moriya K, Suzuki M, Watanabe Y, Takahashi T, Aoki Y, Uchiyama T, Kumaki S, Sasahara Y, Minegishi M, Kure S, Tsuchiya S, Sugamura K, Ishii N. (2012) Development of a Multi-Step Leukemogenesis Model of MLL-Rearranged Leukemia Using Humanized Mice. PLoS One. 7(6):e37892.

[75] Mullighan CG, Downing JR. (2009) Global Genomic Characterization of Acute Lymphoblastic Leukemia. SeminHematol. 46 (1):3–15.

[76] Mullighan CG, Goorha S, Radtke I, Miller CB, Coustan-Smith E, Dalton JD, Girtman K, Mathew S, Ma J, Pounds SB, Su X, Pui CH, Relling MV, Evans WE, Shurtleff SA, Downing JR. (2007) Genome-wide analysis of genetic alterations in acute lymphoblastic leukaemia. Nature.446(7137):758-64.

[77] Nademanee, A. O'Donnell MR, Snyder DS, Schmidt GM, Parker PM, Stein AS, Smith EP, Molina A, Stepan DE, Somlo G, Margolin KA, Sniecinski I, Dagis AC, Niland J, Pezner R, Forrnan SJ. (1995) High- dose chemotherapy with or without total body irradiation followed by autologous bone marrow and/or peripheral blood stem cell transplantation for patients with relapsed and refractory Hodgkin's disease: results in 85 patients with analysis of prognostic factors. Blood. 85(5):1381–1390.

[78] Nazki FH, Masood A, BandayMA,Bhat A, GanaiBA. (2012)Thymidylate synthase enhancer region polymorphism not related to susceptibility to acute lymphoblastic leukemia in the Kashmir population.Genet. Mol. Res. 11 (2): 906-17

[79] Ng A, Taylor GM, Eden OB. (2000) Treatment-related leukemia-a clinical and scientific challenge. Cancer Treatment Rev. 26(5):377–391.

[80] Paietta E. (1995) Proposals for the immunological classification of acute leukemias. Leukemia. 9(12):2147–2148.

[81] Palomero T, Lim WK, Odom DT, Sulis ML, Real PJ, Margolin A, Barnes KC, O'Neil J, Neuberg D, Weng AP, Aster JC, Sigaux F, Soulier J, Look AT, Young RA, Califano A, Ferrando AA. (2006) NOTCH1 directly regulates c-MYC and activates a feed-forward-loop transcriptional network promoting leukemic cell growth. ProcNatlAcadSci USA. 103(48):18261-6.

[82] Pedersen-Bjergaard J, Andersen MK, Christiansen DH, Nerlov C. (2002) Genetic pathways in therapy-related myelodysplasia and acute myeloid leukemia. Blood. 99(6): 1909–1912.

[83] Pendersen-Bjergaard J, Andersen MK, Christiansen DH. (2000) Therapy-related acute myeloid leukemia and myelodysplasia after high-dose chemotherapy and autologous stem cell transplantation. Blood. 95(11):3273–3279.

[84] Pendersen-Bjergaard J, Janssen WG, Lyons J, Philip P, Bartram CR. (1988) Point mutation of the ras protooncogenes and chromosome aberrations in acute nonlymphocytic leukemia and preleukemia related to therapy with alkylating agents. Cancer Res. 48(7): 1812–1817.

[85] Peterson CL, Workman JL. (2000) Promoter targeting and chromatin remodeling by the SWI/SNF complex.CurrOpinGenet. 10(2):187-92.

[86] Pierce BA. (2009) Genética del Cáncer in Genética un enfoque conceptual 3a edición. Ed, Panamericana. 624-44.

[87] Popp HD, Bohlander SK. (2010) Genetic instability in inherited and sporadic leukemias. Genes Chromosomes Cancer. 49(12):1071–1081.

[88] Pui CH, Carroll WL, Meshinchi S, Arceci RJ. (2011) Biology, risk stratification, and therapy of pediatric acute leukemias: an update. J ClinOncol..29(5): 551–65.

[89] Pui CH. (2009) Acute lymphoblastic leukemia: introduction. SeminHematol. 46(1):1-2

[90] Robien K, Ulrich CM. (2003) 5,10-Methylenetetrahydrofolate reductase polymorphisms and leukemia risk: a HuGEminireview. Am J Epidemiol.157(7):571-82.

[91] Rowley JD, Olney HJ. (2002) International workshop on the relationship of prior therapy to balanced chromosome aberrations in therapy-related myelodysplastic syndromes and acute leukemia: overview report. Genes Chromosomes Cancer. 33(4):331–345.

[92] Sanda T, Li X, Gutierrez A, Ahn Y, Neuberg DS, O'Neil J, Strack PR, Winter CG, Winter SS, Larson RS, BoehmerHv, (2010) Look AT. Interconnecting molecular pathways in the pathogenesis and drug sensitivity ofT-cell acute lymphoblastic leukemia.Blood. 115(9):1735-45.

[93] Satter M, James DG. (2003) Molecular Mechanisms of Transformation by the BCR-ABL Oncogene. Sem in Hematol. 40:4-10.

[94] Schnittger S, Kinkelin U, Schoch C, Heinecke A, Haase D, Haferlach T, Büchner T, Wörmann B, Hiddemann W, Griesinger F. (2000) Screening for MLL tandem duplication in 387 unselected patients with AML identify a prognostically unfavorable subset of AML. Leukemia.14(5):796–804.

[95] Sevilla J, Rodriguez A, Hernández Maravor D, de Bustos G, Aguado J, Ojeda E, Arrieta R, Hernández-Navarro F. (2002) Secondary acute myeloid leukemia and myelodisplasia after autologous peripheral blood progenitor cell transplantation. Ann Hematol. 81(1):11–15.

[96] Shaffer LG, Slovak ML, Campbell LJ.Neoplasia in ISCN (2009): An International System for Human Cytogenetic Nomenclature.2009; 88-96.

[97] Sharp L, Little J. (2004) Polymorphisms in genes involved in folate metabolism and colorectal neoplasia: a HuGE review. Am J Epidemiol. 59(5):423-43.

[98] Sheweita SA. (2000) Drug-Metabolizing Enzymes: Mechanisms and functions. Current Drug Metabolism, 1(2):107-32

[99] Skibola CF, Forrest MS, Coppedé F, Agana L, Hubbard A, Smith MT, Bracci PM, Holly EA. (2004) Polymorphisms and haplotypes in folate-metabolizing genes and risk of non-Hodgkin lymphoma. Blood.104(7):2155-62.

[100] Skibola CF, Smith MT, Kane E, Roman E, Rollinson S, Cartwright RA, Morgan G. (1999) Polymorphisms in the methylenetetrahydrofolatereductase gene are associated with susceptibility to acute leukemia in adults. ProcNatlAcadSci U S A. 26;96(22):12810-5.

[101] Smith MA, Rubinstein L, Anderson JL, Arthur D, Catalano PJ, Freidlin B, Heyn R, Khayat A, Krailo M, Land VJ, Miser J, Shuster J, Vena D. (1999) Secondary leukemia or myelodisplastic syndrome after treatament with epypodophillotoxins. J Clin Oncol. 17(2):569–577.

[102] Smith MT, Linet MS, Morgan GJ. (2002) Causative agents in the etiology of the myelodysplastic syndromes and the acute myeloid leukemias. In: Bennett JM (ed). The Myelodysplastic Syndromes, Pathobiology and Clinical Management. New York, NY, USA: Marcel Dekker, Inc. pp. 29–63.

[103] Smith MT. (1996) The mechanism of benzene-induced leukemia: a hypothesis and speculations on the causes of leukemia. Environ Health Perspect. 104 (Suppl 6):1219-25.

[104] Stock W, Tsai T, Golden C, Rankin C, Sher D, Slovak M L, Pallavicini M G,. Radich J P, Boldt DH. (2000) Cell cycle regulatory gene abnormalities are important determinants of leukemogenesis and disease biology in adult acute lymphoblastic leukemia. Blood. 95(7):2364-71.

[105] Stott H, Fox W, Girling DJ, Stephens RJ, Galton DA. (1977) Acute leukemia after busulphan Br Med J. 2(6101):1513–1517.

[106] Strachan DP. Hay fever, hygiene, and household size. BMJ 1989; 299:1259–60.

[107] Tesniere A, Panaretakis T, Kepp O, Apetoh L, Ghiringhelli F, Zitvogel L, Kroemer G. (2008) Molecular characteristics of immunogenic cancer cell death. Cell Death Differ. 5(1):3-12.

[108] Thomsen UL, Madsen HO, Vestergaard TR, Hjalgrim H, Nersting J, Schmiegelow K. (2011) Prevalence of t(12;21) [ETV6-RUNX1] positive cells in healthy neonates. Blood. 117(1):186-189.

[109] Traweek ST, Slovak ML, Nademanee AP, Brynes RK, Niland JC, Forman SJ. (1996) Myelodysplasia and acute myeloid leukemia occurring after autologous bone marrow transplantation for lymphoma. Leuk Lymphoma. 20(5-6):365–372.

[110] Valik D, Radina M, Sterba J, Vojtesek B. (2004)Homocysteine: exploring its potential as a pharmacodynamic biomarker of antifolate chemotherapy. Pharmacogenomics. 5(8): 1151-62.

[111] van Leeuwen FE, Chorus AM, van den Belt-Dusebout AW, Hagenbeek A, Noyon R, van Kerkhoff EH, Pinedo HM, Somers R. (1994) Leukemia risk following Hodgkin's disease: relation to cumulative dose of alkylating agents, treatment with teniposide

combinations, number of episodes of chemotherapy, and bone marrow damage. J Clin Oncol. 1994 May;12(5):1063-73.

[112] Visvader JE. (2011) Cells of origin in cáncer.Nature. 469:314-22.

[113] Yu K, Zhang J, Zhang J, Dou C, Gu S, Xie Y, Mao Y, Ji C. (2010) Methionine synthase A2756G polymorphism and cancer risk: a meta-analysis. Eur J Hum Genet. 18(3):370-8.

[114] Zornoza AV, Agirre X, Palanco VM, Subero JIM, Eneriz ESJ, Garate L, Alvarez S, Miranda E, Otero PR, Rifón J, Torres A, Calasanz MJ, Cigudosa JC, Gómez JR,Prósper F. (2011) Frequent and Simultaneous Epigenetic Inactivation of TP53 Pathway Genes in Acute Lymphoblastic Leukemia. PLoS ONE. 6(2):1-14.

[115] Zuo Z, Jones D, Yao H, Thomas DA, O'Brien S, Ravandi F, Kantarjian HM, Abruzzo LV, Medeiros L J, Chen SS, Luthra R. (2010) A pathway-based gene signature correlates with therapeutic response in adult patients with Philadelphia chromosome-positive acute lymphoblastic leukemia. Modern Pathology. 23(11):1524–34.

Chapter 4

Multi-Role of Cancer Stem Cell in Children Acute Lymphoblastic Leukemia

Dong-qing Wang, Hai-tao Zhu, Yan-fang Liu,
Rui-gen Yin, Liang Zhao, Zhi-jian Zhang,
Zhao-liang Su, Yan-Zhu, Hui-qun Lu,
Juan Hong and Jie Zhang

Additional information is available at the end of the chapter

http://dx.doi.org/10.5772/55075

1. Introduction

Acute lymphoblastic leukemia (ALL) is a malignant proliferation of lymphoid precursor cells in the bone marrow blood. It is an age related tumor, with a peak between the ages of 2 and 10 and a second peak after the age of 5. Among children younger than 15 years, ALL represents 23% of cancer that was diagnosed. The children aged 2 to 3 years were a sharp peak in ALL incidence (>80 per million per year).The rates of the ALL among children aged 8 to 10 years incidence decreasing to 20 per million. Moreover, there has been a gradual increase in the incidence of ALL in the past 25 years.

With the development of the medicine, considerable advances have been made in the treatment of childhood ALL. In the 1980's, relapsed ALL was regarded as an incurable disease. However, about 85% of childhoods ALL can hope to achieve a second remission over the last years. Meanwhile, around 40% of these can hope to achieve long term cure. On the other hand, despite optimal therapy, long term survival rate still limited to 30–40% of patients and about 15-20% children will sustain relapse. Because of the high relapse rate, refractoriness to conventional treatment protocols, the incidence of chemotherapy-related deaths, the complete remission rate, numerous challenges remained in the management of ALL, especially the children with relapsed ALL. Also, the disease mechanism is multi-factorials and involves in different genetic and environmental factors. So, ALL is still a problem that clinic must face up to. However, the emergency of cancer stem cell seems give us a new direction for deeper recognize this disease.

Despite the clone origin of many cancers, a notable characteristic of primary tumors is a marked degree of cellular heterogeneity. The hypothesis that human cancers comprise a heterogeneous population of cells that differ in marker expression, morphology, proliferation, and tumorigenicity has existed for over a century. Every tumor can be viewed as an abnormal organ that harbors a stem cell compartment. Emerging evidence has confirmed that the capacity of a tumor to grow and propagate depends on a small subset of cells within the tumor, which are most specifically referred to as "cancer stem cells" (CSCs), but have also been referred to as "progenitor cells" or "tumor initiating cells" (TICs) to distinguish them from the rest of the neoplastic cells that are unable to regenerate tumors. CSCs are defined to be a distinct population but variable subpopulation of the total tumor mass with stem cell characteristics that are essential for the initiation, development of human cancers, multi-drug resistance and metastases.

In the last two decades, with the wide spread utilization of fluorescence activated cell sorting (FACS) or magnetic activated cell sorting (MACS),the application of these technology to isolate and characterize of distinct cell populations of hematopoietic stem (HSC) or progenitor cell populations has become available. Using the same methodologies that employed to characterize normal hematopoietic stem cells,Cancer stem cells were first identified in haematopoietic malignancies and later in a broad spectrum of solid tumors including those of the breast, pancreatic, colon and brain. So, the malignant stem cell population that has been identified from ALL have been analyzed in most detail. These leukemia initiating, or leukemia stem cells (LSC) reside at the apex of a hierarchy of malignant cells that is analogous to the hierarchy found in normal hematopoietic. Thus, a hierarchical development structure for the leukemic population can be envisaged that originates from the malignant stem cell and is similar to normal hematopoietic processes. Importantly, these subpopulation of leukemic stem cells maintain the key stem cells properties of self-renewal, extensive proliferative potential and differentiate potential, highly resistant to chemo- and radio-therapy, driven metastasis, especially special organ metastases.

Apart from the method of FACS, LSCs may be sorted by various other characteristics.With the characteristic of limit less self-renewal in vitro, LSCs can be enriched in spheres when these cells are cultured in serum-free medium supplemented with the basic fibroblast growth factor (bFGF),epidermal growth factor (EGF),B27, insulin, and transferring. With the characteristic of expressing ABC transporters, these cells are able to pump the fluorescent dye hoechst-33342 out of the cell, namely identify unlabelled "side population" (SP) which highly enriched in stem cells.

With the deeper study of cancer stem cell, the role of it in ALL was believed to be more and more important. These functions include the following aspects.

2. Cancer stem cell may the origination of children Acute lymphoblastic leukemia

The development of the tumour is always believed to be the result of a succession of epigenetic/ genetic alterations and selection steps which leading to the emergence of cells accumulating survival and proliferation advantages. In the primary tumour, selection is proposed to take place continuously which giving rise to heterogeneity that simply reflects the coexistence of cell populations evolving independently and displaying distinct oncogenic potentials. The environment that the tumor exists was thought to be an important factor that impacts the selection procedure. The theory above mentioned denominates the cancer research one century and might be sufficient to interpret the cell diversity observed in tumors. However, it fails to explain how individual disseminated cancer cells escaping from primary tumours yield secondary tumours with similar diversity. An alternative model assumes that primary and secondary tumours arise from cancer cells displaying both self-renewal and differentiation capabilities, namely cancer stem cell. Recently, it became apparent that the different subpopulations have different degrees of proliferative and self-renewing abilities and only a small subpopulation can regenerate all the other tumor cell subpopulations of the original tumor when injected into immuno-compromised mice. This model seems not exclusive of the above theory, but more suitable to explain the origination of the tumor.

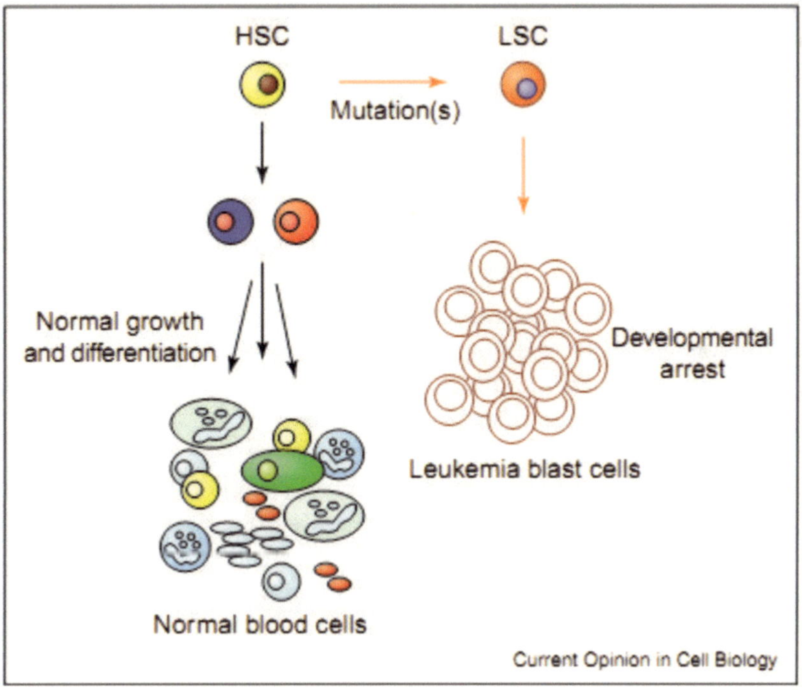

Figure 1. Craig T Jordan.Cancer stem cell biology: from leukemia to solid tumors. Current Opinion in Cell Biology 2004, 16:708–712.

At present, on the basis of expression of a particular cell surface marker, Cancer stem cells that sorted by FACE in children ALL are suggested to be have the most superior ability to form a new tumour in an in vivo xenograft assay and great ability to form cell spheres namely clonogenic when plated at low density in non-adherent culture. These two models were beloved to be the golden standard to test whether the cells own the characteristic of stemness.Meanwhile, it demonstrated that the Leukemic stem cells may be the origination of children ALL.

The Leukemic stem cells (LSCs) appear to retain many characteristics of normal hematopoietic stem cells (HSCs). This observation indicates that the malignant stem cell population can arise in two possible ways. One possibility is that normal HSCs are the direct target of mutations that cause conversion to an LSCs phenotype. Alternatively, more differentiated cell types might acquire mutations that confer stem-cell-like properties on cells that typically would not display stem cell characteristics. Normal stem cells intrinsically possess three hallmark features: first, the potential to undergo self-renewal; second, the potential to undergo extensive proliferation; third, the potential to differentiate into multiple distinct cell types. Like normal stem cells, LSCs own the ability of asymmetric division and symmetric division. Leukemic stem cells undergo symmetric division and expand the stem cell compartment. Conversely, via asymmetric division, CSCs give rise to the variety of differentiated cells in the tumor mass. They are stringently defined by functional attributes including the ability to instigate, maintain and serially propagate leukemia in vivo while retaining capacity to differentiate into committed progeny that lack these properties.

So, LSCs not only sustain the tumor but maintain the number of cancer stem cell in the tumor tissue. One contribution to our understanding of tumor initiation and growth comes from considering the developmental biology of stem cell systems.

3. Cancer stem cells are the main factor of drug resistance and relapse

Subsequent studies have further refined the immunophenotype of ALL stem cells and substantially added to our understanding of their biology. One of the most important characteristics of cancer stem cells is highly resistant to chemo- and radio-therapy. Because of the resistant to chemo- and radio-therapy, cancer stem cells further led to the relapse of the tumor. With the deeper research, it had make out of that resistance could depend on certain features that LSCs share with normal stem cells. First, this property concerns cell proliferation. A lot of research showed that ALL stem cells reside mostly in a quiescent cell cycle state in the absence of specific stimulation from the microenvironment which is analogous to their normal hematopoietic stem cell counterparts. This observation has a great significant in understanding the role of cancer stem cells in drug resistant. Because most therapeutic agents which rely on cycling cells in order to cause lethal cellular damage approaches to leukemia are directed towards actively cycling populations. The quiescent nature of LSCs indicates that standard chemotherapy drugs will not generally be effective against ALL stem cells. Notably, while treatment of ALL children with the drug that specially towards actively cycling sub-populations, it has been highly effective for inducing remission. However, Because of the existence of the quiescent cells, the patients would recurrence in the short time. This evidence indicates the disease is suppressed rather than eradicated. For example, 5-FU which is special for the S stage have obvious effect in the patient who was first diagnose of ALL. However, once the drug was retreat, the tumor may relapse. FACS analyze displayed that the existence cells mostly display the stemness cell characteristic. So, most chemotherapeuticagents,especiallythatarespecialforthecyclepopulationagentswerecytostatic butnotcytotoxictotheLSCs·ThisresultssupportedtheconceptthatablationoftheLSCisnecessary to completely destroy the tumor population permanently.On the other hand, new threpy agent desperatelyneededtobeexploredtopromotethequiescentLSCsintotheactivestate.Second,the second key property of LSCs is their abnormal expression of certain pumps which are absent in their compartment of non-LSC. These proteins included ATP-binding cassette (ABC) transporters super family, multidrug resistance-associated protein (MRP) family, breast cancer resistance protein (BCRP), lung resistance protein (LRP) and so on. They are promiscuous transporters of both hydrophobic and hydrophilic compounds and can help the cell extruding several drugs out of the cells. The exact physiological role of these pumps is not yet fully understood, but it is known that they are involved in cellular protection against exogenous products and in resistance to hypoxic stress, mediated by an increased ability to consume hydrogen peroxide and a reduced accumulation of toxic metabolites.So, with the help of these abnormal proteins, LSCs can display the great ability to promptly eliminate or degrade toxic compounds even though the concentration of the drug at a very high level. Once the treatment stopped, LSCs may self-renewal and differentiate into multiple distinct cell types which led to the relapse. Third, the most important key property is resistance to apoptosis, which can be limited to CSC initially, is often rapidly acquired also by the bulk of tumor cells at relapse, perhaps due to the genetic instability which distinguishes tumor from normal cells. Activation of programmed cell death or apoptosis is a promising strategy for the treatment of cancer, and the balance between anti-apoptotic and pro-apoptotic members is a key factor in the regulation of cell death. In order to maintain the progenitor pool from which differentiated cells derive, cancer stem cells are programmed to be long-lived. For this purpose, cancer stem cells activate some protective mechanisms that protect them from senescence and/or cellular stress. These mechanisms include: (I) The current results showed that cancer stem cells expressed high levels of the anti-apoptotic protein such as Bcl-2, and low levels of the pro-apoptotic protein caspase 3, compared to non cancer stem cells. Enhancement of their anti-apoptosis ability means that tumor cells survival becomes more dependent on anti-apoptotic-pathway activation, and standard therapeutic approaches may thus fail to kill cancer stem cells; (II) activation of some self-renewal pathways, such as TGF-β, Sonic Hedgehog(SHH), Wnt/β-catenin or BMI-1; (III) generation of auto-crine loops through the production of growth factors like epidermal growth factor (EGF), basic fibroblast growth factor (bFGF); and (IV) enhanced capability to repair DNA damage after genotoxic stress.As a consequence of this, chemotherapy invariably causes bone marrow toxicity due to its effects on trans-amplifying, progenitor and even more differentiated cells, whereas tumors may initially regress but subsequently become completely resistant to chemotherapy. By these natures, it was easy found that CSCs are biologically distinct from other cancer cell types. Moreover, certain natural properties of CSCs are likely to increase their resistance to standard chemotherapy agents. So, if cancer therapies do not effectively target the CSC population during initial treatment, then relapse may occur as a consequence of CSC driven tumor expansion. This is almost certainly the case in many instances of ALL, where standard drugs are unlikely to target the LSCs population effectively. Therefore, in developing new cancer therapeutics, analyses that directly assess toxicity towards tumor stem cells are an important priority.

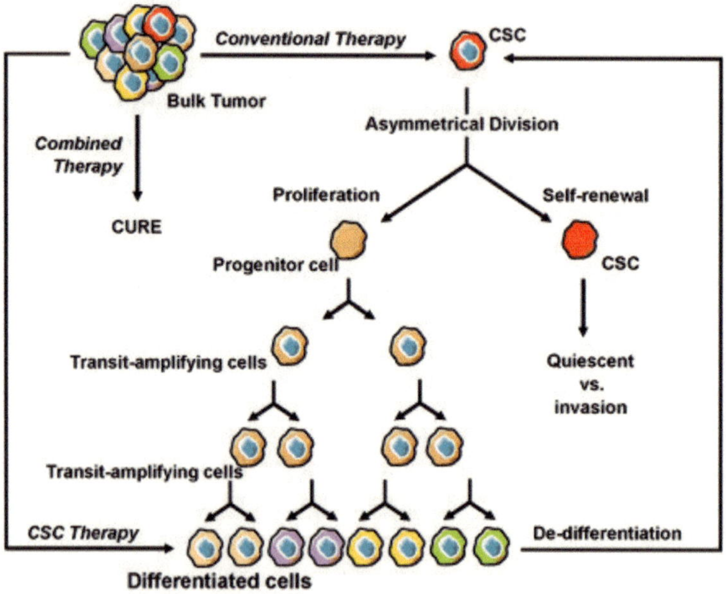

Figure 2. Lara Lacerda,Lajos Pusztai,et al.The role of tumor initiating cells in drug resistance of breast cancer:Implications for future therapeutic approaches. Drug Resistance Updates, 2010,13: 99–108

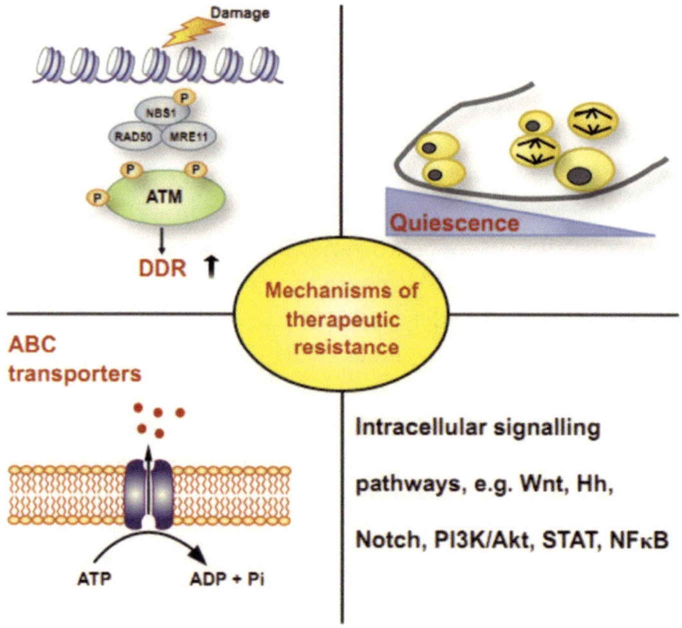

Figure 3. Malcolm R. Alison,Wey-Ran Lin,et al.Cancer stem cells: In the line of fire. Cancer Treatment Reviews, 2012,38:589-598.

http://dx.doi.org/10.5772/55075

4. LSCs solely are capable of driving tumor metastases

With the deeper research, it was well understanding that the cancer metastasis was viewed as a series of distinct steps that comprise the "invasion-metastasis-cascade" on the biological level [30-31]. The first step, cancer cells in the primary tumor acquire the ability to invade into the surrounding tissue such as the basement membrane. Next, tumor cells must gain access to blood and/or lymphatic vessels, enter into these vessels (intravasation), survive transport through these vessels, and exit from the vasculature (extravasation). Finally, small cell clumps or singly disseminated tumor cells must acquire the ability to survive and proliferate in the microenvironment of a foreign tissue in order to form macroscopic metastases, namely colonization or akinosis.

In the procedure of the tumor metastasis, EMT represents a crucial step and plays important role in mediated invasiveness sand metastasis, also is strongly associated with poor clinical outcome in many tumour types [32]. EMT termed epithelio–mesenchymal transformation was first described in a model of chick primitive streak formation. Nowadays, EMT is defined as a biologic process that allows a polarized epithelial cell, which normally interacts with the basement membrane via its basal surface, to undergo multiple biochemical changes that enable it to assume a mesenchymal cell phenotype, which includes enhanced migratory capacity, invasiveness, elevated resistance to apoptosis, and greatly increased production of extracellular matrix components [33-35]. Due to reorganization of epithelial intercellular junctions, EMT weakens cell-cell cohesion. Further-more cell-cell adhesion complexes and their transcriptional repressors are strongly regulated by a number of classical EMT-regulated pathways which including TGF-β, PDGF, Notch, Wnt, many of which also seem to play key role in skeletal metastasis. Moreover,EMT stimulates focal, proteolytic degradation of extracellular natrices, thus favoring invasion of stroma and intravasation. The modification of the cytoskeleton during EMT also contributes to migration. Intermediate filaments of epithelial cells such as cytokeratins are responsible for maintaining cell structure, stiffness and integrity. Apart from invasiveness, EMT also contributes to angiogenesis and intravasation. In addition to stimulating neovascularization, migratory carcinoma cells that have undergone EMT have acquired a number of specific properties that allow them to interact with endothelial cells and to enhance trans-endothelial migration. At last, EMT renders enhanced resistance to apoptotic signals and may contribute to the survival of circulating tumor cells (CTCs) in the hostile bloodstream environment and, eventually formed the second tumor.

It has even been proposed that cancer cells adopt stem cell features only upon undergoing EMT. Indeed, induction of EMT in immortalized human mammary epithelial cells resulted in the expression of stem cell markers, and phenotypes associated with CSCs. These findings illustrated a direct link between EMT and gain of properties characteristic for migratory stem cells. So,it can be concluded that LSCs acquired the property of EMT which is essential for the LSCs to form macroscopic metastases

CD44 has been proposed as one such marker. CD44 may play a crucial role in developing of metastasis in ALL, especially metastasis to special organ. Additionally, LSCs may express higher levels of cell-surface receptors than their non-LSCs counterparts so that they may fully harness the soluble growth factors present at secondary sites, conferring a growth advantage and permitting successful colonization.

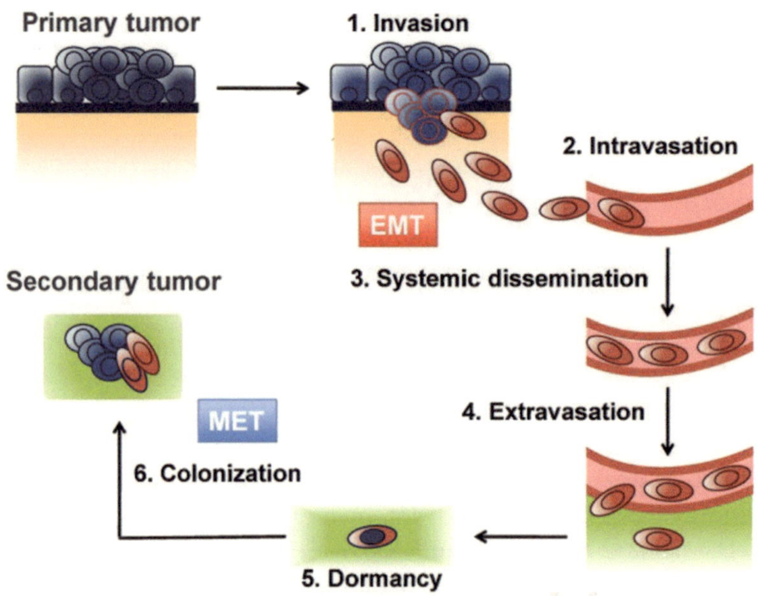

Figure 4. Christina Scheel, Robert A. Weinberg. Cancer stem cells and epithelial–mesenchymal transition: Concepts and molecular links. Seminars in Cancer Biology,2102.

In a world, although LSCs accounting for only a few distinct populations, it is the most important factors that mediated the biology of the ALL. LSCs may play a great role in the origination, drug-resistance and metastases. In the future, LSCs may be the sole target for treatment. A detailed consideration of stem cell biology principles will be useful in better understanding tumor pathogenesis and in designing strategies for more effective therapies.

Acknowledgements

This work was supported by Natural Science Foundation of Jiangsu Province (Grant No. BK2011487) and Social Development Foundation of Zhenjiang City (Grant No. SZC201130128).

Author details

Dong-qing Wang[1], Hai-tao Zhu[1], Yan-fang Liu[2], Rui-gen Yin[1], Liang Zhao[1], Zhi-jian Zhang[3], Zhao-liang Su[3], Yan-Zhu[1], Hui-qun Lu[1], Juan Hong[1] and Jie Zhang[4]

1 Department of Radiology, The Affiliated Hospital of Jiangsu University, Zhenjiang, China

2 Department of Central Laboratory, The Affiliated People's Hospital of Jiangsu University, Zhenjiang, China

3 Department of Immunology & Laboratory Immunology, Jiangsu University, Zhenjiang, China

4 Department of Ultrasound, Xuzhou Children's Hospital, Xuzhou, China

References

[1] Lane, S.W. and D.G. Gilliland, Leukemia stem cells. Semin Cancer Biol, 2010. 20(2): p. 71-6.

[2] Griffin, J.D. and B. Lowenberg, Clonogenic cells in acute myeloblastic leukemia. Blood, 1986. 68(6): p. 1185-95.

[3] Apostolidou, E., et al., Treatment of acute lymphoblastic leukaemia : a new era. Drugs, 2007. 67(15): p. 2153-71.

[4] Kochupillai, V., Emerging concepts in the management of acute lymphoblastic leukaemia. Indian J Med Res, 1993. 98: p. 1-7.

[5] Narayanan, S. and P.J. Shami, Treatment of acute lymphoblastic leukemia in adults. Crit Rev Oncol Hematol, 2012. 81(1): p. 94-102.

[6] McNeer, J.L. and E.A. Raetz, Acute lymphoblastic leukemia in young adults: which treatment? Curr Opin Oncol, 2012. 24(5): p. 487-94.

[7] Wang, X., et al., The role of cancer stem cells in cancer metastasis: New perspective and progress. Cancer Epidemiol, 2012.

[8] Sampieri, K. and R. Fodde, Cancer stem cells and metastasis. Semin Cancer Biol, 2012. 22(3): p. 187-93.

[9] Tsai, R.Y., A molecular view of stem cell and cancer cell self-renewal. Int J Biochem Cell Biol, 2004. 36(4): p. 684-94.

[10] Chu, J.E. and A.L. Allan, The Role of Cancer Stem Cells in the Organ Tropism of Breast Cancer Metastasis: A Mechanistic Balance between the "Seed" and the "Soil"? Int J Breast Cancer, 2012. 2012: p. 209748.

[11] Alison, M.R., et al., Cancer stem cells: in the line of fire. Cancer Treat Rev, 2012. 38(6): p. 589-98.

[12] Lane, S.W., D.T. Scadden, and D.G. Gilliland, The leukemic stem cell niche: current concepts and therapeutic opportunities. Blood, 2009. 114(6): p. 1150-7.

[13] Bonnet, D. and J.E. Dick, Human acute myeloid leukemia is organized as a hierarchy that originates from a primitive hematopoietic cell. Nat Med, 1997. 3(7): p. 730-7.

[14] Al-Hajj, M., et al., Prospective identification of tumorigenic breast cancer cells. Proc Natl Acad Sci U S A, 2003. 100(7): p. 3983-8.

[15] O'Brien, C.A., et al., A human colon cancer cell capable of initiating tumour growth in immunodeficient mice. Nature, 2007. 445(7123): p. 106-10.

[16] Ricci-Vitiani, L., et al., Identification and expansion of human colon-cancer-initiating cells. Nature, 2007. 445(7123): p. 111-5.

[17] Singh, S.K., et al., Identification of human brain tumour initiating cells. Nature, 2004. 432(7015): p. 396-401.

[18] Ponti, D., et al., Isolation and in vitro propagation of tumorigenic breast cancer cells with stem/progenitor cell properties. Cancer Res, 2005. 65(13): p. 5506-11.

[19] Eramo, A., et al., Identification and expansion of the tumorigenic lung cancer stem cell population. Cell Death Differ, 2008. 15(3): p. 504-14.

[20] Alison, M.R., S.M. Lim, and L.J. Nicholson, Cancer stem cells: problems for therapy? J Pathol, 2011. 223(2): p. 147-61.

[21] Coustan-Smith, E. and D. Campana, Immunologic minimal residual disease detection in acute lymphoblastic leukemia: a comparative approach to molecular testing. Best Pract Res Clin Haematol, 2010. 23(3): p. 347-58.

[22] Graham, S.M., et al., Primitive, quiescent, Philadelphia-positive stem cells from patients with chronic myeloid leukemia are insensitive to STI571 in vitro. Blood, 2002. 99(1): p. 319-25.

[23] Huang, Y., Pharmacogenetics/genomics of membrane transporters in cancer chemotherapy. Cancer Metastasis Rev, 2007. 26(1): p. 183-201.

[24] Stavrovskaya, A.A. and T.P. Stromskaya, Transport proteins of the ABC family and multidrug resistance of tumor cells. Biochemistry (Mosc), 2008. 73(5): p. 592-604.

[25] Maciejczyk, A., et al., ABCC2 (MRP2, cMOAT) localized in the nuclear envelope of breast carcinoma cells correlates with poor clinical outcome. Pathol Oncol Res, 2012. 18(2): p. 331-42.

[26] Raghav, P.K., Y.K. Verma, and G.U. Gangenahalli, Peptide screening to knockdown Bcl-2's anti-apoptotic activity: implications in cancer treatment. Int J Biol Macromol, 2012. 50(3): p. 796-814.

[27] Sneddon, J.B. and Z. Werb, Location, location, location: the cancer stem cell niche. Cell Stem Cell, 2007. 1(6): p. 607-11.

[28] Salmaggi, A., et al., Glioblastoma-derived tumorospheres identify a population of tumor stem-like cells with angiogenic potential and enhanced multidrug resistance phenotype. Glia, 2006. 54(8): p. 850-60.

[29] Denissova, N.G., et al., Resveratrol protects mouse embryonic stem cells from ionizing radiation by accelerating recovery from DNA strand breakage. Carcinogenesis, 2012. 33(1): p. 149-55.

[30] Geiger TR. and Peeper DS,Metastasis mechanisms. Biochimica et Biophysica Acta , 2009.10(2):p.293–308.

[31] Fidler IJ. Critical determinants of metastasis. Seminars in Cancer Biology, 2002. 12(2):p .89–96.

[32] Yang J, Weinberg RA. Epithelial–mesenchymal transition: at the crossroads of development and tumor metastasis. Cell,2008.11(14):p.818–29.

[33] Polyak K, Weinberg RA. Transitions between epithelial and mesenchymal states:acquisition of malignant and stem cell traits. Nat Rev Cancer Apr, 2009.9(4):p.265–73.

[34] Kalluri R, Weinberg RA. The basics of epithelial– mesenchymal transition. J Clin Invest Jun, 2009.119(6):p.1420 – 8.

[35] Potenta S, Zeisberg E, Kalluri R. The role of endothelial-to-mesenchymal transition in cancer progression. Br J Cancer Nov,2008.99(9):p.1375-9.

Chapter 5

Adult T-Cell Leukemia/Lymphoma (ATL): Pathogenesis, Treatment and Prognosis

Shoko Kobayashi and Shigeki Iwasaki

Additional information is available at the end of the chapter

http://dx.doi.org/10.5772/54776

1. Introduction

Adult T-cell leukemia/lymphoma (ATL) was first described in 1977 as a distinct clinico-pathological entity with a suspected viral etiology. Subsequently, a RNA retrovirus, human T-cell leukemia /lymphotropic virus type 1 (HTLV-1) was isolated as a carcinogenic pathogens [1].

HTLV-1 infects approximately 15 to 20 million people worldwide, with endemic areas in Japan, the Caribbean, and Africa.

After prolonged latency periods, approximately 3 to 5% of HTLV-1 infected individuals will develop either ATL or other disorders such as HTLV-1-associated myelopathy/tropical spastic paraparesis (HAM/TSP).

2. Transmission and spread

The three major routes of HTLV-1 transmission are, 1)mother-to-child infections via breast milk, 2)sexual intercourse, and 3)blood transfusions. HTLV-1 infection early in life, presumably from breast feeding, is crucial in the development of ATL [2].

3. Initial infection

HTLV-1 infects CD4+ and CD8+ T lymphocytes and can also efficiently infect dendritic cells [3].

The ubiquitous glucose transporter 1 and the neuropilin 1 were identified as members of the HTLV-I receptor complex [4,5].

Moreover, surface heparan sulfate proteoglycans were shown to be required for efficient virus entry [6]. Clonal expansion of HTLV-infected cells mostly relies on the promotion of cycling CD4+ T cells [7].

4. Infected cell types

CD4+ lymphocytes and to a lesser extent CD8+ T cells are considered to be as the main targets of HTLV-1. Plasmacytoid dendritic cells (pDC) were also infected by HTLV-1 in patients. In fact, all types of dendritic cells have been shown to be easily infected by HTLV-1 in vitro and efficiently transmit HTLV-1 to T cells in free viral transmission [8].

The proviral load was higher in isolated pDCs than in T cells. pDCs was found to be stimulated type I interferon α and β which interacted with their cognate receptors on virus infected cells and, through IFN-inducible genes, interfered with viral replication. pDCs from ATL patients were known to be impaired in their production of IFN-α. These observations supported a role for pDC in viral persistence and disease progression [9].

CD4+ T cells can be divided into two major categories: effector T cells and regulatory T cells(Treg). Effector T cells induce the activation of immune responses by secreting proinflammatory cytokines, whereas Treg which express the transcription factor FoxP3, suppress immune responses by both cell-contact dependent and –independent mechanisms. A proportion of HTLV-1 infected CD4+ T cells express FoxP3. It showed that HTLV-1 infection induces the phenotype of FoxP3+CD4+ T cells [7].

5. HTLV-1 virus

5.1. HTLV-1-encoded proteins

The HTLV-1 genome contains typical structural and enzymatic genes (*gag, pro, pol* and *env*) flanked by two long terminal repeats (LTRs). (Fig. 1). The long terminal repeats (LTR) are subdivided into three regions (i.e., U3, R and U5) that contain the *cis*-acting elements essential for viral gene expression: transcription factor-binding sites, transcription start and termination sites, polyadenylation and splicing sites. A region called pX, which is located between the *env* gene and the 3′-LTR, contains at least four partially overlapping reading frames (ORFs) encoding accessory proteins (p12I, p13II, p30II), the post-transcriptional regulator Rex (ORF III) and the Tax transactivator (ORF IV). In addition, HBZ is encoded from the 3′ LTR in the complementary strand of the genome. Among all these regulatory proteins, Tax and HBZ proteins appear to have particularly important roles in viral persistence and pathogenesis [10].

http://dx.doi.org/10.5772/54776

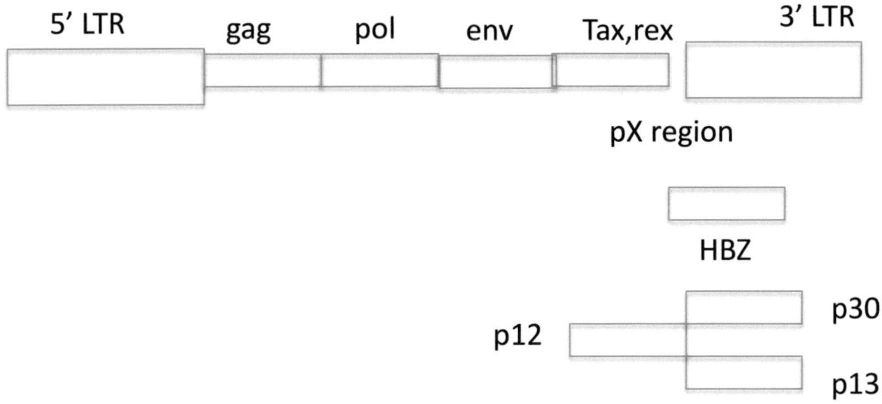

LTR : long terminal repeat
Tax : transcriptional transactivator
HBZ : HTLV-1 bZIP

Figure 1. HTLV-1 proviral gene

5.2. Tax (transcriptional transactivator) (p40)

Tax is a major factor that mediated the following: 1)viral persistence and disease development. 2) oncogenic potential, 3)cell-signalling pathways, 4)interferes with checkpoint control and inhibition of DNA repair, and 5) modulation of the miRNAs environment [11].

Among the cellular pathways activated by Tax, CREB/ATF, NF-κB and AP1 are thought to have predominant roles in T-cell proliferation and transformation.

Tax -mediated NF-κB activation stimulates expression of cytokines and their receptors such as interleukin 2 (IL2)/IL2 receptor (IL2R), IL9, IL13 and IL15/IL15R as well as members of the tumour necrosis factor receptor family.

A major activity of Tax in signaling pathways is the stimulation of G1/S transition. Tax increases the levels of type D cyclin levels in G1 and activates cyclin-dependent kinases (i.e., CDK4 and CDK6) through direct binding, leading to Rb hyperphosphorylation, subsequent release of E2F transcription factor and accelerated transition from G1 to S. Tax also directly interacts with and promotes the degradation of Rb. Furthermore, Tax modulates expression of CDK inhibitors such as p18INK4c, p19INK4d, p21WAF1 and p27KIP1 and inactivates p15INK4b and p16INK4a through direct binding, thereby restraining their inhibitory activity toward CDKs.

Tax stimulate viral production and infection, however, the Tax expression is transient and rapidly turned off (Fig 2). Cells that failed to shut off the Tax are rejected by host immune response, such as cytotoxic T lymphocytes (CTL) and only the cells with latent viral expression should survive. Repeating these cycles for long periods, results in the persistence of infected individuals in a virus carrier state, however Tax-incuced mutaions accumulated in infected cells.

Three mechanisms have been described for inactivating Tax expression in ATL cells have been described: 1) genetic changes (nonsense mutation, deletion, and insertion) in the *tax* gene, 2) deletion of the 5' long terminal repeat (LTR) that contains the viral promoter, and 3) DNA methylation of the 5 ' LTR leading to promoter inactivation.

Tax-mediated mutation would be a critical event in ATL that triggers the clonal selection of infected T cells as malignant leukemia cells [12].

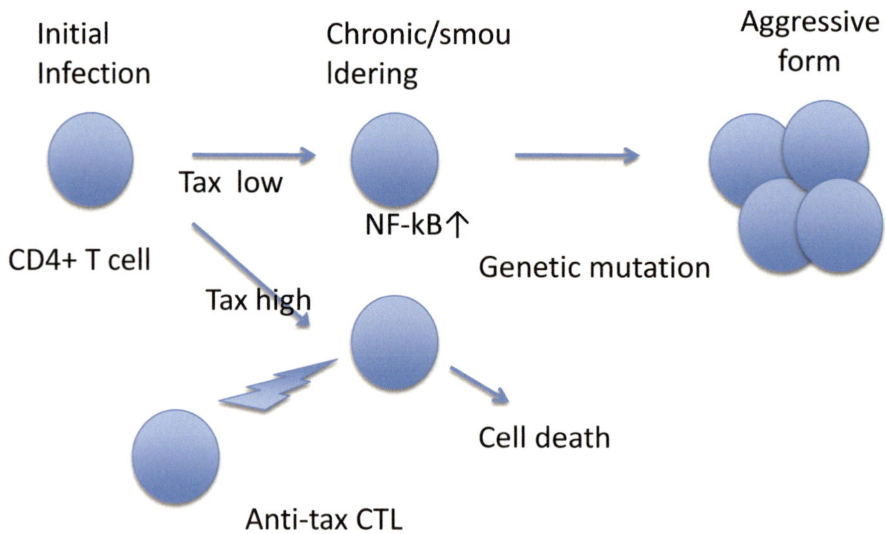

Figure 2. Probable mechanism of pathogenesis in ATL progression

5.3. Other proteins; Rex, p12, p13 and p30

Rex (p27) is an RNA-binding post-transcriptional regulator that binds to its *cis*-acting target sequence, the Rex response element (RRE), located at the 3′-end of sense viral mRNAs.

HTLV-1 contains both regulatory and accessory genes in four pX open reading frames. pX. ORF-II encodes two proteins, p13 and p30.

Proviral clones of HTLV-1 with pX ORF-II mutations diminish the ability of the virus to maintain viral loads in vivo. p30 is acting as a repressor of many genes including Tax, in part by blocking tax/rex RNA nuclear export.

p30 expression results in activation of the G2-M cell cycle checkpoint, events that would promote early viral spread and T-cell survival. [13,14].

The role of four open reading frames (ORFs), located between env and the 3' long terminal repeat of HTLV-1. By differential splicing, ORF II encodes two proteins, p13(II) and p30(II). p13(II) localizes to mitochondria and may alter the configuration of the tubular network of this cellular organelle.

Mutations in pX ORF II diminish the ability of HTLV-1 to maintain high viral loads in vivo and suggest an important function for p13(II) and p30(II) in viral pathogenesis. [15].

The repression in Tax expression is essential to protect infected cells from immune response and to maintain the virus. However, recent studies suggested that a loss of Tax expression also prevents Tax-induced mitotic aberrations that are detrimental to cell proliferation and therefore, to stabilize the karyotype of infected T cells [16].

5.4. HBZ

A recently identified HBZ factor. HTLV-1 bZIP, acts as a negative regulator of Tax-mediated viral transactivation by heterodimerising with CREB, CREB2, and p300/CBP. HBZ RNA expression leads to the upregulation of E2F1 target genes and stimulation of T lymphocyte proliferation [17].

The HBZ protein was first reported to function as a transcription factor that repressed viral expression by competing with Tax-mediated LTR activation.

As previously, Tax is highly immunogenic and its expression induces an immune response that generates CTL primarily directed against this oncoprotein. To escape this CTL-mediated lysis and to maintain viral persistence, HTLV-I infected cells frequently reduce Tax expression by several mechanisms.

HBZ was expected to be responsible for inducing and maintaining the tumor state even after Tax was shut off, which was supported by evidence that *HBZ* transcription was correlated with the proviral load [18-20].

Similar to Tax, HBZ interacts with proteasome subunits and may promote the delivery of cellular factors (such as c-Jun) to the proteasome even in the absence of ubiquitination.

6. Tumor marker

Similar to serum LDH reflecting disease bulk/activity, the soluble form of interleukin-2 receptor α-chain is elevated. [21].

The mean sIL-2R levels of the smoldering, chronic, acute, and lymphoma subtypes of ATL were 1680 U/ml, 6680 U/ml, 45,940 U/ml, and 34,620 U/ml, respectively ($P < 0.01$). The sIL-2R levels of each subtype at the time of diagnosis were more correlated with tumor burden, malignant behavior, and prognosis than LDH levels. In the low, moderate, and high sIL-2R subgroups, the median survival time and percent survival probability at 2 years was 30.2 months (46.0%), 16.5 months (25.0%), and 7.7 months (15.3%), respectively.

These serum markers are useful to detect acute transformation of indolent ATL as well as to detect early relapse of ATL after therapy.

7. Immunophenotype

In most patients, ATL cells exhibit the phenotype of mature CD4+ T cells and express CD2, CD5, CD25, CD45RO, CD29, T-cell receptor αβ, and HLA-DR. Most ATL cells are CD52, CCR4 positive, but occasionally, patients are negative. Immunophenotypic analysis of CD3, CD4, CD7, CD8, and CD25 is the minimum requirement for an ATL diagnosis.

8. Cytogenetics

Karyotypic abnormalities revealed by conventional cytogenetics or comparative genomic hybridization are more common and complex in the acute and lymphoma types compared with the chronic type, with aneuploidy and several hot spots such as 14q and 3p. More sensitive array-comparative genomic hybridization revealed that the lymphoma type had significantly more frequent gains at 1q, 2p, 4q, 7p, and 7q and more losses of 10p, 13q, 16q, and 18p, whereas the acute type showed a gain of 3/3p [22.23].

9. Molecular biology of host genome

Mutation or deletion of tumor suppressor genes, such as *p53* or *p15INK4B/p16INK4A,* is observed in approximately half of ATL patients and is associated with clinical subtypes and prognosis.These new molecular markers may help guide therapeutic decisions. [24].

To predict to respond to antiviral therapy with AZT and IFN-alpha, the expression of proto-oncogene c-Rel and interferon regulatory factor-4 (IRF-4) was examined. Resistant tumors exhibited c-Rel (6 of 10; 60%) more often than did sensitive variants (1 of 9; 11%). This finding was independent of the disease form. Elevated expression of the putative c-Rel target, IRF-4, was observed in 10 (91%) of 11 nonresponders and in all tested patients with c-Rel+ tumors and occurred in the absence of the HTLV-1 oncoprotein Tax. In contrast, tumors in complete responders did not express c-Rel or IRF-4. The expression of nuclear c-Rel and IRF-4 occurs in the absence of Tax in ATLL and is associated with antiviral resistance. [25].

10. Molecular biology of HTLV-1

Monoclonal integration of HTLV-1 proviral DNA is observed in all cases of ATL. Integration of defective HTLV-1 into ATL cells is observed in approximately one-third of ATL patients and is associated with clinical subtypes and prognosis. It is recommended to perform molecular analysis of HTLV-1 integration when possible. Either Southern blotting or polymerase chain reaction for HTLV-1 can be used to identify the presence of viral integration, although

http://dx.doi.org/10.5772/54776

the latter can also be used for quantitative purposes. Clinically, ATL is diagnosed on the basis of seropositivity for HTLV-1 and histologically and/or cytologically proven peripheral T-cell malignancy. [26].

11. Pathogenesis

Tax is a multifunctional protein that affects various cellular machinery and signaling pathways to mediate cellular transformation and viral replication.

The necessity of NF-κB, a transcription factor, in Tax-mediated transformation was confirmed in which a single point mutation in the Tax that disrupts to activate the NFκB pathway also eliminates the viral ability to transform [27].

11.1. Tax-independent NF-κB activation

However, Tax expression is lost in approximately 60% of all ATLs during the late stages of leukemogenesis stages. Notably, NF-κB pathways remain still strongly activated in HTLV-1-infected Tax-negative cells, suggesting the existence of Tax-independent mechanism. Reportedly, Tax-independent NF-κB activation occurs in Tax-positive cells. Several mechanisms are speculated in Tax-independent NF-κB activation, such as IKKB activation and the NF-κB member c-Rel [28-31].

HTLV-1 infection induces expression of many NF-κB stimulators and signaling molecules such as TNF, CD40, CD30, and Bcl-3. TNF is the prototypic stimuli of NF-κB activation, while CD40 and CD30 are potent activators of NF-κB pathways. Bcl-3 binds to p50 or p52 homodimers and transforms them from transcription repressors into activators [32-35].

11.2. Persistent NF-κB activation by HTLV-1

Tax binds to and increases the stability and activity of NF-κB and/or prevents NF-κB from binding to its inhibitors, resulting in a prolonged and elevated activation of NF-κB. NF-κB activation is aberrantly persistent, irrespective of whether it is Tax-dependent or -independent. A main reason for this abnormal activation is the co-existence and cross-activation of different NF-κB and NF-κB-related signaling pathways. [36-40].

In addition to NF-κB, Tax induces many other signaling pathways such as the phosphatidylinositol 3-kinase (PI3K)/AKT and DNA damage signaling pathways, leading to reciprocal enhancement of these pro-oncogenic pathways with NF-κB. Most of the mechanisms activate Tax-independent and -dependent NF-κB pathway. [41.42].

11.3. Differences between tax-dependent and tax-independent NF-κB activation by HTLV-1

NF-κB signaling pathways are persistently activated in HTLV-1-infected cells regardless of Tax expression. Tax-dependent and -independent NF-κB pathways also involve activation of common and distinct NF-κB members. NF-κB members activated in Tax-expressing T cells are predominantly RelA, c-Rel, p50 and p52, and those in Tax-negative T cells are mainly RelA and p50. Consistent with the role of positive feedback mechanisms in persistent NF-κB activation, expression of c-Rel and p100/p52 expression is induced in Tax-expressing cells, whereas p105/p50 mRNA expression is enhanced in ATL cells [43,44].

11.4. NFκB and apoptosis

Lymphoma cell lines including ATL cells, that were constitutively activated NFκB are resistant to various inducers of apoptosis including irradiation, etoposide, and combinations of cycloheximide and TNF or TRAIL, and resist the activation of both the intrinsic and extrinsic apoptotic pathways [45].

Although mutations that delete or inactivate p53 are common in ATLL, Tax can bypass p53-dependent cell-cycle checkpoints.

A Tax transgenic mouse model was analyzed for study the contribution of p53 inactivation to Tax-mediated tumorigenesis. The mice develop primary, peripheral tumors consisting of large granular lymphocytic (LGL) cells, which infiltrate the lymph nodes, bone marrow, spleen, liver, and lungs. Tax-induced tumors exhibited functional inactivation of the p53 apoptotic pathway; such tumors were resistant to an apoptosis-inducing stimulus. Experiments with mating Tax transgenic mice with p53-deficient mice demonstrated minimal tumor acceleration, but significantly accelerated disease progression and death in mice heterozygous for p53. The studies suggest that inactivation of p53 by Tax, whether by mutation or another mechanism, is not critical for initial tumor formation, but contributes to late-stage tumor progression [46,47]..

11.5. Telomerase

Telomerase is compsed of hTR, a 451 nucleotide stretch of RNA, which serves as a template for the RNA-dependent DNA polymerase, telomerase(hTERT).

Telomere length is also regulated by several positive and negative regulators These proteins can them prevent telomerase extension by blocking access of the reverse transcriptase to the now "closed"ends of telomeric DNA.

AZT is a thymidine analog, that has been shown to inhibit cancer growth and telomerase activity. Long-term treatment of HTLV-1 infected cells with AZT inhibits telomerase activity induces telomere attrition and promotes cellular senescence, in absence of apoptosis, due to the reactivation of tumor suppressor p53 transcriptional activities

Analysis of ATLL patients was done to examine the relationship between the responsiveness for antiviral therapy and p53 mutation. Those patients with a mutated p53 did not respond to AZT treatment, demonstrating that AZT treatment causes telomere attrition leading to the reactivation of a functional p53. [48.49].

12. Response criteria

Complete remission (CR) is defined as a normalization of the complete blood count associated with a disappearance of all measurable tumors. The effect has to last for at least 1 month. However, patients with a persistence of < 5% of atypical lymphocytes are considered in CR because this situation may be observed in healthy carriers of HTLV-I. Patients who achieve CR with persistence of > 5% of atypical lymphocytes are considered in very good partial response. Partial response is defined as a decrease of > 50% in the number of leukemic cells and in the size of all measurable tumors. The effect has to last for at least 1 month. No response is defined as < 50% decrease in the number of leukemic cells or in the size of any measurable tumor or as disease progression. Patients who meet the CR or partial-response criteria but with the effect lasting < 1 month are classified as nonresponders.

13. Prognostic factors

Major prognostic indicators for ATL were analyzed in 854 patients; advanced performance status (PS), high LDH level, age ≥ 40 years, more than three involved lesions, and hypercalcemia are prognostic factors that have been identified by multivariate analysis. These factors were used to construct a risk model.5

For the chronic type of ATL, high LDH, high blood urea nitrogen, and low albumin levels have been identified as poor prognostic factors by multivariate analysis. Univariate analysis has revealed that neutrophilia,*p16* deletion, and chromosomal deletion detected by comparative genomic hybridization are associated with poor prognosis in chronic ATL.

In contrast, chronic lymphoid leukemia (CLL)–like morphology of ATL cells was associated with longer transformation-free survival of chronic ATL. Primary cutaneous tumoral type, although generally included among smoldering ATL, was a poor prognostic factor by univariate analyses [50].

The prognosis of acute- and lymphoma-type adult T-cell leukemia/lymphoma (ATL) is poor, but there is marked diversity in survival outcomes.

Data from 807 patients newly diagnosed with acute- and lymphoma-type ATL were evaluated and developed a PI using a multivariable fractional polynomial model. The Ann Arbor stage (I and II v III and IV), performance status (0 to 1 v 2 to 4), and three variables (age, serum albumin, and soluble interleukin-2 receptor [sIL-2R]) were identified as independent prognostic factors. Using these variables, a prognostic model was devised to identify different levels of risk. In the validation sample, MSTs were 3.6, 7.3, and 16.2 months for patients at high, intermediate, and low risk, respectively (P <.001).

A total of 854 ATL patients were analyzed for prognostic factors. Patients were 466 males and 388 females with a mean age of 57.1. A Cox proportional hazards model analysis revealed that five factors, advanced performance status, high lactic dehydrogenase value, age of 40 years or more, increased number of total involved lesions and hypercalcemia, were associated with shortened survival($P<0.01$).

These factors were used to construct a model to identify patients at three different risks for shortened survival. A group of 178 patients (21.8%) with a hazard ratio of less than 0.5 were classified into the low risk (LR) group, 492 (60.4%) with hazard ratio of less than or equal to 0.5 and less than 2.5 into standard high risk (SHR) group, and 145 (17.8%) with hazard ratio of 2.5 or more extremely high risk (EHR) group. MST, and projected 2- and 4-year survival rates were 37 months, 66.3% and 41.2% for LR, 8 months 20.6%, and 4.5% for SHR, and 2.4 months, 5.6% and 0% for EHR, respectively.

14. Classification

The following diagnostic criteria are proposed to classify four clinical subtypes of ATL(Table I); 1) Smouldering type, 2) Chronic type, 3) Lymphoma type, and 4) Acute type.

1. Smouldering type, 5% or more abnormal lymphocytes of T-cell nature in PB, normal lymphocyte level (less than 4 x 10(9)/l), no hypercalcaemia (corrected calcium level less than 2.74 mmol/l), lactate LDH value of up to 1.5 x the normal upper limit, no lymphadenopathy, no involvement of liver, spleen, central nervous system (CNS), bone and gastrointestinal tract, and neither ascites nor pleural effusion. Skin and pulmonary lesion(s) may be present. In case of less than 5% abnormal T-lymphocytes in PB, at least one of histologically-proven skin and pulmonary lesions should be present.
2. Chronic type, absolute lymphocytosis (4 x 10(9)/l or more) with T-lymphocytosis more than 3.5 x 10(9)/l, LDH value up to twice the normal upper limit, no hypercalcaemia, no involvement of CNS, bone and gastrointestinal tract, and neither ascites nor pleural effusion. Lymphadenopathy and involvement of liver, spleen, skin, and lung may be present, and 5% or more abnormal T-lymphocytes are seen in PB in most cases.
3. Lymphoma type, no lymphocytosis, 1% or less abnormal T-lymphocytes, and histologically-proven lymphadenopathy with or without extranodal lesions.
4. Acute type, remaining ATL patients who have usually leukaemic manifestation and tumour lesions, but are not classified as any of the three other types.

A total of 818 ATL patients with a mean age of 57 years, newly diagnosed from 1983 to 1987, were analysed by this criteria. 253 were still alive with a median follow-up time of 13.3 months from diagnosis, while 565 were dead with a median survival time (MST) of 5.4 months. MST was 6.2 months for acute type, 10.2 months for lymphoma type, 24.3 months for chronic type, and not yet reached for smouldering type. 2- and 4-year survival rates were 16.7% and 5.0% for acute type, 21.3% and 5.7% for lymphoma type, 52.4% and 26.9% for chronic type, 77.7% and 62.8% for smouldering type, respectively. Distinct clinical features and laboratory findings of each clinical subtype are described [51].

	Smouldering	Chronic	Lymphoma	Acute
Lymphocyte count	Less than 4	4 or more	less than 4	more than 4
(10 9 lympho/liter)				
% of atypical lympho	5 or more	5 or more	1 or less	more than 5
LDH	1.5x NUL	2x NUL		
Ca	less than 2.74	less than 2.74		more than 2.74
Lyphoadenopathy	No	No	Yes	-
Mean survival time(Mo)		24.3	10.2	6.2
2 year survival (%)	77.7	52.4	21.3	16.7
4 year survival (%)	62.8	26.9	5.7	5
	NUL	Normal upper	limit	

Table 1. Classification of subtypes

15. Treatment options

The treatment of ATL usually depends on the subtype. Patients with aggressive forms have a very poor prognosis due to intrinsic chemoresistance, a large tumor burden, and frequent infectious complications because of immune deficiency.

In multiple Japanese trials for aggressive ATL, data clearly demonstrated that combinations of chemotherapy did not have significant effect on long-term survival. Indolent ATL patients(chronic or smoldering) have a better prognosis. However, recent data from Japanese showed poor long-term results when these patients were managed with a watchful-waiting policy until progression or with chemotherapy [52].

15.1. Conventional chemotherapy

The clinical trials in Japan(protocols LSG1-VEPA and LSG2) demonstrated that first-generation chemotherapy, such as CHOP type, ie, cyclophosphamide, hydroxydaunorubicin, oncovin (vincristine), and prednisone has little impact in ATL, especially in the acute type. Only a 16% to 36% patients achieved CR.

New-generation agents such as deoxycoformycine, a nucleoside analog, irinotecan hydrochloride (CPT-11: a topoisomerase I inhibitor), and MST-16(a topoisomerase II inhibitor), have also been tested in pilot phase II studies of refractory or relapsed ATL patients, however the results have been uniformly disappointing.

A phase III study in Japan demonstrated that the LSG15 regimen consisting of VCAP (vincristine, cyclophosphamide, doxorubicin, prednisolone), AMP (doxorubicin, ranimustine, prednisolone), and VECP (vindesine, etoposide, carboplatin, prednisolone) is superior to biweekly CHOP for newly diagnosed acute, lymphoma, or unfavorable chronic ATL. The CR rate and 3-year overall survival(OS) were greater as 40% vs 25%, 24% vs 13%, respectively, however,the median 13 months survival was disappointing [53].

The poor prognosis of ATL after chemotherapy is probably the consequence of several factors. The cellular immune deficiency observed at the early stages may lead to a high frequency of opportunistic infections. Overexpression of the multidrug resistant gene and p53 gene mutations is a feature of ATL cells and results in intrinsic resistance to chemotherapy.

15.2. Monoclonal antibodies

15.2.1. CC Chemokine Receptor 4 (CCR4)

CC chemokine receptor 4 (CCR4) is a chemokine receptor expressed on T-helper type 2 and regulatory T cells. Because CCR4 is expressed on most ATL cells, KW-0761, a humanized anti-CCR4 monoclonal antibody, which markedly enhances antibody-dependent cellular cytotoxicity, was evaluated in the treatment of patients with relapsed ATL. [54].

A multicenter phase II study of KW-0761 for patients with relapsed, aggressive CCR4-positive ATL. Patients received intravenous infusions of KW-0761 once per week for 8 weeks at a dose of 1.0 mg/kg. Of 28 patients enrolled in this study, responses were noted in 13 of 26 evaluable patients, including CR in 8, with an overall response rate of 50%. The median progression-free time and overall survival were 5.2 and 13.7 months, respectively. The most common adverse events were infusion reactions (89%) and skin rashes (63%), which were manageable and reversible in all the cases.

Because monoclonal antibodies were tried as single agents, trials are needed to define in combination therapies with chemotherapy in the lymphoma form or with antiretroviral therapy in the acute form. Following on a phase III study(JCOG9801(Japan Clinical Oncology Group 9801) for untreated aggressive ATL promote to conduct a randomized trial of VCAP-AMP-VECP chemotherapy with or without KW-0761 for untreated ATL.

15.2.2. CD52

CD52 is also the candidate target. A monoclonal antibody against CD52(Alemtuzumab) has demonstrated good results: however, the results are scanty and limited to case reports. with

http://dx.doi.org/10.5772/54776

or without nucleoside analogs such as pentostatin may be promising. However, the associated immunosuppression is a concern in patients with viral-mediated disease. [55-57].

15.3. HSC transplantation

The several retrospective studies have confirmed that allogeneic SCT(allo SCT) with the use of either myeloablative conditioning or reduced-intensity conditioning conditioning as a promising treatment option for ATL.

The number of ATL patients eligible for allo SCT is quite limited because of the older age at presentation (>60 years), poor performance status, the severe immunosuppression, and the low CR rate, in particular in the acute form.

Although selection criteria for patients and sources of stem cells remain to be resolved, allo-SCT may be considered as a treatment option for patients with aggressive ATL.

For treating aggressive ATL, LSG15 is the standard chemotherapy, however, its efficacy of LSG15 is transient. Improved outcome after allo-SCT, despite a high incidence of graft-versus-host disease, has been reported.

To evaluate whether allo-SCT is more effective than LSG15 for aggressive ATL, an up front phase II clinical trial is now being planned. [1].

15.3.1. Donor selection

Total 386 patients with ATL who underwent allo-SCT using different graft sources were evaluated [58].

154 received human leukocyte antigen (HLA)-matched related marrow or peripheral blood; 43 received HLA-mismatched related marrow or peripheral blood; 99 received unrelated marrow; and 90 received single unit unrelated cord blood. After a median follow-up of 41 months (range, 1.5-102), the 3-year OS for the entire cohort was 33% (95% confidence interval, 28%-38%). Multivariable analysis showed that 4 recipient factors were significantly associated with lower survival rates: older age (> 50 years), male sex, status other than CR, and the use of unrelated cord blood compared with use of HLA-matched related grafts. Treatment-related mortality rate was higher among patients given cord blood transplants; disease-associated mortality was higher among those given transplants not in remission. Among transplants, donor HTLV-I seropositivity adversely affected disease-associated mortality.

15.3.2. Conditioning regimen

A retrospective study of allo SCT for ATL were conducted in Japan for the effects of the preconditioning regimen [59].

The median OS and 3-year OS of bone marrow or peripheral blood transplantation recipients (n=586) were 9.9 months (7.4-13.2 months) and 36% (32-41%), respectively.

The values for recipients of myeloablative conditioning (MAC: n = 280) and reduced-intensity conditioning (RIC: n = 306) were 9.5 months (6.7-18.0 months) and 39% (33-45%) and 10.0 months (7.2-14.0 months) and 34% (29-40%), respectively.

Multivariate analysis showed that 5 variables significantly contributed to poorer OS; older age, male gender, not in CR, poor performance status, and transplantation from unrelated donors. Although no significant difference in OS between MAC and RIC was observed. Regarding mortality, RIC was significantly associated with ATL-related mortality compared with MAC.

15.3.3. Graft-Versus-ATL(GVL) effect

The effects of acute and chronic GVHD on overall survival, disease-associated mortality, and treatment-related mortality among 294 ATL patients who received allo HCT were analyzed [60].

The occurrence of GVHD demonstrated that the development of grade 1-2 acute GVHD (aGVHD) was significantly associated with higher overall survival ($P = 0.018$) compared with the absence of aGVHD. Occurrence of either grade 1-2 or grade 3-4 aGVHD was associated with lower disease-associated mortality compared with the absence of aGVHD, whereas grade 3-4 aGVHD was associated with a higher risk for treatment-related mortality ($P < 0.001$). The development of extensive chronic GVHD (cGVHD) was associated with higher treatment-related mortality ($P = 0.006$) compared with the absence of cGVHD. These results indicate that the development of mild-to-moderate aGVHD attribute a lower risk of disease progression and a beneficial effect on the survival of ATL patients with allografts.

Clinical studies have suggested that allo SCT improves the clinical course of ATL with a graft-versus-ATL effect. It is speculated that donor-derived HTLV-1 Tax-specific CD8(+) cytotoxic T cells (CTLs) contribute to the graft-versus-ATL effect after HSCT.

The frequencies, differentiation, functions and clonal dynamics of Tax-specific CTLs in peripheral blood (PB) and bone marrow (BM) from an ATL patient were analyzed after HSCT [61]. Donor-derived Tax-specific CTLs effectively suppressed HTLV-1 replication in both PB and BM at least during chronic graft-versus-host disease after HSCT.

Tax-specific CTLs persistently existed as less-differentiated CD45RA(-)CCR7(-) effector memory CTLs based on predominant phenotypes of CD27(+), CD28(+/-) and CD57(+/-). Two predominant CTL clones persistently existed and maintained strong cytotoxic activities against HTLV-1 in both PB and BM over three years after HSCT.

To study the GVL effects after allo-HSCT, 21 ATL patients(18 acute, 2 lymphoma and 1 chronic) were examined [62]. allo-HSCT, seven patients were in CR, one was in PR, five had stable disease(SD) and eight had progressive disease(PD). The disease after allo-HSCT was CR in 14, PR in 3, SD in one and PD in 3 patients. Among 15 patients who survived longer than 100 days, ATL relapsed in 10 patients. After the discontinuing of immunosuppressant therapy in these 10 patients, 8 manifested GVHD; ATL was ameliorated to CR in 6 patients. Donor lymphocytes were infused into 2 patients who did not show GVHD; 1 obtained CR. In 5 patients with skin relapse alone, 4 patients achieved CR following the discontinuation of the immunosuppres-

http://dx.doi.org/10.5772/54776

sants. From these results, Gv-ATL effects played an important role in the outcome of allo-HSCT for ATL. [63].

15.4. Antiviral therapy

15.4.1. Zidovudine (AZT) and Interferon(INF)

Zidovudine (AZT) and interferon(INF) are known to be as antiviral agents.

Phase II studies with the combination of AZT and IFN treatment showed a high response rate. For acute ATL, first-line antiviral therapy alone resulted in a significant survival advantage (5-year overall survival [OS] of 28%) compared with first-line chemotherapy with or without maintenance antiviral therapy (5-year OS of 10%). Achieving CR with antiviral therapy resulted in a 5-year survival rate of 82%.

A study of worldwide meta-analysis on 254 ATL survival treated in the United States, the United Kingdom, Martinique, and France (116 acute ATL, 18 chronic ATL, 11 smoldering ATL, and 100 ATL lymphoma) was performed. Five-year OS rates were 46% for 75 patients who received first-line antiviral therapy, 20% for 77 patients who received first-line chemotherapy, and 12% for 55 patients who received first-line chemotherapy followed by antiviral therapy.

Patients with acute, chronic, and smoldering ATL significantly benefited from first-line antiviral therapy, whereas in ATL lymphoma, first-line antiviral therapy resulted in a significant survival disadvantage (median and 5-year OS of 7 months and 0%, respectively) compared with first-line chemotherapy with or without maintenance antiviral therapy (median and 5-year OS of 16 months and 18%, respectively). Finally, a multivariate analysis confirmed that first-line antiviral therapy significantly improves overall survival of ATL patients (hazard ratio 0.47; 95% confidence interval 0.27-0.83; P =.021). [64,65].

Virus expression has been reported to be limited or absent when ATLL is diagnosed, and this has suggested that secondary genetic or epigenetic changes are important in disease pathogenesis.

Nineteen patients were prospectively enrolled in a phase II clinical trial of infusional chemotherapy with etoposide, doxorubicin, and vincristine, daily prednisone, and bolus cyclophosphamide (EPOCH) given for two to six cycles until maximal clinical response, and followed by antiviral therapy with daily zidovudine, lamivudine, and alpha interferon-2a for up to one year [66].

Seven patients were on study for less than one month due to progressive disease or chemotherapy toxicity. Eleven patients achieved an objective response with median duration of response of thirteen months, and two complete remissions. Viral reactivation(median 190-fold) was observed during EPOCH chemotherapy.

Alternative therapies are sorely needed in this disease that simultaneously prevent virus expression.

15.4.2. Arsenic trioxide

Arsenic trioxide synergizes with IFN to induce cell-cycle arrest and apoptosis in HTLV-I–infected and freshly isolated leukemia cells from ATL patients.

The arsenic/IFN combination kills ATL cells through rapid reversal of the constitutive activation of NF-κB and delayed shut down of cell cycle-regulated genes secondary to Tax degradation by the proteasome that was concomitant with cell death induction [67]. It was speculated that that leukemia initiating activity(LIC) is dependent on continuous NF-κB expression. [68]. Other phase II study, the efficacy and safety of the combination of arsenic, IFN, and AZT in 10 newly diagnosed chronic patients was evaluated [69]. 100% response rate was observed, including 7 CR, 2 PR but with > 5% circulating atypical lymphocytes, and 1PR. Side effects were moderate and mostly hematologic.

The addition of arsenic to AZT/IFN, through elimination of LIC activity, may result in long-term disease eradication and potential cure. Treatment of arsenic/IFN/AZT combination was a suboptimal 5-days-per-week treatment, 3 of 6 patients remained in continuous complete remission for 7-18 months after discontinuation of maintenance therapy, whereas 5 patients with chronic ATL previously treated with IFN/AZT alone all relapsed, on average before 5 months. Similarly, in an ongoing trial of ATL lymphoma patients, ie, maintenance therapy with arsenic/IFN after complete remission with chemotherapy, resulted in all assessable patients remaining in complete remission for 23-44 months, a distinctly uncommon finding in these diseases. These observations suggest that in ATL patients arsenic/IFN efficiently targets ATL LIC activity and may be useful as a consolidation therapy.

The results of another phase II trial in which arsenic was added to the combination of AZT and IFN in newly diagnosed chronic ATL were reported. All 10 patients enrolled responded, including seven patients who achieved CR, two patients who achieved very good PR, and one patient achieved PR. Side effects were moderate and no relapse was noted at the time of reporting.

These encouraging results suggest that the triple combination of arsenic, AZT and IFN is a promising even for the first line therapy of ATL.

15.5. Targeting NFκB in ATLL patients

In ATLL cells the NFκB pathway remains activated even after Tax expression is repressed. Thus NFκB remains a therapeutic target even when Tax is not expressed.

To determine if NFκB blockade is tolerated in these patients, and whether or not it improves response rates and overall survival, multicenter trial combines infusional chemotherapy (EPOCH) with bortezomib. This trial includes treatment with integrase inhibitor raltegravir, which was found to inhibit HTLV-1 integration. The addition of an antiviral agent to this ATLL treatment regimen is based clinical trial in which chemotherapy was found to markedly enhance virus expression in a subset of patients.

Bortezomib is another non-specific inhibitor of the NFκB pathway that is capable of inhibiting proliferation of tumors cells [72]. Bay11-7082, an IKK inhibitor, inhibits the NFκB pathway in

ATLL cells and sensitizes HTLV-1 infected cells lines as well as primary ATLL cells to apoptosis [73,74]. Over the past years several additional studies have therapeutically targeted the NFκB pathway in order to kill ATLL cells

Oridonin, NIK-333, curcumin, fucoidan, and histone-deacetylase inhibitors have all been reported to induce apoptosis in ATLL cells by repressing the NFκB pathway. The field now awaits successful clinical trials in vivo [75,76].

15.6. Watch-and-wait policy for indolent ATL

Patients with smoldering or chronic ATL subtypes have a better prognosis than those with aggressive variants of ATL. Therefore, these 2 ATL subtypes were considered indolent and were usually managed with a watchful-waiting policy until disease progression. However, the reported median survival of chronic and smoldering types was only 18 months and 58 months, respectively, and the OS rates were < 20% at 5 years in both types. From Japanese study with longer follow-up period, that indolent ATL had a poor prognosis: patients with smoldering ATL had an estimated 15-year survival rate of 12.7% with a median survival of 2.9 years, whereas patients with chronic ATL had an estimated 15-year survival rate of 14.7% with a median survival of 5.3 years. Importantly, patients who received chemotherapy had a significantly lower survival compared with patients treated on a watch-and-wait policy.

From 1974 to 2003, newly diagnosed indolent ATL in 90 patients (65 chronic type and 25 smoldering type) was analyzed. The median survival time was 4.1 years; The estimated 5-, 10-, and 15-year survival rates were 47.2%, 25.4%, and 14.1%, respectively, with no plateau in the survival curve. Kaplan-Meier analyses showed that advanced PS, neutrophilia, high concentration of lactate dehydrogenase, more than 3 extranodal lesions, more than 4 total involved lesions, and receiving chemotherapy were unfavorable prognostic factors for survival. Multivariate Cox analysis showed that advanced PS was a borderline significant independent factor in poor survival (P =.06). The prognosis of indolent ATL in this study was poorer than expected.

15.7. Telomerase inhibitors

AZT is a thymidine analog that has been shown to inhibit cancer growth and telomerase activity. HTLV-I infected cells undergo senescence during long-term AZT treatment, du to the reactivation of tumor suppressor p53 transcriptional activities. This effect is dependent upon telomere shortening. In vivo patient samples of AZT-treated ATLL patients show decreases in telomerase activity and telomere lengths [48].

16. Treatment strategy

16.1. Acute ATL

As summarized in Fig. 3, in Japan, at present, LSG15 is the standard chemotherapy for the treatment of aggressive ATL, but the efficacy of LSG15 in most patients is transient.

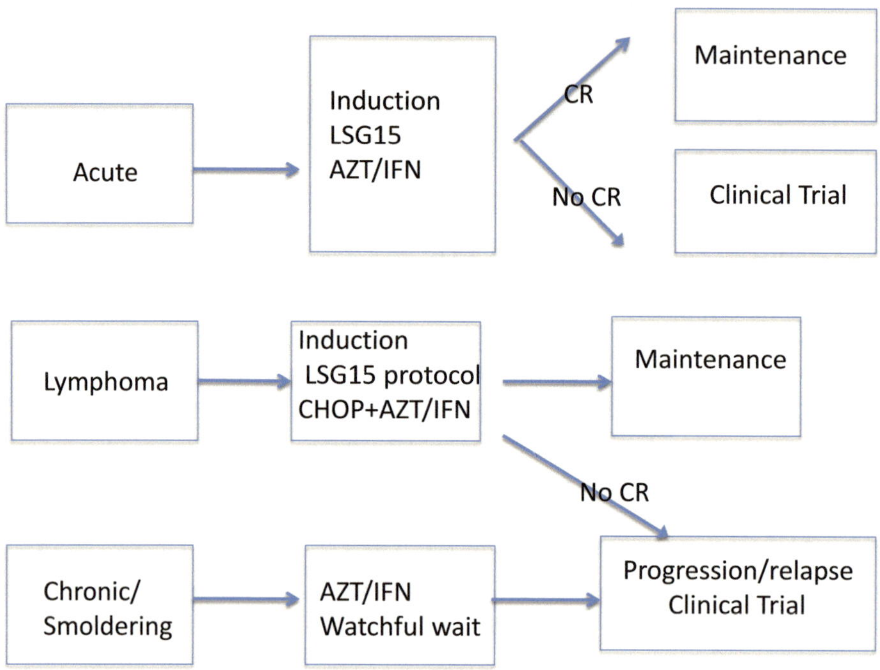

Figure 3. Treatment proposal

To evaluate whether allo-SCT is more effective than the standard chemotherapy (LSG15) for aggressive ATL, clinical trial are needed.

In United States, an antiviral therapy such as AZT+IFN is recommended [1].

16.2. Chronic and smoldering ATL

Although patients with chronic and smoldering ATL have a better prognosis compared with patients with acute ATL and ATL lymphoma, long-term survival is dismal when these patients are managed with a watchful-waiting policy until their disease progresses. Moreover, patients who received chemotherapy alone had even a poorer outcome.

It is one proposal that patients with chronic and smoldering ATL should be treated with antiviral therapy. In the worldwide meta-analysis on ATL survival, patients with chronic/ smoldering ATL who received first-line antiviral therapy only had an excellent survival (100% OS beyond 5 years). The recommended starting dose is AZT 900 mg/d (in 3 divided doses) and IFN-α (5-6 million IU/m2/d). Usually, after 1 month, AZT dose can be titrated down to 600 mg/ d in 2 divided doses, and the IFN dose can be reduced to 3-5 million IU/d or alternatively 1.5 μg/kg of pegylated IFN weekly. The addition of other antiretroviral agents, such as 3TC (lamivudine) or zalcitabine, has been tested by several centers. However, no clinical evidence of added benefit was demonstrated. On the basis of the preclinical data, clinical trials are testing the effect of adding arsenic to the AZT/IFN combination as a consolidation therapy with the aim of then stopping therapy and achieving cure by potential elimination of leukemia-initiating cells.

16.3. Lymphoma

In Japan, LSG protocol is generally tried. When treated with this LSG15 protocol, ATL lymphoma patients achieved a better CR rate (66.7%) than acute type (19.6%) or chronic type (40.0%) patients.

First-line antiviral therapy is less effective than first-line chemotherapy in ATL lymphoma. Probably, the combination of chemotherapy and AZT/IFN is recommended as front-line therapy in ATL lymphoma based on the reactivation of HTLV-1 virues.

Based on encouraging results from Japan, allo SCT is recommended for young patients with ATL lymphoma and sutable donor.

17. Supportive therapy in ATL

Infectious events are often fatal in ATL patients. Sulfamethoxazole-trimethoprim and anti-fungal agents were recommended for the prophylaxis of *Pneumocystis jiroveci* pneumonia and fungal infections, respectively, in the JCOG trials. Although cytomegalovirus infection commonly occurs in ATL patients, ganciclovir is not routinely recommended for prophylaxis. In addition, in patients not receiving chemotherapy, antifungal prophylaxis may not be critical.

18. Prevention

In 1980, investigation of mother-to-child transmission (MTCT) for explaining the infection of HTLV-1. Epidemiological data revealed the MTCT rate at ~20%. Cell-mediated transmission of HTLV-1 without prenatal infection suggested a possibility of milk-borne transmission. A prefecture-wide intervention study to refrain from breast-feeding by carrier fmothers, the ATL Prevention Program Nagasaki revealed a marked reduction of HTLV-1 MTCT by complete bottle-feeding from 20.3% to 2.5%, and a significantly higher risk of short-term breast-feeding (<6 months) than bottle-feeding (7.4% vs. 2.5%, $P < 0.001$) [77].

19. Conclusion

Further investigation on the ATL pathogenesis is crucial for the prevention and treatment of this refractory leukemia/lymphoma. Clinical trials to assess additional targeted therapies such as NF-kB-targeted therapy or monoclonal antibodies are mandatory after achieving CR. Allogeneic BMT with the use of conventional or non-myeloablative conditioning should be considered for suitable patients.

Author details

Shoko Kobayashi* and Shigeki Iwasaki

*Address all correspondence to: qqh558vd@mountain.ocn.ne.jp

Department of Hematology, Seirei Yokohama Hospital, Yokohama city, Japan

References

[1] Bazarbachi, A, Suarez, F, Fields, P, & Hermine, O. How I treat adult T-cell leukemia/ lymphoma. Blood (2011)., 2011, 118-1736.

[2] Yoshida, M. Molecular approach to human leukemia: isolation and characterization of the first human retrovirus HTLV-1 and its impact on tumorigenesis in adult T-cell leukemia. Proc Jpn Acad Ser B Phys Biol Sci. (2010)., 86(2), 117-130.

[3] Journo, C, Douceron, E, & Mahieux, R. HTLV gene regulation: because size matters, transcription is not enough. Future Microbiol. (2009)., 4(4), 425-440.

[4] Manel, N, Kim, F. J, Kinet, S, Taylor, N, Sitbon, M, et al. The ubiquitous glucose transporter GLUT-1 is a receptor for HTLV. Cell. (2003)., 115(4), 449-459.

[5] Ghez, D, Lepelletier, Y, Lambert, S, Fourneau, J. M, Blot, V, et al. Neuropilin-1 is involved in human T-cell lymphotropic virus type 1 entry. J Virol. (2006). Jul;, 80(14), 6844-6854.

[6] Takenouchi, N, Jones, K. S, Lisinski, I, Fugo, K, Yao, K, et al. GLUT1 is not the primary binding receptor but is associated with cell-to-cell transmission of human T-cell leukemia virus type 1. J Virol. (2007)., 81(3), 1506-1510.

[7] Fontenot, J. D, Gavin, M. A, & Rudensky, A. Y. Foxp3 programs the development and function of CD4+CD25+ regulatory T cells. Nat Immunol. (2003)., 4(4), 330-336.

[8] Jones, K. S, Petrow-sadowski, C, Huang, Y. K, & Bertolette, D. C. Ruscetti Cell-free HTLV-1 infects dendritic cells leading to transmission and transformation of CD4(+) T cells. Nat Med (2008).

[9] The 14th International Conference on Human Retrovirology: HTLV and related retroviruses (July(2009). Salvador, Brazil), 1-4.

[10] Boxus, M, & Willems, L. Mechanisms of HTV-I persistence and transformation. Br J Cancer. (2009)., 101(9), 1497-1501.

[11] Boxus, M, & Willems, L. Mechanisms of HTV-I persistence and transformation. Br J Cancer. (2009)., 101(9), 1497-1501.

[12] Yoshida, M. Molecular approach to human leukemia: isolation and characterization of the first human retrovirus HTLV-1 and its impact on tumorigenesis in adult T-cell leukemia. Proc Jpn Acad Ser B Phys Biol Sci. (2010). , 86(2), 117-130.

[13] Taylor, J. M, Ghorbel, S, & Nicot, C. Genome wide analysis of human genes transcriptionally and post-transcriptionally regulated by the HTLV-I protein BMC Genomics. (2009). , 30.

[14] Datta, A, Silverman, L, Phipps, A. J, Hiraragi, H, Ratner, L, et al. Human T-lymphotropic virus type-1 alters cell cycle G2 regulation of T lymphocytes to enhance cell survival. Retrovirology. (2007). , 30.

[15] Bartoe, J. T, Albrecht, B, Collins, N. D, Robek, M. D, & Ratner, L. Functional role of pX open reading frame II of human T-lymphotropic virus type 1 in maintenance of viral loads in vivo. J Virol. (2000). , 74(3), 1094-1100.

[16] Liu, M, Yang, L, Zhang, L, & Liu, B. Merling R Human T-cell leukemia virus type 1 infection leads to arrest in the G1 phase of the cell cycle. J Virol. (2008). , 82(17), 8442-8455.

[17] Nasr, R, El Hajj, H, Kfoury, Y, De Thé, H, Hermine, O, & Bazarbachi, A. Controversies in targeted therapy of adult T cell leukemia/lymphoma: ON target or OFF target effects? Viruses. (2011). , 3(6), 750-769.

[18] Matsuoka, M, & Green, P. L. HBZ gene, a key player in HTLV-I pathogenesis. Retrovirology. (2009).

[19] Usui, T, Yanagihara, K, Tsukasaki, K, Murata, K, & Hasegawa, H. Characteristic expression of HTLV-1 basic zipper factor (HBZ) transcripts in HTLV-1 provirus-positive cells. Retrovirology. (2008).

[20] Saito, M, Matsuzaki, T, Satou, Y, Yasunaga, J, & Saito, K. In vivo expression of the HBZ gene of HTLV-1 correlates with proviral load, inflammatory markers and disease severity in HTLV-1 associated myelopathy/tropical spastic paraparesis (HAM/TSP). Retrovirology. (2009).

[21] Kamihira, S, Atogami, S, Sohda, H, Momita, S, & Yamada, Y. Significance of soluble interleukin-2 receptor levels for evaluation of the progression of adult T-cell leukemia. Cancer. (1994). , 73(11), 2753-2758.

[22] Itoyama, T, Chaganti, R. S, Yamada, Y, Tsukasaki, K, & Atogami, S. Cytogenetic analysis and clinical significance in adult T-cell leukemia/lymphoma: a study of 50 cases from the human T-cell leukemia virus type-1 endemic area, Nagasaki. Blood. (2001). , 97(11), 3612-3620.

[23] Tsukasaki, K, Krebs, J, Nagai, K, Tomonaga, M, & Koeffler, H. P. Comparative genomic hybridization analysis in adult T-cell leukemia/lymphoma: correlation with clinical course. Blood. (2001). , 97(12), 3875-3881.

[24] Oshiro, A, Tagawa, H, Ohshima, K, Karube, K, Uike, N, et al. Identification of subtype-specific genomic alterations in aggressive adult T-cell leukemia/lymphoma. Blood. (2006). , 107(11), 4500-4507.

[25] Ramos, J. C. Ruiz P Jr, Ratner L, Reis IM, Brites C, et al. IRF-4 and c-Rel expression in antiviral-resistant adult T-cell leukemia/lymphoma. Blood. (2007). , 109(7), 3060-3068.

[26] Kimata, J. T, Wong, F. H, Wang, J. J, & Ratner, L. Construction and characterization of infectious human T-cell leukemia virus type 1 molecular clones. Virology. (1994). , 204(2), 656-664.

[27] Robek, M. D, & Ratner, L. Immortalization of CD4(+) and CD8(+) T lymphocytes by human T-cell leukemia virus type 1 Tax mutants expressed in a functional molecular clone. J Virol. (1999). , 73(6), 4856-4865.

[28] Hironaka, N, Mochida, K, Mori, N, Maeda, M, Yamamoto, N, et al. Tax-independent constitutive IkappaB kinase activation in adult T-cell leukemia cells. Neoplasia. (2004). , 6(3), 266-278.

[29] Gupta, N, Delrow, J, Drawid, A, Sengupta, A. M, Fan, G, et al. Repression of B-cell linker (BLNK) and B-cell adaptor for phosphoinositide 3-kinase (BCAP) is important for lymphocyte transformation by rel proteins. Cancer Res. (2008). , 68(3), 808-814.

[30] Weil, R, Levraud, J. P, Dodon, M. D, Bessia, C, Hazan, U, et al. Altered expression of tyrosine kinases of the Src and Syk families in human T-cell leukemia virus type 1-infected T-cell lines. J Virol. (1999). , 73(5), 3709-3717.

[31] Bunting, K, Rao, S, Hardy, K, Woltring, D, Denyer, G. S, et al. Genome-wide analysis of gene expression in T cells to identify targets of the NF-kappa B transcription factor c-Rel. J Immunol. (2007). , 178(11), 7097-7109.

[32] Harhaj, E. W, Harhaj, N. S, Grant, C, Mostoller, K, Alefantis, T, et al. Human T cell leukemia virus type I Tax activates CD40 gene expression via the NF-kappa B pathway. Virology. (2005). , 333(1), 145-158.

[33] Kim, Y. M, Sharma, N, & Nyborg, J. K. The proto-oncogene Bcl3, induced by Tax, represses Tax-mediated transcription via displacement from the human T-cell leukemia virus type 1 promoter. J Virol. (2008). , 300.

[34] Coope, H. J, Atkinson, P. G, Huhse, B, Belich, M, Janzen, J, et al. CD40 regulates the processing of NF-kappaB2 to p52. EMBO J. (2002). , 100.

[35] Miyamoto, S. Nuclear initiated NF-κB signaling: NEMO and ATM take center stage. Cell Res. (2011). , 21(1), 116-130.

[36] Hirai, H, Fujisawa, J, Suzuki, T, Ueda, K, Muramatsu, M, et al. Transcriptional activator Tax of HTLV-1 binds to the NF-kappa B precursor Oncogene. (1992). , 105.

[37] Lanoix, J, Lacoste, J, Pepin, N, Rice, N, & Hiscott, J. Overproduction of NFKB2 (lyt-10) and c-Rel: a mechanism for HTLV-I Tax-mediated trans-activation via the NF-kappa B signalling pathway. Oncogene. (1994). , 9(3), 841-852.

[38] Harhaj, E. W, Harhaj, N. S, Grant, C, Mostoller, K, Alefantis, T, et al. Human T cell leukemia virus type I Tax activates CD40 gene expression via the NF-kappa B pathway. Virology. (2005). , 333(1), 145-158.

[39] Kim, Y. M, Sharma, N, & Nyborg, J. K. The proto-oncogene Bcl3, induced by Tax, represses Tax-mediated transcription via diplacement from the human T-cell leukemia virus type 1 promoter.J Virol. (2008). , 300.

[40] Hirai, H, Fujisawa, J, Suzuki, T, Ueda, K, Muramatsu, M, et al. Transcriptional activator Tax of HTLV-1 binds to the NF-kappa B precursor Oncogene. (1992). , 105.

[41] Arima, N, Molitor, J. A, Smith, M. R, Kim, J. H, Daitoku, Y, et al. Human T-cell leukemia virus type I Tax induces expression of the Rel-related family of kappa B enhancer-binding proteins: evidence for a pretranslational component of regulation.J Virol. (1991). , 65(12), 6892-6899.

[42] Matsuoka, M, & Jeang, K. T. Human T-cell leukaemia virus type 1 (HTLV-1) infectivity and cellular transformation. Nat Rev Cancer. (2007). , 7(4), 270-280.

[43] Li, C. C, Ruscetti, F. W, Rice, N. R, Chen, E, Yang, N. S, et al. Differential expression of Rel family members in human T-cell leukemia virus type I-infected cells: transcriptional activation of c-rel by Tax protein. J Virol. (1993). , 67(7), 4205-4213.

[44] Jeong, S. J, Radonovich, M, Brady, J. N, & Pise-masison, C. A. HTLV-I Tax induces a novel interaction between RelA and p53 that results in inhibition of p53 transcriptional activity. Blood. (2004). , 65.

[45] Bernal-mizrachi, L, Lovly, C. M, & Ratner, L. The role of NF-{kappa}B-1 and NF-{kappa}B-2-mediated resistance to apoptosis in lymphomas. Proc Natl Acad Sci U S A. (2006). , 103(24), 9220-9225.

[46] Portis, T, Grossman, W. J, Harding, J. C, Hess, J. L, & Ratner, L. Analysis of inactivation in a human T-cell leukemia virus type 1 Tax transgenic mouse model.J Virol. (2001). , 53.

[47] Rauch, D. A, & Ratner, L. Targeting HTLV-1 Activation of NFκB in Mouse Models and ATLL Patients. Viru ses. (2011). , 3(6), 886-900.

[48] Bellon, M, & Nicot, C. Telomerase: a crucial player in HTLV-I-induced human T-cell leukemia. Cancer Genomics Proteomics. (2007). , 4(1), 21-25.

[49] Rauch, D. A, & Ratner, L. Controversies in targeted therapy of adult T cell leukemia/ lymphoma ON Target or OFF Target Effects. Viruses. (2011). , 3(6), 750-769.

[50] [No authors listed] Major prognostic factors of patients with adult T-cell leukemia-lymphoma: a cooperative studyLymphoma Study Group ((1984). Leuk Res. 1991;15(2-3):81-90.

[51] Shimoyama M: Diagnostic criteria and classification of clinical subtypes of adult T-cell leukaemia-lymphoma: A report from the Lymphoma Study Group ((1984). Br J Haematol 1991;, 79, 428-437.

[52] Takasaki, Y, Iwanaga, M, Imaizumi, Y, Tawara, M, Joh, T, et al. Long-term study of indolent adult T-cell leukemia-lymphoma. Blood. (2010). , 115(22), 4337-4343.

[53] Tsukasaki, K, Utsunomiya, A, Fukuda, H, Shibata, T, Fukushima, T, et al. Japan Clinical Oncology Group Study JCOG9801. VCAP-AMP-VECP compared with biweekly CHOP for adult T-cell leukemia-lymphoma: Japan Clinical Oncology Group Study JCOG9801. J Clin Oncol. (2007). , 25(34), 5458-5464.

[54] Ishida, T, Joh, T, Uike, N, Yamamoto, K, Utsunomiya, A, et al. Defucosylated anti-CCR4 monoclonal antibody (KW-0761) for relapsed adult T-cell leukemia-lymphoma: a multicenter phase II study. J Clin Oncol. (2012). , 30(8), 837-842.

[55] Zhang, Z, Zhang, M, Ravetch, J. V, Goldman, C, & Waldmann, T. A. Effective therapy for a murine model of adult T-cell leukemia with the humanized anti-CD52 monoclonal antibody, Campath-1H. Cancer Res. (2003). , 63(19), 6453-6457.

[56] Mone, A, Puhalla, S, Whitman, S, Baiocchi, R. A, Cruz, J, et al. Durable hematologic complete response and suppression of HTLV-1 viral load following alemtuzumab in zidovudine/IFN-{alpha}-refractory adult T-cell leukemia. Blood. (2005). , 106(10), 3380-3382.

[57] Ravandi, F, & Faderl, S. Complete response in a patient with adult T-cell leukemia (ATL) treated with combination of alemtuzumab and pentostatin. Leuk Res. (2006). , 30(1), 103-105.

[58] Hishizawa, M, Kanda, J, Utsunomiya, A, Taniguchi, S, Eto, T, et al. Transplantation of allogeneic hematopoietic stem cells for adult T-cell leukemia: a nationwide retrospective study. Blood. (2010). , 116(8), 1369-1376.

[59] Ishida, T, Hishizawa, M, Kato, K, Tanosaki, R, Fukuda, T, et al. Allogeneic hematopoietic stem cell transplantation for adult T-cell leukemia-lymphoma with special emphasis on preconditioning regimen: a nationwide retrospective study. Blood. (2012). , 120(8), 1734-1741.

[60] Kanda, J, Hishizawa, M, Utsunomiya, A, Taniguchi, S, Eto, T, et al. Impact of graft-versus-host disease on outcomes after allogeneic hematopoietic cell transplantation for adult T-cell leukemia: a retrospective cohort study. Blood. (2012). , 119(9), 2141-2148.

[61] Tanaka, Y, Nakasone, H, Yamazaki, R, Wada, H, Ishihara, Y, et al. Long-Term Persistence of Limited HTLV-I Tax-specific Cytotoxic T Cell Clones in a Patient with Adult T Cell Leukemia/Lymphoma after Allogeneic Stem Cell Transplantation. J Clin Immunol. (2012). Jul 5. [Epub ahead of print]

[62] Kanda, J, Hishizawa, M, Utsunomiya, A, Taniguchi, S, Eto, T, et al. Impact of graft-versus-host disease on outcomes after allogeneic hematopoietic cell transplantation for adult T-cell leukemia: a retrospective cohort study. Blood. (2012). Mar 1;, 119(9), 2141-2148.

[63] Yonekura, K, Utsunomiya, A, Takatsuka, Y, Takeuchi, S, Tashiro, Y, et al. Graft-versus-adult T-cell leukemia/lymphoma effect following allogeneic hematopoietic stem cell transplantation. Bone Marrow Transplant. (2008). , 41(12), 1029-1035.

[64] Bazarbachi, A, & Plumelle, Y. Carlos Ramos J, et al. Meta-analysis on the use of zidovudine and interferon-alfa in adult T-cell leukemia/lymphoma showing improved survival in the leukemic subtypes. J Clin Oncol (2010). , 28(27), 4177-4183.

[65] Hermine, O, Dombret, H, Poupon, J, et al. Phase II trial of arsenic trioxide and alpha interferon in patients with relapsed/refractory adult T-cell leukemia/lymphoma. Hematol J (2004). , 5(2), 130-134.

[66] Ratner, L, Harrington, W, Feng, X, Grant, C, Jacobson, S, et al. AIDS Malignancy Consortium. Human T cell leukemia virus reactivation with progression of adult T-cell leukemia-lymphoma. PLoS One. (2009). e4420.

[67] El-Sabban, M. E, Nasr, R, Dbaibo, G, Hermine, O, Abboushi, N, et al. Arsenic-interferon-alpha-triggered apoptosis in HTLV-I transformed cells is associated with tax down-regulation and reversal of NF-kappa B activation. Blood. (2000). , 96(8), 2849-2855.

[68] Nasr, R, Rosenwald, A, Sabban, M. E, Arnulf, B, Zalloua, P, et al. Arsenic/interferon specifically reverses 2 distinct gene networks critical for the survival of HTLV-1-infected leukemic cells. Blood. (2003). , 101(11), 4576-4582.

[69] Kchour, G, Tarhini, M, Kooshyar, M. M, El Hajj, H, Wattel, E, et al. Phase 2 study of the efficacy and safety of the combination of arsenic trioxide, interferon alpha, and zidovudine in newly diagnosed chronic adult T-cell leukemia/lymphoma (ATL). Blood. (2009). , 113(26), 6528-6532.

[70] Seegulam, M. E, & Ratner, L. Integrase inhibitors effective against human T-cell leukemia virus type 1. Antimicrob Agents Chemother. (2011). , 55(5), 2011-2017.

[71] Rauch, D. A, & Ratner, L. Targeting HTLV-1 activation of NF-kB in mouse models and ATLL patients. Viruses. (2011). , 3(6), 886-900.

[72] Mitra-kaushik, S, Harding, J. C, Hess, J. L, & Ratner, L. Effects of the proteasome inhibitor PS-341 on tumor growth in HTLV-1 Tax transgenic mice and Tax tumor transplants. Blood. (2004). , 104(3), 802-809.

[73] Horie, R. NF-kappaB in pathogenesis and treatment of adult T-cell leukemia/lymphoma. Int Rev Immunol. (2007).

[74] Mori, N, Yamada, Y, Ikeda, S, Yamasaki, Y, Tsukasaki, K, et al. Bay 11-7082 inhibits transcription factor NF-kappaB and induces apoptosis of HTLV-I-infected T-cell lines and primary adult T-cell leukemia cells.Blood. (2002). , 100(5), 1828-1834.

[75] Rauch, D. A, & Ratner, L. Targeting HTLV-1 Activation of NFκB in Mouse Models and ATLL Patients. Viruses. (2011). , 3(6), 886-900.

[76] Hasegawa, H, Yamada, Y, Tsukasaki, K, Mori, N, Tsuruda, K, et al. LBH589, a deacetylase inhibitor, induces apoptosis in adult T-cell leukemia/lymphoma cells via activation of a novel RAIDD-caspase-2 pathway. Leukemia. (2011). , 25(4), 575-587.

[77] Hino, S. Establishment of the milk-borne transmission as a key factor for the peculiar endemicity of human T-lymphotropic virus type 1 (HTLV-1): the ATL Prevention Program Nagasaki. Proc Jpn Acad Ser B Phys Biol Sci. (2011). , 87(4), 152-166.

Section 3

Epidemiology of ALL

Chapter 6

Etiological Research of Childhood Acute Leukemia with Cluster and Clustering Analysis

David Aldebarán Duarte-Rodríguez,
Richard J.Q. McNally, Juan Carlos Núñez-Enríquez,
Arturo Fajardo-Gutiérrez and
Juan Manuel Mejía-Arangué

Additional information is available at the end of the chapter

http://dx.doi.org/10.5772/54456

1. Introduction

1.1. The investigation of clusters of diseases

Cluster disease and clustering of diseases is an aggregation of cases of a particular disease that occur within a group of people, a geographic area or a period of time, and which is higher than the researchers would expect considering its natural history, and the chance fluctuations. So far, the study of clusters has led to the identification of health problems that have spatial and temporal dimensions.

According to Elliot and Best, "The study of the geographic patterns of a specific disease is part of the classic triad in descriptive epidemiology characterized for the time, the person, and the place"[1]. Therefore, these studies have been considered as part of *Spatial analysis* in Epidemiology because they can be interpreted in a temporal and spatial context; they should not be confused with an ecological study as commonly happens.

The space-time clustering studies describe populations in historical and geographical contexts, not individuals or population´s particularities, such as risk factors. The results of these studies must be interpreted in terms of period of time and geographic area. The space-time clustering studies are classified as follows:

1. Spatial cluster also named geographic cluster. Is an excess of cases or events in a geographic area, which can range from a small settlement to a large region.

2. Temporal cluster. Is an excess of cases or events observed in a limited period of time. The results of this study must be interpreted chronologically. For example, a cluster composed of unrelated individuals whose dates of birth approximately coincide, would result in a temporary cluster; however, this coincidence do not necessarily is observed in individuals that lived in the same geographic area, they could live distantly. There are clusters which individuals coincide on the time of birth, time of diagnosis, or the period in which they moved to a new city.

3. Space-time cluster. Is an excess of cases or events in both space and time. In other words, a space-time cluster can be observed in cases that are geographically close and are observed in the same period of time.

The more common space-time clustering studies designs are spatial clusters and space-time clustering. Importantly, these types of studies should not be confused with other statistical cluster analysis methods. Both techniques have similarities as they search characteristics of groups or other elements. However, their objectives are different, since the space-time clustering studies search groups of people in both dimensions; while the statistical cluster analysis explores the strength of the relationship between words, ideas or interrelated concepts. The distinction between the two methods is even more ambiguous as is common to find them under the same term [2].

The term spatial dimension is used to refer spatial cluster. The latter research associations between individuals distributed in a geographic space. The spatial cluster involves the presence of an environmental factor or factors in the etiology of the disease. One example worth to mention from veterinary medicine is the exposed by Poljak et al who published a study of influenza in pigs using Cuzick and Edwards method. They searched several clusters, but only found significant results in two strains, for influenza H3N2 Sw/Col/77 and H3N2 Sw/Tex/98 in an area near to a documented region of isolation of avian influenza. From an epidemiological perspective, the source of the spread of these types of influenza in pig herds was an environmental factor. Evidence suggests that the proximity between both types of farms favored the formation of a cluster of swine influenza [3].

There are specific tests for each scenario. The considerations for determining whether a cluster actually exists, or not, depend on the underlying populations. These studies describe the spatial or temporal behavior of a population; making inferences that are able to describe an area or a period. The findings are then extrapolated to the population under study. One of the advantages of these results is that they can be explaining visually when displayed on a map or a time curve.

Moreover, the cluster and the ecological studies differ from the classic major epidemiological studies such as cohort, case-control and cross sectional. However, these studies can be combined with the objective of studying a particular population. For example, information from a cross-sectional study does not require major changes in order to use it for a cluster study. The main objective of a cluster study is the description of the population. The principal objectives of a cross-sectional study are sometimes similar to the objectives of clusters studies. On the other hand, information collected longitudinally, for instance from a cohort study, can

http://dx.doi.org/10.5772/54456

be used for a temporal cluster or space-time cluster. Moreover, data from a cohort study is frequently used for other studies such as temporal cluster studies. For example, Gaudar et al used a cohort study to identify clusters, which allowed them to define an epidemiological surveillance tool [4]. The objective of this research was to identify areas of high risk for malaria using a dynamic cohort from 1996 to 2001. This group of researchers employed a cohort of identification of clusters by Kulldorf's technique. Their results showed an identification of six clusters of high risk of infection by *P. falciparum*, and concluded the advantages of detecting clusters to generate maps of high risk for malaria. A cohort is characterized by collecting data over a period of time. Nonetheless, the passing of time in collecting and analyzing data is not an exclusive characteristic of the cohort study. There are techniques of cluster analysis able to analyze the effect of time on the formation of clusters. Regarding at the studies of clusters, it can be observed that this condition can also occur with temporal data. You can also use data from a case-control research to detect clusters. Alternatively, the case-control studies are generally used to verify the findings of a study of clusters. The techniques that combine case-control studies with clusters studies are currently improving through for example, new scanning techniques [5]; they also can be used to evaluate the mobility of individuals [6]. At the end of this chapter, we present a study of clusters with information from a case-control study.

Historically, studies of clusters were used to know what caused a heterogeneous distribution of cases; in other words to better understand why the incidence of cases were more concentrated in a particular space or time. In fact, with this question in mind the cluster detection studies are conducted. However, on several occasions has taken the initiative to anticipate it and, without waiting for evidencing disease predilection to join an aggregate of cases, the researchers have investigated whether this phenomenon is part of the natural history of the disease.

This difference is related to the distinction between clusters and clustering. By clustering means the overall propensity to form groups of cases. Moreover, clusters are excessive pooling of people, usually in a small and well defined area and generally have a few cases [7]. Thus, with two different approaches, there is another classification of such studies: the *post-hoc*, which is based on observation of past events; and *the priori*, found as a result of a specific statistical exercise. *A priori* investigation of a propensity for the tendency of clustering is relatively new and can be useful in the interpretation of some *post hoc* cluster observations.

The studies of *post hoc* clusters take place because of public concern about a possible cluster. The problem is that the cases have been identified by personal knowledge and therefore may lead to an inherent bias. Indeed cases may not even be from the same disease. The *a priori* surveillance schemes, systematically monitoring a region for geographical or temporal excesses. There are specialized methods for looking for overall clustering (space-time, spatial or temporal) or to find specific clusters. In turn, clusters studies can be classified otherwise, as expressed in the following chart:

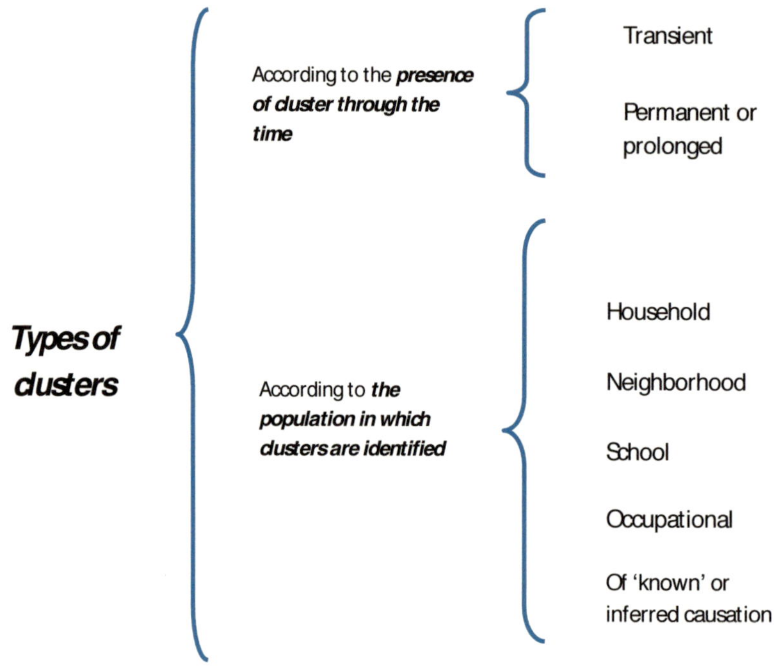

Figure 1. Types of clusters of diseases

The particularity of clusters analysis is that it shows the heterogeneous spatial distribution of cases, or the different behavior of occurrence of cases. It is generally accepted that the explanation of this distinction lies in the unequal distribution of the causal factors of disease in time and space. The underlying causes factors may vary by location, such as city, country, neighborhood, or rural areas. Putative exposures may have changed through time.

The value of a cluster analysis is that they show the hypothetical consequences of any possible factor on the spatial or temporal distribution of the population. If there is a spatial or temporal difference in the incidence of a disease, this could suggest the presence of an environmental factor. When the positive detection of a cluster happens, this suggests that an environmental factor may be involved in the development of this health problem. At the level of individuals, genetic factors are important in determining which people get sick. However, when we need to explain the disease in the population level, environmental factors and lifestyle have a higher relative weight [8]. Given the conclusion, the question is: what are these factors?

2. Spatial epidemiology

2.1. Definition and concepts

Among the various techniques and methods to study epidemiology, there is an area called *Spatial epidemiology* (or *Geographical epidemiology*). The Spatial epidemiology complements other studies that are considered traditional in epidemiology (cross sectional, cohort and case-control studies). The objectives of Spatial epidemiology are two: 1) to identify the possible risk factor that contribute to the spatial variation of the disease, and 2) highlight unusual groups that may say something more, than what is already known through other research channels. Finally in these studies, the clusters are defined as groups of persons [1,9].

Furthermore the study of geographical distribution's patterns of disease depends of the geographic or temporal scale [1]. Of the scale, because, for example, in a big city, one kilometer can be sufficient to determine the presence of a cluster. While on the other hand, if the territory under study is only a section of a city, the assessment may be limited to a few tens of meters. And of the time, since if the health problem is the result of a very clear, and definite exposure, then the clusters of cases may be observable after a few months. One example is the radiation's effects from Chernobyl on the increasing in the prevalence of Down's syndrome in the children of Belarus [10]. This cluster could be related to radiation's exposure, and was confined to a single month. Another example is related to studies that monitoring acute outbreak, which lasted a few days, where a cluster could be detected on a much smaller window of time. E.g., one study, conducted in Hong Kong, illustrates the spatial and temporal dynamics of human influenza A (H1N1). They could detect space-time heterogeneity in the incidence of disease. It is remarkable the chronological description of the spread of disease across the territory of Hong Kong. In this study, were detected space-time clusters of people with the disease from the third week until week 22. It described the cluster transformation weekly. Although researchers have evaluated space-time clustering, rather than temporal clusters, their results demonstrate how can be detected clusters within small periods of weeks, or even in a few days [11].

A study of clusters (or clustering) can support, or not support, an etiological hypothesis. There must be similarities between the premises of the hypothesis and the design principles inherent at the study. For example, in one study of McNally et al, they assumed that, according to the hypothesis put forward by Smith [12] a high incidence of acute leukemia in children is linked with an infectious exposure that occurred *in uterus*. Under this premise, the space-time cluster of children with leukemia should have manifested when it searched according to the place and date of birth, because these are according with assumptions of Smith's hypothesis. If it had, this result could have been interpreted as an indirect support of that acute leukemia in children is linked, in fact, with an infectious exposure *in uterus*, prior to disease development. They did not find this result, so it ended without support the Smith's hypothesis [13]. This is one illustration of how the principles of design of a cluster (or clustering) study, should coincide with the assumptions of a previously stated hypothesis.

The test driver of these studies is derived from other sciences. According to Lawson, Spatial epidemiology concerns the analysis of the spatial-geographical incidence of disease. The Spatial epidemiology keeps a close link with Spatial analysis. Last one forms an entire branch, and a school of thought within the geographical science. Lawson noted that the Spatial epidemiology is a field, or discipline, whose interest concerns the use and interpretation of maps for the location of cases of disease. Also pointed out that all matters related to the production of maps and statistical analysis of mapped data should be dedicated to study in Epidemiology. Furthermore, it pointed out that many epidemiological concepts play an important role in their analysis.

The importance of maps in epidemiological work is clear. However, Spatial epidemiology does not restrict its activity only to such cartographic work. There are a detailed set of tasks for Spatial/Geographical analysis in Epidemiology. There are: cluster (or clustering) studies, models of exposure to sources of risk of disease mapping, field surveys of information, analysis, ecological models of infectious diseases, among other studies [9]. You can do analysis within related areas, comparisons, analysis of surfaces and areas, analysis of lines, and analysis of points. Each category has additional subdivisions into more types of studies [14]. Clustering studies look for general patterns in a region, whereas, in contrast, cluster studies have a focused representation. The study of spatial clusters (or clustering) and spatial-temporal clusters (or clustering) correspond to the study of points and areas, and correspond with focused and general clusters and clustering studies. Both types of studies are having a geographical interpretation. Focused cluster studies actually seek to detect a very specific cluster, e.g., distinctly clustered cases around a defined point localized in a territory. General clustering and focused cluster analyses have their own statistical tests. Also, there are two concepts whose interpretation may be mistaken, and these are cluster and clustering. A cluster is a group of children that arises in a small and well defined area, usually has a few cases. By clustering means the general propensity of cases to form groups [13].

Tango, in his book Statistical Methods for Disease Clustering [15], classified clusters studies according to geographical approach to the problem. If the intention is to recognize the occurrence of conglomerate, over a territory and/or a given time, then this is a general test. If, instead, there is already a predetermined point, as a given event in a defined location, then a test is focused. To further clarify the last point, it is the example of radiation in Chernobyl. The event is the nuclear disaster, the place is the nuclear plant, and the conglomerate is looking around that point, after that event. The cluster, detected in the above example, was a focused cluster.

A focused study of clusters is a specific study of clusters. In these studies, the location of any cluster, if it exists on the map, is a matter of first importance. In these studies there is a source of exposure, which is a fixed place in the territory, and is known incidence of the disease. The search feature is that if any cluster is detected, it should revolve around sources of exposure that are under suspicion. Often this relationship is identified as a causal interaction, i.e., indicate the relationship between nuclear plant exposure and the spatial distribution of sick cases around it. Indirectly, the results of these studies are interpreted as support evidence that an exposure located in one place can generate a disease in the population that is under the effect of exposure. Tango pointed a difference: when the location of possible clusters is expected *a priori*, then it is a specific focusing study; when possible location is unknown, a specific study is not focused [15].

For his part, Lawson, classifies these two ways of approaching with other names: like a general study of clusters, and as specific studies [9]. However, he further detailed definition of both concepts, as he points out the usefulness of studies from a map view. Furthermore, according

http://dx.doi.org/10.5772/54456

to Lawson, a general study of clusters is the valuation of a map of a complete territory, in order to find out if there are clusters in that place. If anything there is no cluster, as proposed by a null hypothesis, the map should not observe any difference in the distribution of the disease. The explanation, in the alternative hypothesis, should then provide some specific mechanisms to understand the grouping that the maps show. It concerns a preconceived notion of how these clusters are given. Such studies may also be called as non-specific, since in reality are not required to identify the place where the clusters are placed, but that really only intended to identify whether there is a pattern, a pattern of grouping into clusters.

It is extremely important, in Spatial epidemiology, which in all the techniques and methods explained, epidemiological considerations, proper exercise of Epidemiology, are taken into account. Elliot and Best, declared that the differences in the distribution of disease incidence, could produce important clues to the etiology of disease research. Then, later studies could be carried out by methods designed to analyze the population at an individual level (e.g. cohort or case-control-control) [1].

The Spatial epidemiological analysis has three peculiarities inherent to the source of their data, which explain the logic of the clusters. First, epidemiological analysis has in statistics and, in particular in spatial statistics, at the core of their method. This is because these data have the property of being geo-referenced (located on a map) and may be interlinked a result of their location. The data can be at the personal level, always associated with it spatial localization. Secondly, in Epidemiology, generally the spatial data are discrete, i.e. they are not quantifiable data on a continuous scale. They are the occurrence of these phenomena is in part a consequence of previous events, and in addition it also depends on an important individual independence, due to random processes. That is, they are stochastic processes. Furthermore, these data (for example, the location of a child with leukemia) behave according to processes associated with discrete probability distributions. Put another way, these are processes whose phenomena are clearly separated values. Finally, the nature of all information used in Spatial epidemiology are linked to conventional studies of Epidemiology, which leads to the derivation of models and methods related to spatial analysis [9]. In these studies a null hypothesis indicates the "normal" variation of sick cases, or with health problems. It is compared against alternative hypothesis, which explains the difference in question

There should be no confusion. This type of study stored multiple matches with other epidemiological studies. For example, the size of the sample examined, studies of clusters also yield less uncertainty when making inferences. Can be made a study of conglomerates stratified, where a disease cases are divided into groups suitable for research purposes. For example, it can do cluster detection between boys and girls or by age groups sensitive to the different susceptibility of some individuals over others. The results of a study of clusters can be enhanced, too, by using more variables. These variables need not be necessarily included in the operations of the proper analysis of the detection of clusters. Its can indicate the environmental conditions of the population. For example, one can know the socioeconomic status of the cases studied the population density of the locality where they live, or industrial activity where they live, just to name a few. Finally, the study outcomes can be explained in light of these variables, also under the logic of stratified analysis, if required. On the other hand, cluster studies are sensitive to data quality. If the database from which the analysis is not good quality, the final conclusion should be taken into account these shortcomings, or even avoid the start of operations. Other deficiencies that also affect the validity of the results include the underestimation a result of misdiagnosis or because of diagnoses made by different methods. Also, excessive division and subdivision into groups or strata of the population under study, can lead to pulverization of the sample into too small sets, unable to be analyzed, without sufficient statistical power. And similarly, these studies are not without the danger of research bias, whether by chance or by a systematic error.

2.2. Limitations

From the epidemiological discipline, two important mistakes could occur in these studies: the fallacy of aggregation, and the ecological fallacy. The concepts are defined, including:

1. Fallacy of aggregation: the misapplication of a causal explanation at the individual, when it was seen as a relation to the group level. It is considered a kind of ecological fallacy [16].

2. Ecological fallacy: it has two meanings. The first sense is very similar to the aforementioned fallacy of aggregation; sometimes it is taken as synonymous with this. The second meaning, more detailed, defines it as an error of inference due to the mistake to distinguish between different levels of organization. "A correlation between variables that are based on characteristics of an group, not necessarily reproduced between variables based on characteristics of individuals; an association that is given at a level could be gone in the other, or even be reversed" [16].

In other words, the conclusions, if not verified by other research designs, should be limited to the population level inferences. For instance, when it is used in conjunction with a case-control study, the formulation of hypotheses that promotes may result in many more immediate applications, like the identification of possible risk factors [17]. Otherwise, any generalization of the results from a study of clusters may be inferred.

A space-time cluster study has the advantage that the associations between cases, being close to both a time and in space, can provide explanations that detail the coincidence of the incidence of leukemia in space and at a time determined. This feature is characteristic also of infectious events. On the other hand, when we only talk about spatial clusters, possible causes of these clusters can potentially just be environmental. The consideration of an infectious cause is harder. The explanations behind their formation must be sought strictly by spatial thought, less specific.

One more limitation is the lack of consistent information between the outcomes of similar studies. Sometimes it is necessary to work with this drawback, in addition to bias influences. This bias can be reported and noted, provided that the information given is somewhat predictable. For example, due to lack of data for workers who arrived in the area of study up before 1983, and the lack of information from other data, the results could be biased [18].

http://dx.doi.org/10.5772/54456

Another limitation is the geographical and historical principles that the researcher must working when making interpretations. Analyzing retrospective data carries uncertainty. For example, using mortality data in children with LA, it seems bias, may not be appropriate for studies of clusters, because the difference between the date of illness onset and date of death are variable among cases, and because people are likely to move between the time of onset and death [19].

If not careful, you can change the unit of analysis, from population to the territory. In itself this is not bad, but the evidence should not be combined. For example, Bellec et al, did a spatial analysis, discarding the population analysis, and results are properly interpreted from a spatial logic, focused on the areas under study [20]. Even after, its meaning was explicated to the people. Related to that, among the challenges to be addressed soon, there are: to study too small areas; to study too large areas; and use biomarkers to check risk factors. An example of the limitations of both geographical and historical boundaries is the definition of significant results for both spatial and temporal dimensions. The danger is that you can led out of the expected results to several other cases are linked. One test, the Knox test shows this disadvantage [21].

One test, known as Moran test, prove test's spatial limits, and how it could produce a bias in the correlation tests. Rogerson's method indicates something similar. These could be due to the difficulty of finding differences in a too small or too large geographic area. This is a disadvantage in cases such as a city, where opportunities for analysis using very large spatial limits potentially could led to finding an enormous variability; but on the other hand, for diseases that are hard to find in general population, like childhood leukemia, to find a cluster in a very large area will be difficult. As shown, also for this reason, is preferable works it with existing cases, and choose a convenient method, or a combination of methods.

Finally, not all studies carried out by detecting the presence of complete clusters. This is in part due to the use of the wrong method, or because the sample size are not adequate. This has been reported with Glass et al [19], and Bellec et al [20]. The work of Birch et al also makes a similar warning [21].

3. Studies of clustering and clusters of children with leukemia

An old idea has always troubled the minds of those who investigate the causes of childhood leukemia. The research regarding the etiology of childhood acute leukemia has a long history of about 100 years, without finding the full factor explaining the origin of the disease. For example, by the results of this research have been identified two risk factors for the development of leukemia: intense ionizing radiation and certain congenital genetic syndromes, which only account for 10% of cases [22]. Amin pointed one factor more: exposure to chemotherapeutic agents. However, these factors explain only a small percentage of all cases of leukemia. He presented several studies that examined the complexity of other risk factors: "early-life exposures to infectious agents, parental, fetal, or childhood exposures to environmental toxins, parental occupational exposures to radiation or chemicals; parental medical conditions during pregnancy or before conception; maternal diet during pregnancy, early postnatal feeding patterns and diet, and maternal reproductive [23]. Finally, he added that environmental factors may play a role in cancer development in children, and too many cases, concentrated in one geographical area, one cluster, could be evidence of that. After all, these sets of studies have supported the etiological investigation of childhood leukemia, especially acute lymphoblastic leukemia. At its completion, attention has been paid to various causes, such as ionizing radiation, contaminated water, petrochemical industry, exposure to agrochemicals [24]. The less controversial idea is that the clusters are evidence that environmental factors are generally involved in the development of cancer, including childhood leukemia.

Ward, for example, since 1917, thought of a theory of infection of childhood acute leukemia [25]. It is a very old hypothesis and, until today, has not been proven or disproved. The study of clustering and clusters is often used to support the ideas developed around the possibility that infections are behind the onset of childhood leukemia. A cluster of children with leukemia has been interpreted as evidence that behind the development of the disease are implicated infections in children's lifetime [7]. Tango, in 2010, said "in the search for evidence of whether a disease such as leukemia, is indeed an infectious disease and, therefore, a viral etiology, the focus will be on whether the cases are grouped into clusters" [15]. Specifically, concerning analysis of space-time clustering McNally and Eden clarified that if the infections were implicated in the etiology of childhood leukemia, then the geographic distribution of these children may show evidence of clustering in space, and under certain conditions may also show space-time clustering [26].

In fact, the presence of a cluster of children with leukemia has been interpreted in a more broad and diverse sense. A cluster of children with leukemia would suggest that since the origin of the disease, one or more factors are involved, not just infection. As already mentioned, genetic predisposition may also play a role. It is very important to reiterate that the results obtained from such studies should be interpreted with special care. The cluster studies, by themselves, do not reveal causal agents in the sense of identifying risk factors involved in a health problem. It should be noted that studies of clustering and clusters are behind the search for relationships that are implicit in theory of the etiology of a disease, but these studies are not used to make formal determinations of risk factors implied. Hence, the inferences developed from the results of these studies are not without controversy.

In a literature review of the last fifteen years (1997-2012), were found more than 20 publications, of which 18 are focused on acute lymphoblastic leukemia (ALL). There are two questions that have been repeatedly proposed to be answered by studies of clusters, the first is whether infections play an important role in the development of childhood acute lymphoblastic leukemia, and the second is whether there are environmental risk factors that are not well specified influence on disease onset. However, some researchers have considered infection like a type of environmental exposure, and therefore the two terms may have been used interchangeably in some research.

The objectives that want to answer research questions of cluster studies are several, for example, the objectives can be descriptive, or may be the result of pose a hypothesis "a priori". Of the 18 studies conducted in children with ALL, eight had a descriptive purpose, proposed a methodological improvement, or only sought to detect at least one cluster in the territory studied [12,26–31]. Also within the objectives of the studies of clusters there are some that are rare but very interesting, such studies have been conducted on exploring the presence of risk factors that could potentially be common between different types of childhood cancer [33]; or studies that are even more specific to look for the presence of a cluster of children, within a particular subtype of leukemia (pre-B ALL) [21]. Moreover cluster studies conducted so far, to consider since the start of the investigation. By contrast, there are publications about where it was proposed as a risk factor that could potentially lead to the development of leukemia, which allowed those jobs also propose a working hypothesis or also called "a priori" with the sole purpose of find scientific evidence [7,17,24,34–38]. As mentioned above, one of the risk factors considered most important, proposed and used in different studies, is related to the role of infections in the development of leukemia, resulting in the so-called infectious hypothesis [17,34–36,39]. Another risk factor that has been considered and that is relevant to this issue is the so-called environmental risk factor (unspecified) [7,37]. For example, in a study conducted by Petridou et al, in the year 1997 was referred on that environmental factors may impact the development of leukemia, but in this study did not specify these environmental factors nor their relationship in a given moment with infections [38].

According to a possible risk factor involved in the development of ALL, referenced within the findings of cluster studies conducted so far, they can be divided into three groups: 1) studies that suggest to infections [17,21,24,29,30,33,34,36,37]; 2) studies proposing an unspecified environmental factor [27,38] and finally 3) studies that consider both factors, infections and unspecified environmental factor [7,13,28].

Likewise cluster studies have favored the generation of new knowledge about how to conduct such studies [21,31], and even both proposals were generated for subsequent original studies as to confirm previous findings [32,35].

A longstanding discussion agreement concerning the definition, existence, frequency and interpretation of clusters of childhood leukemia (CL) remains unresolved [40]. In 2009, zur Hausen et al., said it that is very difficult to understand that mere clusters of cases of leukemia, Hodgkin lymphoma, Hodgkin lymphoma, or even cases of multiple myeloma, are indicating that these tumors have their origin in systemic infections. It has been proposed that viral infections should be revealed in a geographical area according to a random pattern of geographical distribution. The same author argued that if the simple processes in non-infectious disease lead to cancer onset, as further modifications of the genome are needed at the cellular level, caused by viruses. However, he also thought about the possibility that clusters may be the expression of a mutagenic factor in a family or, probably, in a small community or region, exposed to the factor [41].

The debate is not over. The controversies surrounding the usefulness of cluster studies for understanding the leukemia in children are constant. "Most clusters do not have evidence for obvious, prolonged and biologically plausible exposures. The etiology is obscure or unknown. Very rarely they can lead to a better understanding of causation, usually in situations with well-documented and heavy local contamination" [42]. There are intermediate positions, which do not ensure the possibility of a conglomerate but neither discarded. Law, in 2008, setting out "[...] it is difficult to see how these clusters provide evidence for infectious disease being involved in the etiology of childhood leukemia" [43]. But he clarified that the positive results of a study of clusters are used as a proxy, in fact, that its possible etiology. In addition, he relied on evidence generated by other studies, as the peak age between 2 and 5 years, the incidence of disease or increased incidence over time, and seasonal variations in the incidence of leukemia. These studies have been identified as potentially indicative of the role of infections [43].

Perhaps studies of space-time clustering result in less doubt when their results are interpreted. Possibly, they are tremendously bounded by the condition of the two dimensions examined by these techniques. It must be remembered that this type of study seeks to distinguish clustering patterns of cases, both in time and in space, simultaneously. In 2006, McNally, Alexander and Bithell, began a study in the hope of detecting space-time clustering of children with cancer in the United Kingdom. They predicted that if an antecedent infection was involved in cancer development, this type of clusters of children with cancer should be revealed in the territory of the island, if the infection (either viral or bacterial)was not ubiquitous or endemic. Otherwise there could be differences in spatial or temporal dimensions. The authors clarified that, however, this would only occur when the delay time between exposure and cancer diagnosis was short, or at least relatively constant. In the first scenario they wanted to test that, in the etiology of some childhood cancers, the timing of onset of this disease possibly masks the ability to be a rare response to infection [37].

Furthermore, McNally et al., suggested that infections may act in the etiology of certain types of diseases of childhood cancer. Similarly, they relied on the fact that several studies conducted elsewhere in the world, had also found space-time clustering of children with childhood acute leukemia, especially acute lymphoblastic leukemia, with similar conclusions. They began to change their language, from infections to environmental exposures. Three years later, in 2009, they presented a retrospective reflection on the study mentioned in the preceding paragraph, and referred to themselves in the following words: "These findings provided support for the involvement of environmental agents in etiological processes occurring close to diagnosis" [13]. Really, they confirmed a change in favor of extending the suspicion of the sum of environmental factors, rather than just infection.

In that study were found space-time clustering of children with various types of cancer. The children were registered in a database, from 1969 to 1993. Among cancers, they included leukemia. The clusters were searched according to two possible outcomes. The first of these was the phenomenon that presumably finds clusters of children that matched both their place of residence at birth, for the date they were born. The second concerned the possibility of finding these clusters when they seek groups according to place of birth of children and also according to the time of diagnosis, regardless of date of birth. Each result has a different interpretation. By residence and date of birth, there were clusters of cases with Hodgkin lymphoma and central nervous system tumors. When searched according to the residence at birth, but considering the date of diagnosis, there were space-time clusters with leukemia cases (specifically for children aged 1 to 4 years) and also for Wilms tumor and Hodgkin lymphoma.

http://dx.doi.org/10.5772/54456

Interpretations for each type of cancer have its nuances, but the meanings of space-time clusters in the above variables are as follows. When clusters of cases matched both in time and in place of birth, the given interpretation is that this conjunction supports the possible involvement of infections in the etiology of the disease studied. In particular, the space-time clusters of children with Hodgkin lymphoma suggest that a relevant etiological exposure occurred among children at similar ages after birth, or in uterus period. Moreover, since the dates are the time of birth and diagnosis, this would indicate that there was a heterogeneous latent period from the time of exposure until the time of diagnosis. Clusters of children with central nervous system tumors were interpreted with caution. According to the authors, this finding only strengthens the possibility that infections are implicated in the development of tumors mentioned.

On the other hand, when the space-time clusters match the place of birth and date of diagnosis rather than date of birth, the conclusion was different. For example, clusters of cases with NHL suggest that exposure which resulted in the onset of this disease in similar stages, before diagnosis. Childhood leukemia received a special mention. According to McNally et al, in a previous study [37], the authors had found clusters of children with leukemia by place and date of diagnosis, whereas in the study cited here, they found clusters by date of birth more date of diagnosis. In no cases children, clusters were found by location and date of birth. Again, the results supported the hypothesis of infectious childhood leukemia. The result is restricted since, although children with leukemia were between 1 and 4 years of age in the first study, this outcome was found only among children with ALL, the most common; and in the second study, was found among children with overall acute leukemia.

When we talk about leukemia clusters in children, McNally and colleagues reported that there are clusters when they are sought under the variables of time and place of birth [21]. Mulder et al, found clusters around environmental factors: the cases were grouped when analyzed by exposure to petroleum products and pesticides, and even found a link between having swum in a pond contaminated with petrochemical spill in previous years [44]. Petridou's team found correspondence between the ages of cases and their place of residence, while in urban areas had clusters of children between 0 and 4 years, and excluding those over 5 years in rural areas should be age higher [45]. In England, there was found clusters from both the date and place of birth of cases, and between the date and place of diagnosis of the same group [17]. Gustafsson and Carstensen, in contrast, dismissed the clustering according to the place and date of diagnosis, but they found them by date and place [29]. Gilman came to similar results, finding clusters by date and place of diagnosis, and date and place of birth, with the added bonus that also could rule out cancer clusters in solid tumors [46]. Finally, Alexander, who sought and found clusters with defined variables from another perspective: cases susceptible and infected cases [47].

There are also studies of clustering and clusters with negative outcomes. In France, Bellec not found clusters in a study which used data from the national registry, notwithstanding they used many different methods to detect clusters: Potthoff-Whittinghill, Moran, Knox and Kulldorff [20]. Dockerty and colleagues [48], and Alexander et al [49], found nothing when only raw data were based on geographic, demographic and diagnostic information. There are certainly limitations to this type of study, but, specifically, since 1970, it warned that a number of cases over a long period could lead to detection of artificial nature [50].

The infectious etiology of acute leukemia has been revised, too, from other study designs. Wartenberg et al, in 2004, sought to study the infectious origin of leukemia, testing a hypothesis developed for this purpose (Kinlen hypothesis). The study was conducted from an ecological point of view. This type of study is characterized in that its inferences can only be applied to the ambient, and cannot be categorical causal statements about the population being studied [51]. Another ecological study, carried out by Knox [52], revealed an association between the prevalence of childhood cancers (including leukemia) with the geographic distribution of air pollutants. In a third study, also ecological [53], there was a comparison between cases of people with different cancers (and ages), in a city of Wales. Hypothetically they expected that the prevalence of cancers decrease as people were found at greater distances from a source of pollution (petrochemical industry). There was an inverse correspondence between the distance and the incidence of some cancers, but not the incidence or mortality of leukemia.

The relationship between environmental factors and the development of cancer, including leukemia, has been extensively studied, and the outcomes, far from discouraging the search, prompt further investigation.

Studies of Lehtinen et al [54], Bogdanovic et al [55], Roman et al [56], Gilham et al [57], looked for associations between viral agents and the development of leukemia. These studies used a case-control design. Lehtinen hypothesized about *in utero* infection with Epstein-Barr virus and human herpes virus. There were no significant results. Bogdanovic analyzed the relationship between the Epstein-Barr virus and its reactivation in the mother, showing a possible association with childhood acute lymphoblastic leukemia. Roman found positive relationships between the incidences of disease by these viruses generated with leukemia. Gilham assumed that a large exposure to infection, when the child lives in day care, was associated with protection that reduced the development of childhood leukemia; his results led to conclude that reduced exposure to infections during the first months of the child's life increases the risk of developing acute lymphoblastic leukemia.

The study of clusters suggests possible etiologies. The interest is that these putative risk factors can be assessed in more detail. For example, the study of cluster analysis is often combined with a case-control study. This gives more relevant results, as measured relationships between risk factors and disease [44,48,58–61]. In addition, cluster detection techniques can be compared with other techniques, using the same data, allowing comparisons [20,62,63].

When spatial distributions are unusual, it is possible to speculate on the etiological implications [49]. A study of clusters can evaluate multicausal factors. Bellec's findings supported the hypothesis that a community's geographic isolation and low density, possibly combined with the mixture of different populations, may play an important role in the etiology of leukemia. It could not been possible to consider the geographic isolation as a risk factor using any other technique. However, the same author suggests that a new research question should be to determine whether this phenomenon was specific to one age group or diagnosis; and proposes that future statistical models could allow further

http://dx.doi.org/10.5772/54456

investigation and better understanding of these findings, especially with respect to the role of population density and population mixing [20].

4. Analysis of data from Mexico City

Acute leukemia among children in Mexico City has been studied for over a decade. Through these studies, we know well that its incidence is among the highest in the world. In 2011 Pérez Saldívar et al., reported an incidence of 57.6 cases/million children [64]. This high incidence, coupled with the large population of the city—more than eight million in 2010 in the territory of the Federal District, and more than 20 million people in the metropolitan area of Mexico City, in the same year—are expressed in more than 200 children with childhood leukemia each year. These children and adolescents are treated in nine tertiary hospitals, the highest rank of specialist medical care in the Mexican health system. It has been estimated that these hospitals serve approximately 97.5% of the cases of childhood acute leukemia in Mexico City [65].

For over ten years it was suspected that the spatial distribution of children with leukemia in Mexico City was heterogeneous. In 2000, in a descriptive longitudinal study, conducted by researchers at the Instituto Mexicano del Seguro Social [66], were found morbidity standardized rates (MSR), that suggest a spatial concentration of cases of childhood leukemia. For acute lymphoblastic leukemia (ALL), the MSR were highest at south of Mexico City; for acute myeloblastic leukemia (AML), the MSR were highest in the west. In addition, from further investigations, some matches attracted the attention: it was found that among patients with acute leukemia (AL), some of them were immediate neighbors, suggesting that behind the development of the disease there is an environmental factor that could promote it [67]. It was, therefore, decided to make a study of spatial clustering in Mexico City, to confirm the hypothesis that children with leukemia are grouped into clusters that reflect the aforementioned heterogeneous spatial distribution.

Information was extracted on individuals aged 0-14 years, diagnosed with ALL between 2006 and 2007, who were resident in Mexico City (Federal District). A total of 224 incident cases were identified. We also included 224 children without leukemia (controls), nor other cancers, genetic malformation or asthma. The controls were matched by sex, age and health institution of origin. We located the addresses of the homes, with an accuracy of 0.1 km, from where children residing at diagnosis of leukemia, or the time of the interview, in those without the disease. The cases were recruited between the years 2006 and 2007, and for the controls needed a much larger period, from 1998 to 2011. Due to this discrepancy, we discard the detection of clusters according to the temporal dimension. We used the Kullorff's scan statistic, which is based on a Bernoulli model, to identify individual clusters. The complete study region was scanned by construction of a two-dimensional circular window. The window was varied so at most it included 50% of the entire geographical area. The variable circular window is centered on the geo-reference of each case [68]. The method has been used previously in an analysis of leukaemia in Sweden [69]. Statistical significance ($P<0.05$) was evaluated using one-sided tests and 99999 simulations. Only one large statistically significant cluster was identified (see Fig.

2) (O=98, E=74.66, O/E=1.313, p=0.01325). There were no statistically significant secondary clusters. This finding indicates that locally varying environmental factors may be implicated in the origin of ALL in Mexico City. However, the possibility of chance may play a role, cannot be excluded.

Although we cannot exclude the effect of chance on these results, nor forget the fact of that the periods of data collection between cases and controls are different, these results are remarkable. For comparison, in a study conducted in Ohio [62], also carried out with SaTScan, the most significant data were found for the group of children aged 10-14 years, with a value p=0.33, and only three cases formed part of cluster. When all the data were analyzed together, including all types of leukemia and all ages, the most likely cluster had 43 cases, with p=0.81. As we can see, none of the clusters is statistically significant. The author of the paper commented that these results were not entirely surprising, considering that the study area is very large and diverse (the state of Ohio). He argued that in a large area, it is doubtful that a particular risk factor going to have a consistent and sustained effect through space. It's unlikely to see a cluster in a large geographical area. And again, in other study, Wheeler repeated the same sentence with another argument: the results are consistent with the literature worldwide, because it is difficult to find statistically significant clusters. Wheeler used several tests of clusters (K-function, Cuzick & Edward's, kernel intensity function) plus SaTScan, without finding significant associations with any of them.

Apparently the cluster analysis is most effective for small-area spatial analysis [31], on the scale of a city, and not in an area as large as a U.S. state, or in a entire country. Goujon-Bellec et al, concluded that very few cluster detection techniques have enough power to scan large areas, as a large country like France [70]. It has also been observed that when the unit of geographic analysis is very large, such as an aggregate of municipalities (about 30 × 30 Km) or cantons, the sensitivity of a technique for detecting clusters is diminished; it is as though the proximity between the cases are "diluted" among these geographical units, and the cluster simply "does not appear". Studies of Germany [7] and France [20] seem to confirm it. Therefore, differences in surface between the territories of Ohio, in the United States, and Mexico City, in the Mexican capital (116,096 Km^2 vs. 1,485 Km^2, respectively), could be one reason why we detected a cluster in the city. However, the number of clster's children (98 cases), and a value of p = 0.01325, is not commonly reported. In addition, the data collection period of the cases was two years, against eight of Ohio study.

When the geographic location of the children who make up the cluster is mappeding, it can be seen that this spatial cluster is located to the east of Mexico City (Federal District), slightly to the northeast. Indeed, about half of all children with leukemia investigated are part of this cluster. The conglomerate is clearly excluded from west and southwest of Mexico City. The extent of the surface cluster includes the territories of some of the boroughs of the Mexican Federal District. The hypothetical explanations for this cluster are the following.

Industrial establishments located in the environment of a child have been considered as risk factors for developing cancer. Sans et al, in 1995, expected the prevalence of cancers, including childhood acute leukemia, decrease as people were found farther from the petrochemical industry plant, as in Britain [53]. According to data from the National Institute of Statistics,

Geography and Informatics (INEGI by its Spanish acronym), the two main boroughs by number of economic units of industrial activity are Azcapotzalco and Miguel Hidalgo. In fact, these two areas form the most industrialized landscape of Mexico City, for over half a century. There was an old oil refinery, an auto plant, dozens of railways and many other industries. Contradictorily, these delegations are not part of the cluster found on the east of Mexico City. At first glance, this suggests that the spatial cluster detected in this study is not related to large industrial facilities. However, to be more careful, we can see that the phenomenon probably does have a relationship but more nuanced. In third place for the number of industrial establishments, appears Iztapalapa borough, which is included within the area of spatial cluster. When comparing those boroughs, Azcapotzalco and Miguel Hidalgo, against the latter, Iztapalapa, we note that the average personnel employed in industrial establishments is very different. While the staff working at the Miguel Hidalgo and Azcapotzalco boroughs is 32.01 and 31.29 workers per economic unit, respectively comparatively, in the Iztapalapa borough would, there are on average, 11.19 workers per industrial unit. This suggests that facilities most prevalent in the spatial cluster detected include small establishments such as family workshops. If so, the work on these workshops can be an important parental exposure.

Another consideration is air pollution, which is a risk factor that has been studied. Knox suggested an association between the prevalence of cancer in the geographical distribution of air pollutants [71]. According to National Institute of Ecology (INE by its Spanish acronym), the impact of air pollution in Mexico City generates 4,000 premature deaths per year and 2.5 million lost work days [72]. EMBARQ states that, with about 18 million people and 6 million cars, Mexico City's metropolitan area is one of the largest and busiest cities in the world. Around 600 new cars come into service each day, and in 2007 it sold just over 300,000 cars this year. Most alarming is that, according to the same place, less than 4% of vehicles, trucks and buses, generated in 2002, about 70% of air pollution. The other 30 percent is allocated to factories, small cars and motorcycles [73]. Air pollution is thus mainly attributed to heavy cars. The smog of Mexico City is concentrated in the southern part of it, and the children of the conglomerate are located mainly to the east. With the evidence found, it is difficult to ensure that the cause of spatial cluster is due, mainly, to the atmospheric concentration of pollution in the city. If so, we would have expected a spatial cluster in the south-southwest of Mexico City, instead of having appeared in the east.

In an earlier study, which also uses the information from the same database of this study, we measured the relationship between socioeconomic status and the development of childhood acute leukemia. The study, conducted by Perez-Saldivar et al, considered the problem according to three indicators [64]. The first is indirect and only represents the existing agricultural activity in each delegation of Mexico [74]. The second used the information developed by the United Nations to measure human development, the Human Development Index by municipalities, published to Mexico in 2005 [75]. The third sought to relate the average number of people per household [76]. The results only showed a relationship between the incidences of ALL with the number of people per household, in Pre-B ALL. For none of the other two indicators found a significant relationship. In this study, the detected cluster is located in an area of relatively low economic level, with several boroughs suffering from poverty problems in Mexico City and higher number of people per household. However, given the information that it has, we cannot explain a relationship between socioeconomic status and the cluster reported in the study. Further studies are needed to investigate this point.

In summary, we can say that the investigation of spatial clusters in geographic areas of a relatively small size, as a city with a high population density and a high incidence of childhood acute leukemia, is favorable for the detection of clusters.

Unfortunately we do not have a longer register of children with leukemia, so that the interpretation of the results is inconclusive. The results of this study support the involvement of environmental factors in the development of childhood acute lymphoblastic leukemia.

these studies, we know well that its incidence is among the highest in the world. In 2011 we reported an incidence of 57.6 cases/million children [64]. This high incidence, coupled with the large population of the city—more than eight million in 2010 in the territory of the Federal District, and more than 20 million people in the metropolitan area of Mexico City, in the same year—are expressed in the more than 200 children with childhood leukemia incidents each year. These children and adolescents are treated in nine tertiary hospitals, the highest rank of specialist medical care in the Mexican health system. It has been estimated that these hospitals serve approximately 97.5% of the cases of childhood acute leukemia Mexico City [65].

For over ten years it was suspected that the spatial distribution of children with leukemia in Mexico City was heterogeneous. In 2000, in a descriptive longitudinal study, conducted by researchers at the Mexican Social Security Institute [66], were found morbidity standarized rates (MSR), that suggest a spatial concentration of cases of childhood leukemia. For acute lymphoblastic leukemia (ALL), the MSR were highest at south of Mexico City; for acute myeloblastic leukemia (AML), the MSR were highest in the west. In addition, from further investigations, some matches attracted the attention: it was found that among patients with acute leukemia (AL), some of them were immediate neighbors, suggesting that behind the development of the disease; there is an environmental factor that could promote it [67]. It was, therefore, decided to make a study of spatial clustering in Mexico City, to confirm the hypothesis that children with leukemia are grouped into clusters that reflect the aforementioned heterogeneous spatial distribution.

Information was extracted on individuals aged 0-14 years, diagnosed with ALL between 2006 and 2007, who were resident in Mexico City. A total of 224 incident cases were identified. We also included 224 children without leukemia, nor other cancers, genetic malformation or asthma. Were matched by sex, age and health institution of origin. We located the addresses of the homes, with an accuracy of 0.1 km, from where children residing at diagnosis of leukemia, or the time of the interview, in those without the disease. The cases were collected between 2006 and 2007, and for the controls needed a much larger period, from 1998 to 2011. Due to this discrepancy, we discard the detection of clusters according to the temporal dimension. We used Kullorff´s scan statistic based on a Bernoulli model to identify individual clusters. The complete study region was scanned by construction of a two-dimensional circular window. The window was varied so at most it included 50% of the entire geographical area.

http://dx.doi.org/10.5772/54456

The variable circular window is centered on the geo-reference of each case [68]. The method has been used previously in an analysis of leukaemia in Sweden [69]. Statistical significance ($P<0.05$) was evaluated using one-sided tests and 99999 simulations. Only one large statistically significant cluster was identified (see Fig. 2) (O = 98, E = 74.66, O/E = 1.313, P = 0.01325). There were no statistically significant secondary clusters. This finding indicates that locally varying environmental factors may be implicated in the origin of ALL in Mexico City. However, the possibility that variable levels of ascertainment may play a role cannot be excluded.

Although we cannot exclude the effect of chance on these results, or forget the fact of that the periods of data collection between cases and controls are different, these results are remarkable. For comparison, in a study conducted in Ohio [62], also carried out with SaTScan, the most significant data were found for the group of children aged 10-14 years, with a value $p = 0.33$, and only three cases formed part of cluster. When all the data were analyzed together, including all types of leukemia and all ages, the most likely cluster had 43 cases, with $p = 0.81$. As we can see, none of the clusters is statistically significant. The author of the paper commented that these results were not entirely surprising, considering that the study area is very large and diverse (the state of Ohio). He argued that in a large area, it is doubtful that a particular risk factor going to have a consistent and sustained effect through space. It's unlikely to see a cluster in a large geographical area. And again, Wheeler repeated the same sentence with another argument: the results are consistent with the literature worldwide, because it is difficult to find statistically significant clusters. Wheeler used several tests of clusters (K-function, Cuzick & Edward's, kernel intensity function) plus SaTScan without finding significant associations with any of them.

Apparently the cluster analysis is most effective for small-area spatial analysis [31], on the scale of a city, and not in an area as large as a U.S. state. Goujon-Bellec et al, concluded that very few cluster detection techniques have enough power to scan large areas, as a large country like France [70]. It has also been observed that when the unit of geographic analysis is very large, such as a county or a municipality, or an aggregate of these, the sensitivity of a technique for detecting clusters is diminished; it is as though the proximity between the cases are "diluted" among these geographical units, and the cluster simply "does not appear". Studies of Germany [7] and France [20] seem to confirm it. Therefore, differences in surface between the territories of Ohio, in the United States, and Mexico City, in the Mexican capital (116.096 km^2 vs. 1485 km^2, respectively), could be one reason why we detected a cluster in the city. However, many children (98 cases), and a value of $p = 0.01325$, statistically significant, is not commonly reported. In addition, the data collection period of the cases was two years, against eight of Ohio study.

When the geographic location of the children who make up the cluster is mapped, it can be seen that this spatial cluster is located to the east of Mexico City (Federal District), slightly to the northeast. Indeed, about half of all children with leukemia investigated are part of this cluster. The conglomerate is clearly excluded from west and southwest of Mexico City. The extent of the surface cluster includes the territories of some of the boroughs of the Mexican Federal District. The hypothetical explanations for this cluster are the following.

Industrial establishments located in the environment of a child have been considered as risk factors for developing cancer. Sans et al, in 1995, expected the prevalence of cancers, including childhood acute leukemia, decrease as people were found farther from the petrochemical industry plant, as in Britain [53]. According to data from the National Institute of Statistics, Geography and Informatics (INEGI by its Spanish acronym), the two main boroughs by number of economic units of industrial activity are Azcapotzalco and Miguel Hidalgo. In fact, these two areas form the most industrialized landscape of Mexico City, for over half a century. There was an old oil refinery, an auto plant, dozens of railways and many other industries. Contradictorily, these delegations are not part of the cluster found on the east of Mexico City. At first glance, this suggests that the spatial cluster detected in this study is not related to large industrial facilities. However, to be more careful, we can see that the phenomenon probably does have a relationship but more nuanced. In third place for the number of industrial establishments, appears Iztapalapa borough, which is included within the area of spatial cluster. When comparing those boroughs, Azcapotzalco and Miguel Hidalgo, against the latter, Iztapalapa, we note that the average personnel employed in industrial establishments is very different. While the staff working at the Miguel Hidalgo and Azcapotzalco boroughs is 32.01 and 31.29 workers per economic unit, respectively. Comparatively in the Iztapalapa borough would, on average, 11.19 workers per industrial unit. This suggests that facilities most prevalent in the spatial cluster detected include more small establishments such as family workshops. If so, the work on these workshops can be an important parental exposure.

Another consideration is air pollution, which is a risk factor that has been studied. Knox suggested an association between the prevalence of cancer in the geographical distribution of air pollutants [71]. According to National Institute of Ecology (INE by its Spanish acronym), the impact of air pollution in Mexico City generates 4,000 premature deaths per year and 2.5 million lost work days [72]. EMBARQ states that, with about 18 million people and 6 million cars, Mexico City is one of the largest and busiest cities in the world. Around 600 new cars come into service each day, and in 2007 it sold just over 300,000 cars this year. Most alarming is that, according to the same place, less than 4% of vehicles, trucks and buses, generated in 2002, about 70% of air pollution. The other 30 percent is allocated to factories, small cars and motorcycles [73]. Air pollution is thus mainly attributed to heavy cars. The smog of Mexico City is concentrated in the southern part of it, and the children of the conglomerate are located mainly to the east. With the evidence found, it is difficult to ensure that the cause of spatial cluster is due, mainly, to the atmospheric concentration of pollution in the city. If so, we would have expected a conglomerate in the south-southwest of Mexico City, instead of having appeared in the east.

In an earlier study, which also uses the information from the same database of this study, we measured the relationship between socioeconomic status and the development of childhood acute leukemia. The study, conducted by Perez-Saldívar et al, considered the problem according to three indicators [64]. The first is indirect and only represents the existing agricultural activity in each delegation of Mexico [74]. The second used the information developed by the United Nations to measure human development, the Human Development Index by municipalities, published from Mexico in 2005 [75]. The third sought to relate the average

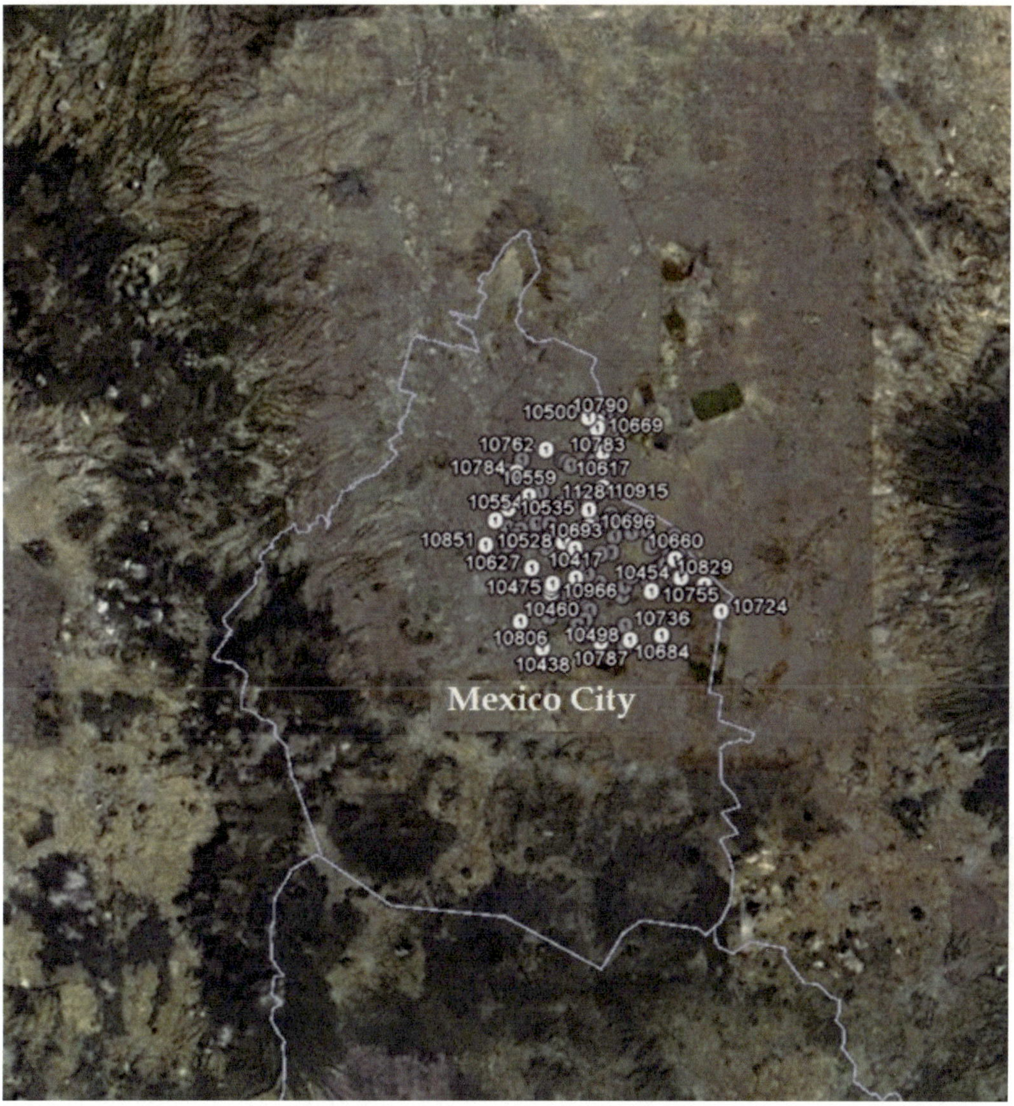

Figure 2. Location of spatial cluster of childhood acute leukemia cases in Mexico. The numbers are the identification of each case into the cluster

number of people per household [76]. The results only showed a relationship between the incidences of ALL with the number of people per household, in Pre-B ALL. For none of the other two indicators found a significant relationship. In this study, the detected cluster is located in an area of relatively low economic level, with several boroughs suffering from poverty problems in Mexico City. However, given the information that it has, we cannot explain a relationship between socioeconomic status and the cluster reported in the study. Further studies are needed to investigate this point.

Acknowledgements

This work was funded by the Consejo Nacional de la Ciencia y la Tecnología (CONACYT) through its program, Fondo Sectorial de Investigación en Salud y Seguridad Social (SALUD 2007-1-71223/FIS/IMSS/PROT/592); the Fondo Sectorial de Investigación para la Educación (CB-2007-1-83949/FIS/IMSS/PROT/616) and by Instituto Mexicano del Seguro Social (FIS/IMSS/PROT/G10/846).

Author details

David Aldebarán Duarte-Rodríguez[1], Richard J.Q. McNally[2], Juan Carlos Núñez-Enríquez[1], Arturo Fajardo-Gutiérrez[1] and Juan Manuel Mejía-Aranguré[3]

1 Unidad de Investigación en Epidemiología Clínica, Hospital de Pediatría, Centro Médico Nacional Siglo XXI, Instituto Mexicano del Seguro Social (IMSS), México

2 Institute of Health and Society, Newcastle University, UK

3 Coordinación de Investigación en Salud, Centro Médico Nacional Siglo XXI, Instituto Mexicano del Seguro Social (IMSS), México

References

[1] Elliot, P. NB. Geographic patterns of disease. In: Armitage P, Colton T, editors. International Encyclopaedia of Biostatistics. 2nd ed. Chichester: Wiley; (1998).

[2] Mejía-arangure, J. Pe´rez-Saldivar M, Rosana Pelayo-Camacho R, Fuentes-Panana´ E, Bekker-Mendez C, Morales-Sa´nchez A, et al. Childhood Acute Leukemias in Hispanic Population: Differences by Age Peak and Immunophenotype. In: Faderl S, editor. Novel Aspects in Acute Lymphoblastic Leukemia [Internet]. InTech; (2011). cited 2012 Aug 15]. Available from: http://intechopen.com/books/novel-aspects-in-acute-lymphoblastic-leukemia/childhood-acute-leukemias-in-hispanic-population-differences-by-age-peak-and-immunophenotype

[3] Poljak, Z, Dewey, C. E, Martin, S. W, Christensen, J, Carman, S, & Friendship, R. M. Spatial clustering of swine influenza in Ontario on the basis of herd-level disease status with different misclassification errors. Preventive Veterinary Medicine [Internet]. (2007). Oct 16 [cited 2012 Aug 15];Available from: http://www.ncbi.nlm.nih.gov/pubmed/17531333, 81(4), 236-49.

[4] Gaudart, J, Poudiougou, B, Dicko, A, Ranque, S, Toure, O, Sagara, I, et al. Space-time clustering of childhood malaria at the household level: a dynamic cohort in a Mali

village. BMC Public Health [Internet]. (2006). Jan [cited 2012 Nov 7];6:286. Available from: http://www.pubmedcentral.nih.gov/articlerender.fcgi?artid=1684261&tool=pmcentrez&rendertype=abstract

[5] Duczmal, L. H, Moreira, G. J, Burgarelli, D, Takahashi, R. H, Magalhães, F. C, & Bodevan, E. C. Voronoi distance based prospective space-time scans for point data sets: a dengue fever cluster analysis in a southeast Brazilian town. International Journal of Health Geographics [Internet]. (2011). Jan [cited 2012 Nov 14];10:29. Available from: http://www.pubmedcentral.nih.gov/articlerender.fcgi?artid=3118312&tool=pmcentrez&rendertype=abstract

[6] Meliker, J. R, & Jacquez, G. M. Space-time clustering of case-control data with residential histories: insights into empirical induction periods, age-specific susceptibility, and calendar year-specific effects. Stochastic Environmental Research and Risk Assessment [Internet]. (2007). Aug [cited 2012 Nov 14];Available from: http://www.pubmedcentral.nih.gov/articlerender.fcgi?artid=2430065&tool=pmcentrez&rendertype=abstract, 21(5), 625-34.

[7] Schmiedel, S, Blettner, M, Kaatsch, P, & Schüz, J. Spatial clustering and space-time clusters of leukemia among children in Germany, 1987-2007. European Journal of Epidemiology [Internet]. (2010). Sep [cited 2012 Aug 15];Available from: http://www.ncbi.nlm.nih.gov/pubmed/20623321, 25(9), 627-33.

[8] Rose, G. Sick individuals and sick populations. International Journal of Epidemiology [Internet]. (1985). Mar [cited 2012 Aug 23];Available from: http://www.ncbi.nlm.nih.gov/pubmed/3872850, 14(1), 32-8.

[9] Lawson, A. B. Statistical Methods in Spatial Epidemiology. Wiley, editor. West Sussexs; (2001). , 277.

[10] Zatsepin, I, Verger, P, Robert-gnansia, E, Gagnière, B, Tirmarche, M, Khmel, R, et al. Down syndrome time-clustering in January 1987 in Belarus: link with the Chernobyl accident? Reproductive toxicology (Elmsford, N.Y.) [Internet]. (2007). cited 2012 Aug 15];24(3-4):289-95. Available from: http://www.ncbi.nlm.nih.gov/pubmed/17706919

[11] Lee, S. S, & Wong, N. S. The clustering and transmission dynamics of pandemic influenza A (H1N1) 2009 cases in Hong Kong. The Journal of Infection [Internet]. (2011). Oct [cited 2012 Aug 23];Available from: http://www.ncbi.nlm.nih.gov/pubmed/21601284, 63(4), 274-80.

[12] Smith, M. Considerations on a possible viral etiology for B-precursor acute lymphoblastic leukemia of childhood. Journal of Immunotherapy [Internet]. (1997). Mar [cited 2012 Aug 15];Available from: http://www.ncbi.nlm.nih.gov/pubmed/9087381, 20(2), 89-100.

[13] McNally RJQBithell JF, Vincent TJ, Murphy MFG. Space-time clustering of childhood cancer around the residence at birth. International Journal of Cancer [Internet].

(2009). Jan 15 [cited 2012 Aug 15];Available from: http://www.ncbi.nlm.nih.gov/pubmed/18844236, 124(2), 449-55.

[14] Albert, D. P, Gesler, W. M, & Levergood, B. Spatial Analysis, GIS, and Remote Sensing Applications in the Health Sciences. Chelsea, Michigan: Ann Arbor Press; (2000). , 221.

[15] Tango, T. Statistical Methods for Disease Clustering. 1st ed. New Yory: Springer; (2010). , 248.

[16] Porta, M. A Dictionary of Epidemiology. 5th ed. Porta M, editor. Oxford University Press; (2008). , 320.

[17] Birch, J. M, Alexander, F. E, Blair, V, Eden, O. B, Taylor, G. M, & Mcnally, R. J. Space-time clustering patterns in childhood leukaemia support a role for infection. British Journal of Cancer [Internet]. (2000). May;Available from: http://www.pubmedcentral.nih.gov/articlerender.fcgi?artid=2363399&tool=pmcentrez&rendertype=abstract, 82(9), 1571-6.

[18] Boutou, O, Guizard, A-V, Slama, R, Pottier, D, & Spira, A. Population mixing and leukaemia in young people around the La Hague nuclear waste reprocessing plant. British Journal of Cancer [Internet]. (2002). Sep 23 [cited 2012 Aug 15];Available from: http://www.pubmedcentral.nih.gov/articlerender.fcgi?artid=2364264&tool=pmcentrez&rendertype=abstract, 87(7), 740-5.

[19] Glass, A. G, & Mantel, N. Lack of time-space clustering of childhood leukemia in Los Angeles County, 1960-1964. Cancer Research [Internet]. (1969). Available from: http://www.ncbi.nlm.nih.gov/pubmed/5358216, 29(11), 1995-2001.

[20] Bellec, S, Hémon, D, Rudant, J, Goubin, A, & Clavel, J. Spatial and space-time clustering of childhood acute leukaemia in France from 1990 to 2000: a nationwide study. British Journal of Cancer [Internet]. (2006). Mar 13 [cited 2012 Aug 15];Available from: http://www.pubmedcentral.nih.gov/articlerender.fcgi?artid=2374236&tool=pmcentrez&rendertype=abstract, 94(5), 763-70.

[21] McNally RJQAlexander FE, Birch JM. Space-time clustering analyses of childhood acute lymphoblastic leukaemia by immunophenotype. British Journal of Cancer [Internet]. (2002). Aug 27 [cited 2012 Aug 15];Available from: http://www.pubmedcentral.nih.gov/articlerender.fcgi?artid=2376144&tool=pmcentrez&rendertype=abstract, 87(5), 513-5.

[22] Wiemels, J. Perspectives on the causes of childhood leukemia. Chemico-Biological Interactions [Internet]. (2012). Apr 5 [cited 2012 Oct 22];Available from: http://www.ncbi.nlm.nih.gov/pubmed/22326931, 196(3), 59-67.

[23] Amin, R, Bohnert, A, Holmes, L, Rajasekaran, A, & Assanasen, C. Epidemiologic mapping of Florida childhood cancer clusters. Pediatric Blood & Cancer [Internet]. (2010). Available from: http://www.ncbi.nlm.nih.gov/pubmed/20054842, 54(4), 511-8.

[24] Alexander, F. E, Chan, L. C, Lam, T. H, Yuen, P, Leung, N. K, Ha, S. Y, et al. Clustering of childhood leukaemia in Hong Kong: association with the childhood peak and common acute lymphoblastic leukaemia and with population mixing. British Journal of Cancer [Internet]. (1997). Jan;Available from: http://www.pubmedcentral.nih.gov/articlerender.fcgi?artid=2063384&tool=pmcentrez&rendertype=abstract, 75(3), 457-63.

[25] Ward, G. The infective theory of acute leukemia. British Journal of Childhood's Disease. (1917). , 14, 10-20.

[26] McNally RJQAlston RD, Eden TOB, Kelsey AM, Birch JM. Further clues concerning the aetiology of childhood central nervous system tumours. European Journal of Cancer [Internet]. (2004). Dec [cited 2012 Aug 15];Available from: http://www.ncbi.nlm.nih.gov/pubmed/15571959, 40(18), 2766-72.

[27] Demoury, C, Goujon-bellec, S, Guyot-goubin, A, Hémon, D, & Clavel, J. Spatial variations of childhood acute leukaemia in France, 1990-2006: global spatial heterogeneity and cluster detection at "living-zone" level. European Journal of Cancer Prevention [Internet]. (2012). Jul [cited 2012 Oct 26];Available from: http://www.ncbi.nlm.nih.gov/pubmed/22108445, 21(4), 367-74.

[28] Gilman, E. A. McNally RJQ, Cartwright RA. Space-time clustering of Hodgkin's Disease in parts of the UK, Leukemia & Lymphoma [Internet]. (1999). Available from: http://www.ncbi.nlm.nih.gov/pubmed/10613453, 1984-1993.

[29] Gustafsson, B, & Carstensen, J. Evidence of space-time clustering of childhood acute lymphoblastic leukaemia in Sweden. British Journal of Cancer [Internet]. (1999). Feb; 79(3-4):655-7. Available from: http://www.pubmedcentral.nih.gov/articlerender.fcgi?artid=2362409&tool=pmcentrez&rendertype=abstract

[30] Gustafsson, B, & Carstensen, J. Space-time clustering of childhood lymphatic leukaemias and non-Hodgkin's lymphomas in Sweden. European Journal of Epidemiology [Internet]. (2000). Jan [cited 2012 Oct 25];Available from: http://www.ncbi.nlm.nih.gov/pubmed/11484799, 16(12), 1111-6.

[31] Kaatsch, P, & Mergenthaler, A. Incidence, time trends and regional variation of childhood leukaemia in Germany and Europe. Radiation Protection Dosimetry [Internet]. (2008). Jan [cited 2012 Aug 15];Available from: http://www.ncbi.nlm.nih.gov/pubmed/18996968, 132(2), 107-13.

[32] Kulkarni, K, Stobart, K, Witol, A, & Rosychuk, R. J. Leukemia and lymphoma incidence in children in Alberta, Canada: a population-based 22-year retrospective study. Pediatric Hematology and Oncology [Internet]. (2011). Nov [cited 2012 Oct 26];Available from: http://www.ncbi.nlm.nih.gov/pubmed/21981741, 28(8), 649-60.

[33] McNally RJQEden TOB, Alexander FE, Kelsey AM, Birch JM. Is there a common aetiology for certain childhood malignancies? Results of cross-space-time clustering analyses. European Journal of Cancer [Internet]. (2005). Dec [cited 2012 Oct 25];Available from: http://www.ncbi.nlm.nih.gov/pubmed/16243517, 41(18), 2911-6.

[34] Alexander, F. E, Boyle, P, Carli, P. M, Coebergh, J. W, Draper, G. J, Ekbom, A, et al. Spatial temporal patterns in childhood leukaemia: further evidence for an infectious origin. EUROCLUS project. British Journal of Cancer [Internet]. (1998). Mar;Available from: http://www.pubmedcentral.nih.gov/articlerender.fcgi?artid=2149966&tool=pmcentrez&rendertype=abstract, 77(5), 812-7.

[35] Alexander, F. E, Boyle, P, Carli, P. M, Coebergh, J. W, Draper, G. J, Ekbom, A, et al. Spatial clustering of childhood leukaemia: summary results from the EUROCLUS project. British Journal of Cancer [Internet]. (1998). Mar;Available from: http://www.pubmedcentral.nih.gov/articlerender.fcgi?artid=2149947&tool=pmcentrez&rendertype=abstract, 77(5), 818-24.

[36] Francis, S. S, Selvin, S, Yang, W, Buffler, P a, & Wiemels, J. L. Unusual space-time patterning of the Fallon, Nevada leukemia cluster: Evidence of an infectious etiology. Chemico-Biological Interactions [Internet]. Elsevier Ireland Ltd; (2012). Apr 5 [cited 2012 Aug 15];Available from: http://www.ncbi.nlm.nih.gov/pubmed/21352818, 196(3), 102-9.

[37] McNally RJQAlexander FE, Bithell JF. Space-time clustering of childhood cancer in great Britain: a national study, 1969-1993. International Journal of Cancer [Internet]. (2006). Jun 1 [cited 2012 Aug 15];Available from: http://www.ncbi.nlm.nih.gov/pubmed/16381003, 118(11), 2840-6.

[38] Petridou, E, Alexander, F. E, Trichopoulos, D, Revinthi, K, Dessypris, N, Wray, N, et al. Aggregation of childhood leukemia in geographic areas of Greece. Cancer Causes & Control [Internet]. (1997). Mar;Available from: http://www.ncbi.nlm.nih.gov/pubmed/9134248, 8(2), 239-45.

[39] Staines, a, Bodansky, H. J, Mckinney, P a, Alexander, F. E, Mcnally, R. J, Law, G. R, et al. Small area variation in the incidence of childhood insulin-dependent diabetes mellitus in Yorkshire, UK: links with overcrowding and population density. International Journal of Epidemiology [Internet]. (1997). Dec;Available from: http://www.ncbi.nlm.nih.gov/pubmed/9447411, 26(6), 1307-13.

[40] MacMahon BIs acute lymphoblastic leukemia in children virus-related? American Journal of Epidemiology [Internet]. (1992). Oct 15;Available from: http://www.ncbi.nlm.nih.gov/pubmed/1456268, 136(8), 916-24.

[41] Zur Hausen HChildhood leukemias and other hematopoietic malignancies: interdependence between an infectious event and chromosomal modifications. International Journal of Cancer [Internet]. (2009). Oct 15 [cited 2012 Aug 15];Available from: http://www.ncbi.nlm.nih.gov/pubmed/19330827, 125(8), 1764-70.

[42] McNally RJQLecture for master's Newcastle university. Newcastle; (2012)., 96.

[43] Law, G. R. Host, family and community proxies for infections potentially associated with leukaemia. Radiation Protection Dosimetry [Internet]. (2008). Jan [cited 2012

Aug 15];Available from: http://www.ncbi.nlm.nih.gov/pubmed/18945723, 132(2), 267-72.

[44] Mulder, Y. M, Drijver, M, & Kreis, I a. Case-control study on the association between a cluster of childhood haematopoietic malignancies and local environmental factors in Aalsmeer, The Netherlands. Journal of Epidemiology and Community Health [Internet]. (1994). Apr;Available from: http://www.pubmedcentral.nih.gov/articlerender.fcgi?artid=1059926&tool=pmcentrez&rendertype=abstract, 48(2), 161-5.

[45] Petridou, E, Revinthi, K, Alexander, F. E, Haidas, S, Koliouskas, D, Kosmidis, H, et al. Space-time clustering of childhood leukaemia in Greece: evidence supporting a viral aetiology. British Journal of Cancer [Internet]. (1996). May;Available from: http://www.pubmedcentral.nih.gov/articlerender.fcgi?artid=2074508&tool=pmcentrez&rendertype=abstract, 73(10), 1278-83.

[46] Gilman, E. A, & Knox, E. G. Childhood cancers: space-time distribution in Britain. Journal of Epidemiology and Community Health [Internet]. (1995). Apr [cited 2012 Aug 15];Available from: http://www.pubmedcentral.nih.gov/articlerender.fcgi?artid=1060101&tool=pmcentrez&rendertype=abstract, 49(2), 158-63.

[47] Alexander, F. E. Space-time clustering of childhood acute lymphoblastic leukaemia: indirect evidence for a transmissible agent. British Journal of Cancer [Internet]. (1992). Apr;Available from: http://www.pubmedcentral.nih.gov/articlerender.fcgi?artid=1977570&tool=pmcentrez&rendertype=abstract, 65(4), 589-92.

[48] Dockerty, J. D, Sharples, K. J, & Borman, B. An assessment of spatial clustering of leukaemias and lymphomas among young people in New Zealand. Journal of Epidemiology and Community Health [Internet]. (1999). Mar;Available from: http://www.pubmedcentral.nih.gov/articlerender.fcgi?artid=1756850&tool=pmcentrez&rendertype=abstract, 53(3), 154-8.

[49] Alexander, F, Cartwright, R, Mckinney, P a, & Ricketts, T. J. Investigation of spacial clustering of rare diseases: childhood malignancies in North Humberside. Journal of Epidemiology and Community Health [Internet]. (1990). Mar;Available from: http://www.pubmedcentral.nih.gov/articlerender.fcgi?artid=1060595&tool=pmcentrez&rendertype=abstract, 44(1), 39-46.

[50] Klauber, M. R, & Mustacchi, P. Space-Time Clustering of Childhood Leukemia in San Francisco Space-Time Clustering of Childhood Leukemia in San Francisco. Cancer Research. (1970). , 30, 1969-73.

[51] Wartenberg, D, Schneider, D, & Brown, S. Childhood leukaemia incidence and the population mixing hypothesis in US SEER data. British Journal of Cancer [Internet]. (2004). May 4 [cited 2012 Nov 15];Available from: http://www.pubmedcentral.nih.gov/articlerender.fcgi?artid=2409734&tool=pmcentrez&rendertype=abstract, 90(9), 1771-6.

[52] Knox, E. G, & Gilman, E. Leukaemia clusters in Great Britain. 1. Space-time interactions. Journal of Epidemiology and Community Health [Internet]. (1992). Dec;Availa-

ble from: http://www.pubmedcentral.nih.gov/articlerender.fcgi?artid=1059670&tool=pmcentrez&rendertype=abstract, 46(6), 566-72.

[53] Sans, S, Elliott, P, Kleinschmidt, I, Shaddick, G, Pattenden, S, Walls, P, et al. Cancer incidence and mortality near the Baglan Bay petrochemical works, South Wales. Occupational and Environmental Medicine [Internet]. (1995). Apr;Available from: http://www.pubmedcentral.nih.gov/articlerender.fcgi?artid=1128198&tool=pmcentrez&rendertype=abstract, 52(4), 217-24.

[54] Lehtinen, M. Maternal Herpesvirus Infections and Risk of Acute Lymphoblastic Leukemia in the Offspring. American Journal of Epidemiology [Internet]. (2003). Aug 1 [cited 2012 Aug 15];Available from: http://aje.oxfordjournals.org/cgi/content/abstract/158/3/207, 158(3), 207-13.

[55] Bogdanovic, G, Jernberg, A. G, Priftakis, P, Grillner, L, & Gustafsson, B. Human herpes virus 6 or Epstein-Barr virus were not detected in Guthrie cards from children who later developed leukaemia. British Journal of Cancer [Internet]. (2004). Aug 31 [cited 2012 Aug 15];Available from: http://www.pubmedcentral.nih.gov/articlerender.fcgi?artid=2409878&tool=pmcentrez&rendertype=abstract, 91(5), 913-5.

[56] Roman, E, Simpson, J, Ansell, P, Kinsey, S, Mitchell, C. D, Mckinney, P. A, et al. Childhood acute lymphoblastic leukemia and infections in the first year of life: a report from the United Kingdom Childhood Cancer Study. American Journal of Epidemiology [Internet]. (2007). Mar 1 [cited 2012 Aug 15];Available from: http://www.ncbi.nlm.nih.gov/pubmed/17182983, 165(5), 496-504.

[57] Gilham, C, Peto, J, Simpson, J, & Roman, E. Eden TOB, Greaves MF, et al. Day care in infancy and risk of childhood acute lymphoblastic leukaemia: findings from UK case-control study. BMJ (Clinical research ed.) [Internet]. (2005). Jun 4 [cited 2012 Aug 15];330(7503):1294. Available from: http://www.pubmedcentral.nih.gov/articlerender.fcgi?artid=558199&tool=pmcentrez&rendertype=abstract

[58] Knox, E. G. Leukaemia clusters in childhood: geographical analysis in Britain. Journal of Epidemiology and Community Health [Internet]. (1994). Aug;Available from: http://www.pubmedcentral.nih.gov/articlerender.fcgi?artid=1059986&tool=pmcentrez&rendertype=abstract, 48(4), 369-76.

[59] Williams EH (Kuluva HSmith PG (DHSS CE and CTU, Day NE (WHO IA for R on C, Geser A (East AVRI, Ellice J, Tukei P. Space-time clustering of Burkitt's Lymphoma in the West Nile District of Uganda: 1961-1975. British Journal of Cancer. (1978)., 37, 109-22.

[60] Smith, P. G. Case-control studies of leukaemia clusters. BMJ (Clinical research ed.) [Internet]. (1991). Mar 23 [cited 2012 Aug 15];Available from: http://www.pubmedcentral.nih.gov/articlerender.fcgi?artid=1669108&tool=pmcentrez&rendertype=abstract, 302(6778), 672-3.

[61] Morris, V. Space-time interactions in childhood cancers. Journal of Epidemiology and Community Health [Internet]. (1990). Mar;Available from: http://www.pubmedcen-

tral.nih.gov/articlerender.fcgi?artid=1060598&tool=pmcentrez&rendertype=abstract, 44(1), 55-8.

[62] Wheeler, D. C. A comparison of spatial clustering and cluster detection techniques for childhood leukemia incidence in Ohio, International Journal of Health Geographics [Internet]. (2007). Jan [cited 2012 Aug 15];6(13). Available from: http://www.pubmedcentral.nih.gov/articlerender.fcgi?artid=1851703&tool=pmcentrez&rendertype=abstract, 1996-2003.

[63] Bithell, J. F, Dutton, S. J, Draper, G. J, & Neary, N. M. Distribution of childhood leukaemias and non-Hodgkin's lymphomas near nuclear installations in England and Wales. BMJ (Clinical research ed.) [Internet]. (1994). cited 2012 Aug 15];Available from: http://www.pubmedcentral.nih.gov/articlerender.fcgi?artid=2542713&tool=pmcentrez&rendertype=abstract, 309(6953), 501-5.

[64] Pérez-saldivar, M. L, Fajardo-gutiérrez, A, Bernáldez-ríos, R, Martínez-avalos, A, Medina-sanson, A, Espinosa-hernández, L, et al. Childhood acute leukemias are frequent in Mexico City: descriptive epidemiology. BMC Cancer [Internet]. (2011). Jan [cited 2012 Aug 16];11:355. Available from: http://www.pubmedcentral.nih.gov/articlerender.fcgi?artid=3171387&tool=pmcentrez&rendertype=abstract

[65] Fajardo-gutiérrez, A, Sandoval-mex, A. M, Mejía-aranguré, J. M, & Rendón-macías, M. E. Martínez-García M del C. Clinical and social factors that affect the time to diagnosis of Mexican children with cancer. Medical and Pediatric Oncology [Internet]. (2002). Jul [cited 2012 Jul 16];Available from: http://www.ncbi.nlm.nih.gov/pubmed/12116075, 39(1), 25-31.

[66] Mejía-aranguré, J. M, Fajardo-gutiérrez, A, Bernáldez-ríos, R, Paredes-aguilera, R, Flores-aguilar, H, & Martínez-garcía, M. C. Incidencia de las leucemias agudas en niños de la ciudad de México, de 1982 a 1991. Salud Pública de México [Internet]. (2000). cited 2012 Aug 16];Available from: http://www.ncbi.nlm.nih.gov/pubmed/11125628, 42(5), 431-7.

[67] Duarte Rodríguez DAConglomerados espaciales de niños con leucemia aguda infantil en la Ciudad de México. Universidad Nacional Autónoma de México; (2012). , 104.

[68] Kulldorff, M, & Nagarwalla, N. Spatial disease clusters: detection and inference. Statistics in Medicine [Internet]. (1995). Apr 30 [cited 2012 Aug 23];Available from: http://www.ncbi.nlm.nih.gov/pubmed/7644860, 14(8), 799-810.

[69] Hjalmars, U, Kulldorff, M, Gustafsson, G, & Nagarwalla, N. Childhood leukaemia in Sweden: using GIS and a spatial scan statistic for cluster detection. Statistics in Medicine [Internet]. (1996). Available from: http://www.ncbi.nlm.nih.gov/pubmed/9132898

[70] Goujon-bellec, S, Demoury, C, Guyot-goubin, A, Hémon, D, & Clavel, J. Detection of clusters of a rare disease over a large territory: performance of cluster detection methods. International Journal of Health Geographics [Internet]. (2011). Jan;10:53.

Available from: http://www.pubmedcentral.nih.gov/articlerender.fcgi?artid=3204219&tool=pmcentrez&rendertype=abstract

[71] Knox, E. G, & Gilman, E a. Hazard proximities of childhood cancers in Great Britain from 1953-80. Journal of Epidemiology and Community Health [Internet]. (1997). Apr;Available from: http://www.pubmedcentral.nih.gov/articlerender.fcgi?artid=1060437&tool=pmcentrez&rendertype=abstract, 51(2), 151-9.

[72] Dirección General de Investigaciones sobre la Contaminación Urbana Regional y Globall/Instituto Nacional de Ecología/Secretaría del Medio Ambiente del Gobierno del Distrito FederalMovilidad en la ciudad, transporte y calidad de vida [Internet]. Mexico City: Instituto Nacional de Ecología; (2005). cited 2012 Nov 15]. Available from: http://www.ine.gob.mx/descargas/calaire/folleto_mov_urbana.pdf, 20.

[73] EMBARQMexico City, Mexico [Internet]. [cited (2011). Nov 22]. Available from: http://www.embarq.org/en/city/mexico-city-mexico

[74] INEGICensos económicos (2009). Ciudad de México: INEGI; 2009.

[75] Programa de las Naciones Unidas para el Desarrollo MéxicoÍndice de Desarrollo Humano Municipal en México 2005 [Internet]. Programa de las Naciones Unidas para el Desarrollo. (2005). cited 2010 Nov 9]. Available from: http://www.undp.org.mx/spip.php?

[76] INEGIII Conteo de Población y Vivienda 2005. Ciudad de México: INEGI; (2005).

Chapter 7

Sociodemographic and Birth Characteristics in Infant Acute Leukemia: A Review

ML Pérez-Saldivar, JM Mejía-Aranguré,
A Rangel-López and A Fajardo Gutiérrez

Additional information is available at the end of the chapter

http://dx.doi.org/10.5772/54457

1. Introduction

Acute leukemias are cancers of the hematopoietic system that involve, in the majority of cases, a malignant transformation of myeloid and lymphoid progenitor cells [1]. Acute leukemias represent the most common type of childhood cancer [2,3]. Acute lymphoblastic leukemia (ALL) has a frequency of five times greater than that of acute myeloblastic leukemia (AML) and is the most common cancer in children, representing 25% to 35% of all childhood cancers [3,4]. The incidence of ALL varies significantly among developed and developing countries. With a reported annual incidence of 20-45 cases per million children, the highest incidence rates are recorded in the Hispanic population in California, Texas and Florida and in Costa Rica and the City of Mexico [4-7]. Despite advances in therapy and improvements in survival, acute leukemia represents one of the main causes of morbidity and mortality in children. The etiology of this disease remains unknown. Only Down syndrome and ionizing radiation have been recognized as risk factors for the development of childhood acute leukemia [8]. However, the risk attributable to these factors is very small. Epidemiological studies exploring different environmental exposures along with advances in cytogenetics and immunophenotyping have identified different subgroups of the disease that must be considered separately. Such is the case of infantile leukemia. Although it is a rare disease in this group, the molecular characteristics and survival are different in infants than in older children, suggesting that the etiology is distinct and most likely involves prenatal factors. The purpose of this chapter is to introduce the reader to a systematic review of the current literature on reported risk factors for childhood acute leukemia (AL). This review reports what is currently known about acute leukemia in infants and future directions.

2. Descriptive epidemiology

Leukemia in infants (<1 year) is an extremely rare disease, and few studies exist that explore the incidence of leukemia in this age group. Parkin et al., reporting incidence rates for this age group in different regions of the world, determined that Mexico recorded the highest incidence rate in children <1 year for the study period, exceeding the rates of the United States, some countries in Latin America, Europe, Asia and Oceania [5]. However, United States, Great Britain, and Australia have some of the highest incidence rates for infantile ALL, with approximately 20-40 cases per million children, whereas countries like Brazil and Cuba have reported rates of approximately 8-12 cases per million children. The Hispanic population of infants in Los Angeles, Japan and Australia has been reported to have the highest AML incidence rates of approximately 10-12 cases per million children. As with ALL, Brazil and Cuba have some of the lowest incidence rates, with approximately 3-5 cases per million children [6].

Descriptive epidemiological studies conducted in Mexico City on acute leukemia and childhood cancer have consistently identified a significant incidence for AL in the infant population. In the 1980-1992 study period, in newborns population ALL occupied the third place as the main type of cancer and the second place in the infant population and after 2 years of age, a very important peak in AL development is observed [9]. For the period 1996-2002, the incidence of AL in infants was 37.5 per 10^6 children [10,11], and between 1996 and 2006 another study reported an incidence of 33.0 ALL cases per 10^6 children < 1 year of age [12]. The most recent survey of childhood AL in 2006-2007 in Mexico City reported an incidence rate of ALL and AML of 24.3 and 4.1 per 10^6 infants, respectively [7].

Epidemiological studies in infants are rare. However, there is a predominance of females in infants with ALL, whereas in children older than 1 year, male are more frequently diagnosed [13]. Because of the young age of presentation of infantile leukemia, studies are focused specifically on pre-conception exposures during pregnancy as potentially relevant exposures that occur *in utero* or shortly before pregnancy. That is, the window of study for the disease in this cohort is very short – approximately 9 months. Therefore, the study of this group can provide essential information not only for this group but also for the development of childhood AL [14,15]. The epidemiological studies have evaluated maternal exposure during pregnancy to different risk factors that could be associated with the development of leukemia in infants. These studies are presented in table 1 and include the publication of epidemiological studies in the last 12 years in the infant population and its association with AL. Although the studies are interesting and provide important information, some studies have failed to find significant associations because they have some methodological limitations, such as sample size (small number of exposed individuals among subgroups) or incomplete and biased exposure assessment (not validated). In some cases they have a low response rates between cases and controls. It is important to consider these aspects for future association studies. Despite these limitations, these studies provide an important contribution to the limited amount of existing studies linking infants with AL and risk factors.

Variables studied	Study design	Cases analyzed	OR (95% CI)	Conclusions	Author and year
Maternal exposure to household chemicals	Case-control	264 ALL 172 AML 7 Other	Petroleum products Any ALL OR 1.56 (0.90-2.70); AML OR 2.33 (1.30-4.18); MLL+ OR 1.38 (0.77-2.48) Month before pregnancy ALL OR 1.31 (0.71-2.41); AML OR 1.42 (0.71-2.83); MLL+ OR 1.14 (0.58-2.21) During pregnancy ALL OR 1.60 (0.90-2.83); AML OR 2.54 (1.40-4.62); MLL- 2.69 (1.47-4.93)	Gestational exposure to petroleum products was associated with infant leukemia, particularly AML and MLL-.	Slater et al., 2011[23]
Analgesic use during pregnancy	Case-control	262 ALL 172 AML	Before knowledge pregnancy Any use Aspirin ALL OR 1.03 (0.58-1.85) AML OR 0.55 (0.24-1.26) Non-aspirin non-steroidal anti-inflammatory drugs (NSAID) ALL OR 1.15 (0.80-1.67) AML OR 0.60 (0.37-0.97) Acetaminophen ALL OR 1.16 (0.80-1.68) AML OR 0.66 (0.43-1.01) After knowledge pregnancy Any use Aspirin ALL OR 1.21 (0.48-3.05) AML OR 0.96 (0.32-2.92) NSAID ALL OR 1.33 (0.75-2.37) AML OR 0.81 (0.36-1.83) Acetaminophen ALL OR 1.03 (0.70-1.53) AML OR 0.79 (0.50-1.24)	Analgesic use during pregnancy was not significantly associated with the risk of infant leukemia.	Ognjanovic et al., 2011[24]
Maternal prenatal cigarette, alcohol and illicit drug use	Case-control	264 ALL 172 AML 7 Other	During pregnancy Cigarette use OR 0.80 (0.52-1.24) ALL OR 0.87 (0.54-1.40)	Cigarette smoking was not associated with childhood leukemia; alcohol and illicit drug use were not consistent with prior reports.	Slater et al., 2011[25]

Variables studied	Study design	Cases analyzed	OR (95% CI)	Conclusions	Author and year
			AML OR 0.74 (0.40-1.35)		
			Alcohol use		
			OR 0.64 (0.43-0.94)		
			ALL OR 0.64 (0.43-0.94)		
			Illicit drug use		
			OR 0.69 (0.40-1.18)		
			ALL OR 0.84 (0.47-1.51)		
			AML OR 0.52 (0.23-1.16)		
Maternal vitamin and iron supplementation	Case-control	264 ALL 172 AML	Prenatal	The authors did not observe a prenatal vitamin-infant leukemia association.	Linabery et al., 2010 [26]
			Vitamins		
			OR 0.79 (0.44-1.42)		
			ALL OR 0.63 (0.34-1.18)		
			AML OR 1.20 (0.53-2.75)		
			Iron supplements		
			OR 1.07 (0.75-1.52)		
			ALL OR 1.22 (0.82-1.80)		
			AML OR 0.82 (0.51-1.33)		
			Periconceptional		
			Vitamins		
			OR 0.89 (0.64-1.24)		
			ALL OR 0.77 (0.54-1.11)		
			AML OR 1.05 (0.68-1.61)		
			Iron supplements		
			OR 1.23 (0.63-2.38)		
			ALL OR 1.30 (0.62-2.72)		
Continued...			AML OR 0.77 (0.46-1.27)		
			During pregnancy		
			Vitamins		
			OR 0.78 (0.48-1.28)		
			ALL OR 0.66 (0.39-1.11)		
			AML OR 1.05 (0.55-2.04)		
			Iron supplements		
			OR 1.06 (0.74-1.53)		

Variables studied	Study design	Cases analyzed	OR (95% CI)	Conclusions	Author and year
			ALL OR 1.22 (0.81-1.84) AML OR 0.77 (0.46-1.27)		
Congenital abnormalities	Case-control	264 ALL 172 AML 7 Other	Congenital abnormality (CA) OR 1.2 (0.8-1.9) Birthmarks OR 1.3 (0.7-2.4) Urogenital abnormalities OR 0.7 (0.2-2.0) Other CA OR 1.4 (0.7-2.8)	The authors did not find evidence for a link between CAs and infant leukemia	Johnson et al., 2010 [27]
Parental infertility and infertility treatment	Case-control	264ALL 172 AML	Women not trying to conceive OR 1.62 (1.01-2.59) ALL OR 2.50 (1.36-4.61) AML OR 1.17 (0.61-2.22) Women with ≥1 year of trying OR 0.99 (0.47-2.07) ALL OR 2.01 (0.85-4.78) AML 0.35 (0.09-1.27)	There were no positive associations between parental infertility or infertility treatment and infant leukemia.	Puumala et al., 2010 [28]
Dipyrone	Case-control	132 Acute leukemia	N-Acetyltransferase 2 (NAT2) dipyrone during pregnancy OR 5.19 (1.86-14.5)	NAT2 slow-acetylation profiles associated with infant leukemia &dipyrone	Zanrosso et al., 2010 [29]
Birth weight	Case-control	148 ALL 53 AML	Birth weight >3999 g OR 1.59 (0.79-3.17) ALL OR 2.28 (1.08-4.75) MLL+ OR 2.68 (0.99-7.15)	The results suggest that high birth weight is associated with an increased risk of infant leukemia.	Koifman et al., 2008 [30]
Birth characteristics and maternal reproductive history	Case-control	149 ALL 91 AML	Birth weight ≥4,000 g OR 1.09 (0.67-1.79) Gestational age <37 weeks OR 0.74 (0.32-1.70) Birth order 2nd OR 0.60 (0.40-0.91) Maternal age ≥35 years OR 0.75 (0.46-1.23)	Maternal history of fetal loss and other birth characteristics were not related to infant leukemia.	Spector et al., 2007 [31]

Variables studied	Study design	Cases analyzed	OR (95% CI)	Conclusions	Author and year
			Prior fetal loss Any OR 1.04 (0.70-1.55) Pre-pregnancy BMI 25-29.9 OR 1.61 (1.04-2.48) Weight gain during pregnancy (kg)>18.14 OR 1.50 (0.84-2.68)		
Maternal anemia	Case-control	178 Acute leukemia	Anemia during pregnancy (<11 g dl^{-1}) OR 0.93 (0.57-1.53) ALL OR 1.14 (0.65-2.01) AML OR 0.67 (0.32-1.37) ALL/MLL+ OR 0.98 (0.50-1.91) AML/MLL- OR 0.57 (0.16-2.07)	The authors did not find evidence for an increased risk of leukemia in the offspring of mothers with hemoglobin <11 g dl^{-1} during pregnancy.	Peters et al., 2006 [32]
Maternal illicit drugs, pain medication, vitamins/iron supplement, folic acid, hormones, abortive drugs, herbal infusions, pesticides during pregnancy	Case-control	202 Acute leukemia	TobaccoORa 0.89 (0.63-1.25) MarijuanaORa 0.87 (0.63-1.20) DipyroneORa 1.45 (1.02-2.06) Amoxicillin ORa 0.88 (0.63-1.25) Folic acid ORa 1.22 (0.73-2.05) MetronidazoleORa 1.39 (0.82-2.34), MisoprostolORa 1.23 (0.38-4.02) Hormones ORa 8.76 (2.85-26.93) Herbal infusions ORa 1.93 (0.49-7.58) Pesticides ORa 2.18 (1.53-2.13) Hormones intake: Preconception OR 2.26 (1.21-4.21); MLL+ OR 3.34 (1.51-7.36) 1st trimester OR 11.35 (3.20-40.20); MLL+ OR 10.57 (2.33-47.91) 2nd trimester OR 4.49 (1.07-18.87); MLL + OR 2.62 (0.15-17.56) 3rd trimester OR 2.32 (0.60-8.98); MLL+ 1.02 (0.10-9.93)	A statistically significant association between the maternal use of hormones during pregnancy and infant leukemia.	Pombo-de Oliveira et al., 2006 [33]
Maternal diet (DNA topoisomerase II	Case-control	149 ALL 91 AML	DNAt2 inhibitor with MLL+ Quartile 4 OR 0.7 (0.4-1.5)	Maternal consumption of vegetables and fruits were associated	Spector et al., 2005 [34]

Variables studied	Study design	Cases analyzed	OR (95% CI)	Conclusions	Author and year
inhibitor)			ALL OR 0.5 (0.2-1.1) AML OR 3.2 (0.9-11.9) Vegetable and fruits plus index Quartile 4 OR 0.6 (0.3-1.1) ALL OR 0.5 (0.2-0.9) AML OR 1.1 (0.4-2.9)	with a decreased risk of infant leukemia, particularly MLL+. DNAt2 inhibitors increase the risk of AML (MLL+).	
Maternal smoking, alcohol, DNA damaging drugs, herbal medicines, pesticides, Dipyrone, insecticides	Case-control	49 ALL (19 MLL+) 74 AML (29 MLL+) 13 Other (2 MLL+)	Smoking ALL OR 1.59 (0.82-3.07); AML OR 1.33 (0.63-2.80); MLL+ OR 0.98 (0.46-2.09) Alcohol ALL OR 0.63 (0.25-1.60); AML OR 1.92 (0.90-4.10); MLL+ OR 0.74 (0.29-1.90) DNA Damaging drugs ALL OR 1.78 (0.95-3.34); AML OR 2.28 (1.10-4.71); MLL+ OR 2.31 (1.06-5.06) Herbal medicines ALL OR 4.45 (2.06-9.63); AML OR 2.09 (0.89-4.92); MLL+ OR 3.00 (1.38-6.54) Maternal Pesticide ALL OR 2.53 (0.71-8.97); AML OR 5.08(1.84-14.04); MLL+ OR 4.96 (1.71-14.43) Dipyrone ALL OR 3.13 (1.02-9.57); AML OR 3.01 (0.93-9.79); MLL+ OR 5.84 (2.09-16.30) Insecticides ALL OR 4.30 (0.66-28.08); AML OR 7.82 (1.73-35.39); MLL+ OR 9.68 (2.11-44.40)	The data suggest that specific chemical exposures of the fetus during pregnancy may cause MLL gene fusions.	Alexander et al., 2001 [35]

Table 1. Risk factors for infant leukemia studied in the last 12 years.

3. Clinical characteristics

Infants with leukemia possess different molecular genetics features, immunophenotypes and cytogenetic characteristics with respect to older children. Infants with ALL have a very high leukocyte count (hyperleukocytosis); the median of leukocyte count in infants with ALL was recorded as 100 x 10^9 L. Infants with ALL also often exhibit hepatosplenomegaly, widened mediastinum, and compromise of the central nervous system (CNS) in approximately 15% of cases. In addition, 13% of male infants exhibit infiltrated testes [16,17]. The ratio ALL/AML in infants is approximately 1.5-2.0, and the M4 or M5 morphology predominates in infants diagnosed with AML [5,18,19].

A significant proportion of infants diagnosed with ALL are characterized by a very immature precursor B-lineage ALL – pro B CD-10. The mature B-lineage ALL is very rare and only 4% of cases are of T-lineage [13]. The leukemic cells of infants with ALL express myeloid antigens, which may indicate that this type of leukemia is generated in immature precursor cells that have no lymphoid differentiation [17]. Unlike older children diagnosed with ALL, with a 5-year survival rate of 80%, infants with leukemia have a very poor 5-year survival rate of 50% or less. The 5-year survival rate for infants with AML is 40%, similar to that reported in older children [20-22].

4. Genetic characteristics in infants

Both ALL and AML in infants are frequently associated with abnormalities (genetic rearrangements) involving the Mixed Lineage Leukemia (MLL) gene, also called Htrx, ALL-1 or HRX, which is located on chromosome 11 band q23 [36-38]. This gene is fused promiscuously with different pairs of chromosomes; up to 70 partners have been reported in human leukemia [39]. The most common fusion partners include chromosome 4, reported in 50% of cases; chromosome 11, with a frequency of 20%; and chromosome 9, present in 10% of cases. Fusions of chromosome 9 are presented in older infants, unlike fusions of chromosomes 4 or 11 [40,41]. The ENL chromosome has also been found fused with MLL, although at a lower frequency [38]. Infants with the MLL gene have a very poor prognosis compared with older children with the disease [13,42,43].

MLL translocations are present in 75-85% of ALL infants less than 1 year and in 60% of infant AML casesMLL translocations are found in older children and are reported in 5% of cases of childhood AL and 85% of leukemias secondary to treatment with topoisomerase II inhibitors, which are usually AMLs [37,42,44,45]. This last frequency is very important because it has implications for the etiology of leukemia in infants.

5. Structure of the MLL gene

The MLL gene is located on chromosome 11q23 just after the repressor domain. The MLL gene is 90 kb, consists of 38 exons, and produces a 12-kb mRNA that encodes a 430-kDa protein of 3969 amino acids in a complex structure. This protein is widely expressed in the developing embryo, where it functions as a regulator of nuclear transcription. In adult tissues, the protein is only minimally expressed [38,41,46,47].

The MLL protein is normally cleaved in the cytoplasm by caspasa 1 at amino acids 2666 (cleavable site 1 or CS1) and 2718 (cleavable site 2 or CS2), generating two subunits: the 300-kDa MLL-N and the 180-kDa MLL-C. MLL functions to acetylate, deacetylate and methylate the histones of nucleosomes [40,46]. The mature protein contains a 8.3-kb breakpoint cluster region between exons 5 and 11, and multiple protein domains have been identified: AT hooks, a DNA methyltransferase domain (transcriptional repression domain, TRD), a Plant homology domain (PHD), a transcription activator domain (TA) and Su (var) 3-9 enhancer of zest trithorax (SET) domain [38,47,48].

MLL gene alterations include deletions, duplications, inversions and reciprocal translocations. In reciprocal translocations, the fusion proteins are generated by interactions with the C-termini of other genes to replace the transcriptional repression and nuclear signaling domains located at the N-terminus of the MLL protein [49,50].

These fusion proteins have been postulated to be involved in leukemogenesis by increasing the expression of the HOXA9 gene during embryo development. The HOXA9 gene encodes a transcription factor, and the increased expression of this gene could represent a critical mechanism for MLL-related leukemia [46,49,51]. Another mechanism by which these fusion proteins promote leukemia is to increase the expression of FLT3 tyrosine kinase [41,52].

6. Prenatal origin

Numerous molecular biology studies have been conducted in twins with blood samples collected at birth from newborns (Guthrie cards) and with blood samples from the umbilical cord to detect inborn metabolic problems and other problems that could occur in newborns. Neonatal blood samples are stored, and thereafter the samples of a child with a diagnosis of leukemia are examined to understand the patient's genetic abnormalities at birth. These abnormalities are compared with those reported in the diagnosis of the patient. In a large proportion of neonatal blood samples, studies have concluded that the leukemia likely started *in utero* during fetal hematopoiesis, although this is not true for all chromosomal abnormalities [14,53,54].

Monozygotic and dizygotic twins have also been studied to determine the heritable fraction of childhood leukemia. More than 50% of twins share a placenta (monozygotic), which allows blood exchange. In these cases, it is likely that if one of the twins had a leukemic clone, it may have an intraplacentarian metastasis through which the clone could be transmitted to the other twin [37,53]. This hypothesis has been demonstrated through studies in twins with leukemia using translocation markers for unique genetic breakpoints, especially in TEL-AML1 and MLL rearrangements [14,53-55].

In twin infants with a diagnosis of leukemia, the concordance rate was approximately 100% among those twins who shared the placenta [53]. An explanation for this is that the MLL gene is sufficient to cause leukemia, which could happen if the protein has an overall effect on the structure of chromatin or on the stability of gene expression [37,56]. It is likely that the effect of the MLL gene in DNA repair or cell cycle regulation facilitates additional genetic changes caused by continuous exposure to genotoxic chemicals *in utero* [14]. However, some authors have noted that the MLL gene is not sufficient to generate leukemogenesis and that additional secondary genetic events are necessary in the development of the disease [57,58]. More so when it has reported the presence of this rearrangement in children over 1 year of age which raises the possibility that the relation of this rearrangement to the development of ALL is similar to that of the TEL-AML1 rearrangement; that is, it is an essential cause, but it is indispensable that another environmental factor be involved in order for children with this rearrangement (acquired at birth or not) to develop the disease [59].

Unlike infant leukemias, acute leukemias in older children exhibit a concordance rate between identical twins who share the same placenta of only 10%. This finding, together with transgenic models, indicates that post-natal events are necessary to produce sufficient genetic changes to develop leukemia. This finding explains why leukemia in infants is a different entity than that of older children, and attention must be paid to transplacental exposure *in utero* during embryonic development and fetal hematopoiesis [37,60].

7. Enzyme DNA topoisomerase II

The function of the enzyme DNA topoisomerase II (DNAt2) is to relax the DNA strands that are tightened and knotted during cell replication [61]. DNAt2 generates a break in the double strands of DNA that are then re-sealed, causing a relaxation of the DNA. Some drugs used in the treatment of leukemia, such as the epidofilotoxinas and anthracyclines, have apoptotic effects by inhibiting DNAt2. These drugs interfere with the normal function of DNAt2 by stabilizing the break-cleavable complex, which is the DNAt2 enzyme complex responsible for breaking the double-stranded DNA, slowing the ligation of the strands and leaving free the single-stranded DNA ends that can lead to chromosomal abnormalities. These chromosomal abnormalities have been observed in leukemias secondary to the treatment of epidofilotoxins and anthracyclines in children and adults [62,63], and patients treated with these drugs have a greater likelihood of developing secondary AML with MLL translocations [64]. Several chemical compounds are able to inhibit DNAt2, including chemotherapeutic drugs containing quinone substances [65,66]. The enzyme NAD(P)h:quinone oxidoreductase 1 (NQO1) is involved in the metabolism of chemicals that inhibit DNAt2. The functional polymorphism C609T reduces the activity of NQO1 and exhibits a phenotypic dose-gene effect [67,68]. Several studies have assessed the associated risk of possessing the variant allele T at locus NQO1 C609T in patients with childhood AL and MLL rearrangement. The results are mixed; only some studies observed an increased risk with NQO1 C609T in infants with leukemia and MLL [66,69,70].

However, there are other sources of exposure to DNAt2 inhibitors that may increase the risk of acute leukemia in infants [42]. These DNAt2 inhibitors are found in some drugs, substances derived from benzene and naturally in some foods that contain flavonoids [71].

http://dx.doi.org/10.5772/54457

8. Therapy-related secondary leukemias

The growing use of intensive therapies in the treatment of patients with cancer has caused an increase in the incidence of secondary neoplasms. The complexity of anti-cancer treatments makes it difficult to know what agents are more leucemogenous and which act more quickly in the leukemic transformation of the hematopoiesis progenitor cells. The term secondary leukemia is usually employed to indicate both forms of AML evolving from previous myelodysplasia and forms of acute leukemia developing after exposure to environmental or therapeutic toxins or radiation (therapy-related). Secondary leukemias account for 10-30% of all AML. The majority of secondary leukemias resulting from the use of cytotoxic drugs can be divided into two well defined groups depending on whether the patient has received: 1) alkylating agents or 2) drugs binding to the enzyme DNA-topoisomerase II.

Alkylating agents related leukemias are very similar to post myelodysplasia leukemias being characterized frequently by a preleukemic phase, trilineage dysplasia, frequent cytogenetic abnormalities involving chromosomes 5 and 7 and a poor prognosis. Secondary leukemias related to therapy with topoisomerase II inhibitors are not preceded by a preleukemic phase and show frequently balanced translocations involving chromosome 11q23. Among therapy-related leukemias, AML is generally a second neoplasm, thus a predisposition to malignancy, independently from previous chemotherapy, cannot be excluded. It has been mentioned that the incidence of secondary leukemias increases with age [72] and leukemic cells predominantly exhibit a monocytic or myelomonocytic phenotype and balanced chromosomal translocations including 11q23 and 21q22 rearrangements or abnormalities such as t(15;17)(q22;q12) and inv(16)(p13q22). A history of previous treatment with topoisomerase-II-inhibitors is common in these individuals. However, as many patients have received multiple lines of treatment including several classes of chemotherapy compounds, both structural and balanced chromosomal aberrations are frequently observed in the leukaemic clone. The World Health Organization (WHO) has therefore abandoned its former classification into alkylating agent or topoisomerase-II-inhibitor associated therapy-related disease. As a conservative estimate, about 10% of cases of AML and myelodysplastic syndrome (MDS) are therapy related [73].

Alkylating agents

Alkylating agents were the first chemotherapeutic compounds to be associated with leukaemia development after successful treatment of solid and haematological cancers [74-78]. They comprise a large group of anti-cancer drugs with clinical application across almost all cancer types. Alkylating agents induce DNA damage by transferring alkyl groups – such as -CH3 or -CH2-CH3 – to oxygen or nitrogen atoms of DNA bases, resulting in highly mutagenic DNA base lesions, such as O6-methylguanine and N3-methylcytosine [79-82].

Drugs binding to the enzyme DNA-topoisomerase II (topoisomerase inhibitors)

While alkylating agents associated with therapy-related myeloid neoplasms (t-MNs) are characterized by a complex karyotype often featuring partial or complete loss of chromosomes 5 and/or 7, exposure to topoisomerase inhibitors leads to the development of leukaemias with balanced translocations involving MLL at 11q23, RUNX1 at 21q22 and RARA at 17q21 [83-85]. MLL fusion genes are also MLL fusion genes are also common in secondary acute myeloid leukemia (usually French-American-British (FAB) M4/M5) associated with prior therapeutic exposure to topoisomerase-II inhibiting anthracyclines or epidophyllotoxins [62]. These observations have prompted speculation on possible exposure to topoisomerase-II inhibiting substances during pregnancy that might give rise to MLL fusions during fetal hematopoiesis [86].

DNA topoisomerases are critical enzymes responsible for unknotting and relaxing supercoiled DNA, thus allowing DNA replication to occur. To relax supercoiled DNA, topoisomerases bind covalently to the DNA strand and create transient single (type I topoisomerases) and DSBs (type II topoisomerases). These DNA strand breaks are readily religated after topoisomerases are released from the DNA [87]. As these ubiquitous enzymes are essential to cell survival, DNA topoisomerases have become a valuable target for several cytostatic drugs, such as epipodophyllotoxins and anthracyclines. Topoisomerase inhibitors block the release of topoisomerases from cleaved DNA, preventing religation of the DNA strands [88]. Thus, topoisomerase inhibitors lead to the generation of permanent DNA DSBs that trigger DSB-induced apoptosis. However, persistent DNA DSBs are also highly mutagenic and can result in chromosomal deletions, insertions, inversions and translocations, all of which are characteristic of the leukaemic cell clone in t-MNs. The exact molecular effects of these inhibitors on the acquisition of chromosomal aberrations and the development of this t-MN subtype have recently been reviewed in detail [89].

Dexrazoxane – a bisdioxopiperazine iron chelator used to reduce cardiopulmonary toxicity in patients treated with anthracyclines – also interferes with topoisomerase II in its dimerized state by bridging and stabilizing the ATPase region. In a randomized phase III study in paediatric patients treated with chemo- and radiotherapy for Hodgkin´s disease, dexrazoxane was associated with a cumulative incidence of MDS/AML of 2.5% - 1.0% as compared with 0.85% - 0.6% for the non-dexrazoxane group (P = 0.16). This trend towards an increased risk of secondary neoplasms associated with dexrazoxane was subsequently confirmed in patients with childhood acute lymphoblastic leukaemia [90]. In children cured of ALL, the risk of a therapy-related acute myeloid leukaemia (t-AML) has been evaluated in different series to be between 3.8% at 6 years and 5.9% at 4 years [64,91-96]. The risk of secondary acute myeloid leukemia (sAML) was higher among ALL children who received a high cumulative dose of epipodophyllotoxins (>4,000 mg/m2) and prolonged epipodophyllotoxin therapy in weekly or twice-weekly doses. In adults a GIMEMA study demonstrated a low incidence of t-AML, which could be explained by the lower doses of epipodophyllotoxins administered in the various therapeutic approaches used for the treatment of adult ALL [96].

MLL gene has been involved in secondary leukemias treatment, mainly of the type AML in patients treated with inhibitors of topoisomerase II as a primary cancer treatment. It has been postulated the presence of similar mechanisms for Leukemia in infants whose mothers had exposure to native II topoisomerases [97].

http://dx.doi.org/10.5772/54457

9. Diet and infant leukemia

Studies on environmental risk factors related to AL with MLL rearrangements have focused on maternal diet effects on *in utero* exposure. Dietary compounds exists that can inhibit the function of DNAt2, thereby posing a potential leukemogenesis threat in infants [43,64]. DNAt2 is critical in cellular processes such as replication, where transiently breaks down and subsequently seals the DNA strand [37]. DNAt2 is able to rapidly increase its activity during cell division [98]. Diet is a natural source of DNAt2 inhibitors, including flavonoids [71,99].

Flavonoids are a very large group of Polyphenolic compounds found in foods of plant origin. Polyphenols are involved in the development and reproduction of plants, and they provide resistance against pathogens, plagues and protect crops from diseases that inhibit the germination of their seeds [100]. Flavonoids are divided into 6 subgroups: flavones, flavanols, flavanones, catechins, anthocyanidins and isoflavones [71] (see table 2); in the last decade, more than 5000 subclasses have been identified [101,102]. Importantly, several biological effects have been observed in in vitro studies of flavonoids, including its antioxidant activity, modulation of enzyme activity, inhibition cell proliferation and use as antibiotics, anti-allergy, anti-diarrhea, anti-ulcer and anti-inflammatory agents [103-106].

The properties attributed to flavonoids have prompted increased interest in alternative medicine and herbal remedies. Numerous foods, beverages and supplements exist on the market that contains high levels of flavonoids. Therefore, it is likely that the amount of flavonoids in the typical diet is presently increasing [102].

The study the consumption of DNAt2 inhibitors during pregnancy in women who have children who develop leukemia is founded on the idea that foods containing natural DNAt2 inhibitors cause damage to DNA, much in the same way as the epidofilotoxinas. There have been several bioavailability studies on flavonoids that have demonstrated that there are differences in their absorption, depending on the source of food. The accumulation of these compounds in blood has been measured [107]. Some studies in animals and in vitro have demonstrated that flavonoid DNAt2 inhibitors are capable of crossing the placenta and damaging DNA [108,109]. One study reported the flavonoids can cause a break in the MLL gene in hematopoietic progenitor cells, which was reversible when the exposure was removed. The site of disruption caused by the flavonoids was co localized with the same site associated with the epidofilotoxinas [37,60,99]. All of these findings provide evidence for epidemiological studies in the pursuit of this association with leukemia in infants.

Studies of maternal diets during pregnancy and their association with childhood AL have been led by Ross JA. [110], who through a case-control study in infants and a questionnaire for maternal exposure to dietary DNAt2 inhibitors and drugs in pregnancy observed a statistically significant association between AML and the medium and high consumption of DNAt2 inhibitors (OR 9.8; 95% confidence interval [CI] 1.1-84.8; OR 10.2; 95% CI 1.1-96.4). However, this study observed no association with ALL. Ross JA intends to continue studying infants with AL and stresses the importance of incorporating molecular markers that could provide more information.

Flavones (Apigenin, luteolin, diosmetin)	Flavonols (Quercetin, myrecetin, kaempferol)	Flavanones (Naringenin, hesperidin)	Catechins or Flavanols (Epicatechin, gallocatechin)	Anthocyanidins (Pelargonidin, malvidin, cyanidin)	Isoflavones (Genistein, daidzein)
Parsley	Onions	Citrus foods	Tea	Cherries	Soya beans
Thyme	Kale	Prunes	Apples	Grapes	Legumes
Celery	Broccoli		Cocoa		
Sweet red	Apples				
pepper	Cherries				
	Fennel				
	Sorrel				
	Berries				
	Tea				

Table 2. Major subgroups of flavonoids and food sources.

Later, Jensen CD et al. [111] studied maternal diet and its association with childhood ALL through a food frequency questionnaire, observing a protective effect with the consumption of vegetables, protein and fruits (OR 0.53; 95% CI 0.33-0.85; OR 0.40; 95% CI 0.18-0.90; OR 0.71; 95% CI 0.49-1.04, respectively). In 2005s Spector et al. [34] published the results of a case-control study in infants in which they proposed that exposure to high levels of DNAt2 inhibitors in the diet was associated with the risk of MLL+ leukemia in infants. The authors observed a non-significant association between MLL+ AML but a trend among the second and fourth quartiles of DNAt2 inhibitor consumption (OR 1.9; 95% CI 0.5-7.0; OR 2.1; 95% CI 0.6-7.7; OR 3.2; 95% CI 0.9-11.9). A non-significant inverse association was observed with MLL+ ALL. Another study conducted by Petridou et al. [112] in children ≤4 years old diagnosed with ALL asked about the mothers' diets during pregnancy and found that the consumption of fruits (OR 0.72; 95% CI 0.57-0.91), vegetables (OR 0.76; 95% CI 0.60-09) and fish/seafood (OR 0.72; 95% CI 0.59-0.89) decreased the risk for ALL. However, the consumption of sugar/honey and meat/derivatives increased the risk for ALL (OR 1.32; 95% CI 1.05-1.67; OR 1.25; 95% CI 1.00-1.57, respectively). The most recent study on maternal diet and childhood ALL was undertaken by Kwan ML et al., [113] who applied a food-frequency questionnaire about food consumed 1 year before pregnancy. The results of their study indicate that the risk for ALL was inversely associated with maternal consumption of vegetables (OR 0.65; 95% CI 0.50-0.84), sources of protein (OR 0.55; 95% CI 0.32-0.96), fruits (OR 0.81; 95% CI 0.65-1.00) and legume food groups (OR 0.75; 95% CI 0.59-0.95).

http://dx.doi.org/10.5772/54457

Thus far, epidemiological studies have identified the protective effect of fruits and vegetables consumption during pregnancy against infantile ALL. These results are not observed in AML with the exception of the studies of Ross et al., in which the authors identified a positive association between the high intake of DNAt2 inhibitors in foods and AML/MLL+ in infants. These results confirm that AL in children is composed of different subgroups with different disease etiologies [37,42].

The most recent epidemiological study in infants is the one published by the group of Ross et al., [114] with a significant number of cases (374). In this study, the authors describe some of the demographic factors and the MLL gene status in infants with leukemia. They generally reported a higher frequency of females (50.8%), and the most common ethnic group was Caucasian (70%), followed by Hispanics (27.8%). The most frequent age of diagnosis was 4-6 months (27.8%), and 51.5% of cases were MLL+, 33.0% were MLL-, and 15.6% were undetermined. The chromosome most frequently found fused to the MLL gene was chromosome 4 [t (4; 11)]. Interestingly, the black ethnic group had a lower risk of MLL+ leukemia (OR 0.27; 95% CI 0.11-0.70), and a protective effect was observed in infants 10-12 months old (OR 0.39; 95% CI 0.21-0.73). Cases of ALL and t(9;11) were diagnosed at older ages than cases with t(4;11) or other translocations (P = 0.01). These findings provide important information of the biology of the disease. Undoubtedly, this study necessitates future publications to report socio-economic data, exposure to DNAt2 inhibitors and other maternal risk factors during pregnancy and their association with leukemia in infants.

Another study is currently being conducted by our research group in Mexico City. This study emerged because Mexico City has a high incidence rate of acute leukemia in infants. In addition, a previous study observed that the frequency of MLL/AF4 rearrangements in patients diagnosed with childhood leukemia was high [59]. This is an epidemiological case-control study in infants; the objectives are to identify the relationship between *in utero* exposure to environmental factors inhibiting DNAt2 that are present in the maternal diet during pregnancy, including drugs and benzene derivatives. Biological samples of patients are being analyzed to detect the MLL/AF4 gene rearrangement in infants. In addition, we will know the frequencies of exposure to environmental factors that inhibit DNAt2 in the mothers of infants with MLL+ AL. Nine hospitals that belong to the most important public health institutions in our country are participating in this study. These hospitals diagnose and treat 97.5% of all leukemia cases in Mexico City [7]. The results obtained from this study will be very relevant to one of the cities with the highest incidence rates for childhood AL.

10. Future directions

Due to the findings reported thus far, the authors have recommended carrying out studies in infants that are focused on different biological strata like female/male rations because hormonal differences could indicate an important predisposition to the presence of MLL+ rearrangement. Another suggestion is to study different ethnic groups, where the genetic involvement can provide substantial information about this cohort [112]. For future studies, one must consider the importance of a big sample size, questionnaires validated and, when possible to incorporate biological or environmental samples that enhance the exposure information, such as pre-diagnostic biological samples. In addition to considering collaborative studies between epidemiologists, clinicians, biologists, and others will enrich the results of these studies.

11. Conclusion

There is sufficient evidence to indicate that acute leukemia in infants is initiated *in utero* with MLL rearrangements. Epidemiological studies have demonstrated that flavonoids and some benzene derivatives present in the maternal diet during pregnancy can act as inhibitors of DNAt2 and are associated with the development of AML in infants with MLL+. This association has not been observed for ALL in infants, although an inverse association with the consumption of vegetables and fruits has been reported for ALL. Is a priority to identify environmental or other types of factors that could be contributing to the greater presence of this type of rearrangement during pregnancy and their association with leukemia in infants.

Acknowledgements

Supported by CONSEJO NACIONAL DE CIENCIA Y TECNOLOGIA (CONACYT), Grant 2010-1-141026, IMSS/FIS/PROT 895; CB-2007-1-83949; 2007-1-18-71223, IMSS/FIS/PROT 056.

Author details

ML Pérez-Saldivar[1*], JM Mejía-Aranguré[2], A Rangel-López[2] and A Fajardo Gutiérrez[1]

*Address all correspondence to: maria_luisa_2000_mx@yahoo.com

1 Unidad de Investigación en Epidemiología Clínica, Unidad Médica de Alta Especialidad UMAE Hospital de Pediatría, Centro Médico Nacional (CMN) Siglo XXI, México

2 Coordinación de Investigación en Salud, Instituto Mexicano de Seguridad Social (IMSS), México D.F., México

References

[1] Greaves, M. (1996). The New biology of leukemia, In: Henderson ES, Lister TA, Greaves MF. (Eds) Leukemia. Philadelphia: WB Saunders. , 34-45.

[2] Parkin, D. M. International variation. Oncogene (2004). , 23(38), 6329-6340.

[3] Stiller, C. A. Epidemiology and genetics of childhood cancer. Oncogene (2004). , 23(38), 6429-6444.

[4] Lightfoot, T. J, & Roman, E. Causes of childhood leukaemia and lymphoma. Toxicology and Applied Pharmacology (2004). , 199(2), 104-117.

[5] Parkin, D. M, Stiller, C. A, Draper, G. J, & Bieber, C. A. The international incidence of childhood cancer. International Journal of Cancer (1988). , 42(4), 511-520.

[6] Parkin, D. M, Kramárová, E, Draper, G. J, Masuyer, E, Michaelis, J, & Neglia, J. Qureshi S & Stiller CA (Eds.). International Incidence of Childhood Cancer: IARC Scientific Publications International Agency for Research on Cancer; (1998). , 2(144)

[7] Pérez-saldivar, M. L, Fajardo-gutiérrez, A, Bernáldez-ríos, R, Martínez-avalos, A, Medina-sanson, A, & Espinosa-hernández, L. Flores-Chapa Jde D, Amador-Sánchez R, Peñaloza-González JG, Alvarez-Rodríguez FJ, Bolea-Murga V, Flores-Lujano J, Rodríguez-Zepeda Mdel C, Rivera-Luna R, Dorantes-Acosta EM, Jiménez-Hernández E, Alvarado-Ibarra M, Velázquez-Aviña MM, Torres-Nava JR, Duarte-Rodríguez DA, Paredes-Aguilera R, Del Campo-Martínez Mde L, Cárdenas-Cardos R, Alamilla-Galicia PH, Bekker-Méndez VC, Ortega-Alvarez MC, Mejia-Arangure JM. Childhood acute leukemias are frequent in Mexico City: descriptive epidemiology. BMC Cancer (2011).

[8] Eden, T. Aetiology of childhood leukaemia. Cancer Treatment Reviews (2010). , 36(4), 286-297.

[9] Mejía Aranguré JMFlores Aguilar H, Juárez Muñoz I, Vázquez Langle J, Games Eternod J, Pérez Saldívar ML, Ortega Alvarez MC, Rendón Macías ME, Gutiérrez AF. Age of onset of different malignant tumors in childhood. Revista Médica del Instituto Mexicano del Seguro Social (2005). , 43(1), 25-37.

[10] Fajardo-gutiérrez, A, Juárez-ocaña, S, González-miranda, G, Palma-padilla, V, Carreón-cruz, R, Ortega-alvárez, M. C, & Mejía-arangure, J. M. Incidence of cancer in children residing in ten jurisdictions of the Mexican Republic: importance of the Cancer registry (a population-based study). BMC Cancer (2007).

[11] Rendón-macías, M. E, Mejía-aranguré, J. M, Juárez-ocaña, S, & Fajardo-gutiérrez, A. Epidemiology of cancer in children under one year of age in Mexico City. European Journal of Cancer Prevention (2005). , 14(2), 85-89.

[12] Bernaldez-rios, R, Ortega-alvarez, M. C, Perez-saldivar, M. L, & Alatoma-medina, N. E. Del Campo-Martinez Mde L, Rodriguez-Zepeda Mdel C, Montero-Ponce I, Franco-Ornelas S, Fernandez-Castillo G, Nuñez-Villegas NN, Taboada-Flores MA, Flores-Lujano J, Argüelles-Sanchez ME, Juarez-Ocaña S, Fajardo-Gutierrez A, Mejia-Arangure JM. The age incidence of childhood B-cell precursor acute lymphoblastic leukemia in Mexico City. Journal of pediatric hematology/oncology (2008). , 30(3), 199-203.

[13] Pieters, R. Biology and treatment of infant leukemias, In: Ching-Hon Pui. (ed.) Treatment of acute leukemias: New Directions for Clinical Research. Totowa, New Jersey: Humana Press; (2003). , 61-73.

[14] Greaves, M. In utero origins of childhood leukaemia. Early human development (2005). , 81(1), 123-129.

[15] Ross, J. A. Environmental and genetic susceptibility to MLL-defined infant leukemia. Journal of the National Cancer Institute Monographs (2008).

[16] Ross, J. A, Davies, S. M, Potter, J. D, & Robison, L. L. Epidemiology of childhood leukemia, with a focus on infants. Epidemiologic reviews (1994). , 16(2), 243-272.

[17] Pieters, R. Infant acute lymphoblastic leukemia: Lessons learned and future directions. Current hematologic malignancy reports (2009). , 4(3), 167-174.

[18] Cimino, G, Rapanotti, M. C, Elia, L, Biondi, A, Fizzotti, M, Testi, A. M, Tosti, S, Croce, C. M, Canaani, E, & Mandelli, F. and Lo Coco F. ALL-1 gene rearrangements in acute myeloid leukemia: association with M4-M5 French-American-British classification subtypes and young age. Cancer research (1995). , 55(8), 1625-1628.

[19] Gurney, J. G, Ross, J. A, Wall, D. A, Bleyer, W. A, Severson, R. K, & Robison, L. L. Infant cancer in the U.S.: histology-specific incidence and trends, 1973 to 1992. Journal of pediatric hematology/oncology (1997). , 19(5), 428-432.

[20] Hilden, J. M, Dinndorf, P. A, Meerbaum, S. O, Sather, H, Villaluna, D, Heerema, N. A, Mcglennen, R, Smith, F. O, Woods, W. G, Salzer, W. L, Johnstone, H. S, & Dreyer, Z. Reaman GH; Children's Oncology Group. Analysis of prognostic factors of acute lymphoblastic leukemia in infants: report on CCG 1953 from the Children's Oncology Group. Blood (2006). , 108(2), 441-451.

[21] Ries LAGEisner MP, Kosary CL, Hankey BF, Miller BA, Clegg L, Mariotto A, Fay MP, Feuer EJ, Edwards BK (eds). SEER Cancer Statistics Review, National Cancer Institute. Bethesda, MD, http://seer.cancer.gov/csr/1975_2000/,(2003). accesed 10 July 2012)., 1975-2000.

[22] Ries, L. A. G, Smith, M. A, Gurney, J. G, Linet, M, Tamra, T, Young, J. L, & Bunin, G. R. Cancer incidence and survival among children and adolescents: United States SEER Program (1999). , 1975-1995.

[23] Slater, M. E, Linabery, A. M, Blair, C. K, Spector, L. G, Heerema, N. A, Robison, L. L, & Ross, J. A. Maternal prenatal cigarette, alcohol and illicit drug use and risk of infant leukaemia: a report from the Children's Oncology Group. Paediatric and perinatal epidemiology (2011). , 25(6), 559-565.

[24] Ognjanovic, S, Blair, C, Spector, L. G, Robison, L. L, Roesler, M, & Ross, J. A. Analgesic use during pregnancy and risk of infant leukaemia: a Children's Oncology Group study. British journal of cancer (2011). , 104(3), 532-536.

[25] Slater, M. E, Linabery, A. M, Blair, C. K, Spector, L. G, Heerema, N. A, Robison, L. L, & Ross, J. A. Maternal prenatal cigarette, alcohol and illicit drug use and risk of infant leukaemia: a report from the Children's Oncology Group. Paediatric and perinatal epidemiology (2011). , 25(6), 559-565.

[26] Linabery, A. M, Puumala, S. E, Hilden, J. M, Davies, S. M, Heerema, N. A, & Roesler, M. A. Ross JA; Children's Oncology Group. Maternal vitamin and iron supplementation and risk of infant leukaemia: a report from the Children's Oncology Group. British journal of cancer (2010). , 103(11), 1724-1728.

[27] Johnson, K. J, Roesler, M. A, Linabery, A. M, Hilden, J. M, Davies, S. M, & Ross, J. A. Infant leukemia and congenital abnormalities: a Children's Oncology Group study. Pediatric blood & cancer (2010). , 55(1), 95-99.

[28] Puumala, S. E, Spector, L. G, Wall, M. M, Robison, L. L, Heerema, N. A, Roesler, M. A, & Ross, J. A. Infant leukemia and parental infertility or its treatment: a Children's Oncology Group report. Human reproduction (2010). , 25(6), 1561-1568.

[29] Zanrosso, C. W, Emerenciano, M, Gonçalves, B. A, Faro, A, Koifman, S, & Pombo-de-oliveira, M. S. N-a. c. e. t. y. l. t. r. a. n. s. f. e. r. a. s. e. polymorphisms and susceptibility to infant leukemia with maternal exposure to dipyrone during pregnancy. Cancer epidemiology, biomarkers & prevention (2010). , 19(12), 3037-3043.

[30] Koifman, S. Pombo-de-Oliveira MS; Brazilian Collaborative Study Group of Infant Acute Leukemia. High birth weight as an important risk factor for infant leukemia. British journal of cancer (2008). , 98(3), 664-667.

[31] Spector, L. G, Davies, S. M, Robison, L. L, Hilden, J. M, Roesler, M, & Ross, J. A. Birth characteristics, maternal reproductive history, and the risk of infant leukemia: a report from the Children's Oncology Group. Cancer epidemiology, biomarkers & prevention (2007). , 16(1), 128-134.

[32] Peters, A. M, Blair, C. K, Verneris, M. R, Neglia, J. P, Robison, L. L, Spector, L. G, Reaman, G. H, & Felix, C. A. Ross JA; Children's Oncology Group. Maternal haemoglobin concentration during pregnancy and risk of infant leukaemia: a children's oncology group study. British journal of cancer (2006). , 95(9), 1274-1276.

[33] Pombo-de-oliveira, M. S. Koifman S; Brazilian Collaborative Study Group of Infant Acute Leukemia. Infant acute leukemia and maternal exposures during pregnancy. Cancer epidemiology, biomarkers & prevention (2006). , 15(12), 2336-2341.

[34] Spector, L. G, Xie, Y, Robison, L. L, Heerema, N. A, Hilden, J. M, Lange, B, Felix, C. A, Davies, S. M, Slavin, J, Potter, J. D, Blair, C. K, Reaman, G. H, & Ross, J. A. Maternal diet and infant leukemia: the DNA topoisomerase II inhibitor hypothesis: a report from the children's oncology group. Cancer epidemiology, biomarkers & prevention (2005). , 14(3), 651-655.

[35] Alexander, F. E, Patheal, S. L, Biondi, A, Brandalise, S, Cabrera, M. E, Chan, L. C, Chen, Z, Cimino, G, Cordoba, J. C, Gu, L. J, Hussein, H, Ishii, E, Kamel, A. M, Labra, S, Magalhães, I. Q, Mizutani, S, Petridou, E, De Oliveira, M. P, Yuen, P, Wiemels, J. L, & Greaves, M. F. Transplacental chemical exposure and risk of infant leukemia with MLL gene fusion. Cancer research (2001). , 61(6), 2542-2546.

[36] Brassesco, M. S, Montaldi, A. P, Gras, D. E, Camparoto, M. L, Martinez-rossi, N. M, Scrideli, C. A, Tone, L. G, & Sakamoto-hojo, E. T. Cytogenetic and molecular analysis of MLL rearrangements in acute lymphoblastic leukaemia survivors. Mutagenesis (2009)., 24(2), 153-60.

[37] Greaves, M. F, & Wiemels, J. Origins of chromosome translocations in childhood leukaemia. Nature reviews Cancer (2003)., 3(9), 639-649.

[38] Krivtsov, A. V, & Armstrong, S. A. MLL translocations, histone modifications and leukaemia stem-cell development. Nature reviews Cancer (2007)., 7(11), 823-833.

[39] Meyer, C, Schneider, B, Jakob, S, Strehl, S, Attarbaschi, A, Schnittger, S, Schoch, C, Jansen, M. W, & Van Dongen, J. J. den Boer ML, Pieters R, Ennas MG, Angelucci E, Koehl U, Greil J, Griesinger F, Zur Stadt U, Eckert C, Szczepański T, Niggli FK, Schäfer BW, Kempski H, Brady HJ, Zuna J, Trka J, Nigro LL, Biondi A, Delabesse E, Macintyre E, Stanulla M, Schrappe M, Haas OA, Burmeister T, Dingermann T, Klingebiel T, Marschalek R. The MLL recombinome of acute leukemias. Leukemia (2006)., 20(5), 777-784.

[40] Daser, A, & Rabbitts, T. H. Extending the repertoire of the mixed-lineage leukemia gene MLL in leukemogenesis. Genes & development (2004)., 18(9), 965-974.

[41] Chowdhury, T, & Brady, H. J. Insights from clinical studies into the role of the MLL gene in infant and childhood leukemia. Blood cells, molecules & diseases (2008)., 40(2), 192-199.

[42] Ross, J. A. Maternal diet and infant leukemia: a role for DNA topoisomerase II inhibitors? International journal of cancer Supplement (1998).

[43] Pui, C. H, Carroll, W. L, Meshinchi, S, & Arceci, R. J. Biology, risk stratification, and therapy of pediatric acute leukemias: an update. Journal of clinical oncology (2011)., 29(5), 551-565.

[44] Ross, J. A. Environmental and genetic susceptibility to MLL-defined infant leukemia. Journal of the National Cancer Institute Monographs (2008).

[45] Brassesco, M. S, Montaldi, A. P, & Sakamoto-hojo, E. T. Preferential induction of MLL(Mixed Lineage Leukemia) rearrangements in human lymphocyte cultures treated with etoposide. Genetics and molecular biology (2009)., 32(1), 144-150.

[46] Slany, R. K. The molecular biology of mixed lineage leukemia. Haematologica (2009)., 94(7), 984-993.

[47] Wiederschain, D, Kawai, H, Shilatifard, A, & Yuan, Z. M. Multiple mixed lineage leukemia (MLL) fusion proteins suppress response to DNA damage. The Journal of biological chemistry (2005)., 53.

[48] Hess, J. L. MLL: a histone methyltransferase disrupted in leukemia. Trends in molecular medicine (2004)., 10(10), 500-507.

[49] Aplan, P. D. Chromosomal translocations involving the MLL gene: molecular mechanisms. DNA Repair (Amst) (2006).

[50] Rubnitz, J. E, Behm, F. G, & Downing, J. R. q23 rearrangements in acute leukemia. Leukemia (1996). , 10(1), 74-82.

[51] Bach, C, Buhl, S, Mueller, D, García-cuéllar, M. P, Maethner, E, & Slany, R. K. Leukemogenic transformation by HOXA cluster genes. Blood (2010). , 115(14), 2910-2918.

[52] Armstrong, S. A, Kung, A. L, Mabon, M. E, Silverman, L. B, & Stam, R. W. Den Boer ML, Pieters R, Kersey JH, Sallan SE, Fletcher JA, Golub TR, Griffin JD, Korsmeyer SJ. Inhibition of FLT3 in MLL. Validation of a therapeutic target identified by gene expression based classification. Cancer Cell (2003). , 3(2), 173-183.

[53] Greaves, M. F, Maia, A. T, Wiemels, J. L, & Ford, A. M. Leukemia in twins: lessons in natural history. Blood (2003). , 102(7), 2321-2333.

[54] Maia, A. T, Van Der Velden, V. H, Harrison, C. J, Szczepanski, T, Williams, M. D, Griffiths, M. J, Van Dongen, J. J, & Greaves, M. F. Prenatal origin of hyperdiploid acute lymphoblastic leukemia in identical twins. Leukemia (2003). , 17(11), 2202-2206.

[55] Hong, D, Gupta, R, Ancliff, P, Atzberger, A, Brown, J, Soneji, S, Green, J, Colman, S, Piacibello, W, Buckle, V, Tsuzuki, S, Greaves, M, & Enver, T. Initiating and cancer-propagating cells in TEL-AML1-associated childhood leukemia. Science (2008). , 319(5861), 336-339.

[56] Ayton, P. M, & Cleary, M. L. Molecular mechanisms of leukemogenesis mediated by MLL fusion proteins. Oncogene (2001). , 20(40), 5695-5707.

[57] Bueno, C, Montes, R, Catalina, P, Rodríguez, R, & Menendez, P. Insights into the cellular origin and etiology of the infant pro-B acute lymphoblastic leukemia with MLL-AF4 rearrangement. Leukemia (2011). , 25(3), 400-410.

[58] Eguchi, M, Eguchi-ishimae, M, & Greaves, M. Molecular pathogenesis of MLL-associated leukemias. International journal of hematology (2005). , 82(1), 9-20.

[59] Daniel-cravioto, A, Gonzalez-bonilla, C. R, Mejia-arangure, J. M, Perez-saldivar, M. L, Fajardo-gutierrez, A, Jimenez-hernandez, E, Hernandez-serrano, M, & Bekker-mendez, V. C. Genetic rearrangement MLL/AF4 is most frequent in children with acute lymphoblastic leukemias in Mexico City. Leukemia & lymphoma (2009). , 50(8), 1352-1360.

[60] Ford, A. M, Ridge, S. A, Cabrera, M. E, Mahmoud, H, Steel, C. M, Chan, L. C, & Greaves, M. In utero rearrangements in the trithorax-related oncogene in infant leukaemias. Nature (1993). , 363(6427), 358-360.

[61] Wang, J. C. DNA topoisomerases. Annual review of biochemistry (1996).

[62] Felix, C. A. Secondary leukemias induced by topoisomerase-targeted drugs. Biochimica et biophysica acta (1998).

[63] Rowley, J. D, & Olney, H. J. International workshop on the relationship of prior therapy to balanced chromosome aberrations in therapy-related myelodysplastic syndromes and acute leukemia: overview report. Genes Chromosomes Cancer (2002). , 33(4), 331-345.

[64] Pui, C. H, Behm, F. G, Raimondi, S. C, Dodge, R. K, George, S. L, & Rivera, G. K. Mirro J Jr, Kalwinsky DK, Dahl GV, Murphy SB. Secondary acute myeloid leukemia in children treated for acute lymphoid leukemia. The New England journal of medicine (1989). , 321(3), 136-142.

[65] Chen, H, & Eastmond, D. A. Topoisomerase inhibition by phenolic metabolites: a potential mechanism for benzene's clastogenic effects. Carcinogenesis (1995). , 16(10), 2301-2307.

[66] Wiemels, J, Wiencke, J. K, Varykoni, A, & Smith, M. T. Modulation of the toxicity and macromolecular binding of benzene metabolites by NAD(P)H:Quinone oxidoreductase in transfected HL-60 cells. Chemical research in toxicology (1999). , 12(6), 467-475.

[67] Siegel, D, Mcguinness, S. M, Winski, S. L, & Ross, D. Genotype-phenotype relationships in studies of a polymorphism in NAD(P)H:quinone oxidoreductase 1.Pharmacogenetics (1999). , 9(1), 113-121.

[68] Ross, D, & Siegel, D. NAD(P)H:quinone oxidoreductase 1 (NQO1, DT-diaphorase), functions and pharmacogenetics. Methods in enzymology (2004).

[69] Eguchi-ishimae, M, Eguchi, M, Ishii, E, Knight, D, Sadakane, Y, Isoyama, K, Yabe, H, Mizutani, S, & Greaves, M. The association of a distinctive allele of NAD(P)H:quinone oxidoreductase with pediatric acute lymphoblastic leukemias with MLL fusion genes in Japan. Haematologica (2005). , 90(11), 1511-1515.

[70] Krajinovic, M, Sinnett, H, Richer, C, Labuda, D, & Sinnett, D. Role of NQO1, MPO and YP2E1 genetic polymorphisms in the susceptibility to childhood acute lymphoblastic leukemia. International journal of cancer (2002). , 97(2), 230-236.

[71] Ross, J. A, & Kasum, C. M. Dietary flavonoids: bioavailability, metabolic effects, and safety. Annual review of nutrition (2002).

[72] Hann, I. M, Stevens, R. F, Goldstone, A. H, Rees, J. K, Wheatley, K, Gray, R. G, & Burnett, A. K. Randomized comparison of DAT versus ADE as induction chemotherapy in children and younger adults with acute myeloid leukemia. Results of the Medical Research Council's 10th AML trial (MRC AML10). Adult and Childhood Leukaemia Working Parties of the Medical Research Council. Blood (1997). , 89(7), 2311-2318.

[73] Leone, G, Fianchi, L, Pagano, L, & Voso, M. T. Incidence and susceptibility to therapy-related myeloid neoplasms. Chemico-biological interactions (2010).

[74] Kyle, R. A, Pierre, R. V, & Bayrd, E. D. Multiple myeloma and acute myelomonocytic leukemia. The New England journal of medicine (1970). , 283(21), 1121-1125.

[75] Kyle, R. A, Pierre, R. V, & Bayrd, E. D. Primary amyloidosis and acute leukemia associated with melphalan therapy. Blood (1974). , 44(3), 333-337.

[76] Rosner, F, & Grünwald, H. Hodgkin's disease and acute leukemia. Report of eight cases and review of the literature. The American journal of medicine (1975). , 58(3), 339-353.

[77] Reimer, R. R, Hoover, R, Fraumeni, JF Jr, & Young, RC. . Acute leukemia after alkylating-agent therapy of ovarian cancer. The New England journal of medicine (1977). , 297(4), 177-181.

[78] Rowley, J. D, Golomb, H. M, & Vardiman, J. W. Nonrandom chromosome abnormalities in acute leukemia and dysmyelopoietic syndromes in patients with previously treated malignant disease. Blood (1981). , 58(4), 759-767.

[79] Saffhill, R, Margison, G. P, & Connor, O. PJ. Mechanisms of carcinogenesis induced by alkylating agents. Biochimica et biophysica acta (1985). , 823(2), 111-145.

[80] Horsfall, M. J, Gordon, A. J, Burns, P. A, Zielenska, M, Van Der Vliet, G. M, & Glickman, B. W. Mutational specificity of alkylating agents and the influence of DNA repair. Environmental and molecular mutagenesis (1990). , 15(2), 107-122.

[81] Shulman, L. N. The biology of alkylating-agent cellular injury. Hematology/oncology clinics of North America (1993). , 7(2), 325-335.

[82] Drabløs, F, Feyzi, E, Aas, P. A, Vaagbø, C. B, Kavli, B, Bratlie, M. S, Peña-diaz, J, Otterlei, M, Slupphaug, G, & Krokan, H. E. Alkylation damage in DNA and RNA-repair mechanisms and medical significance. DNA Repair (Amst) (2004). , 3(11), 1389-1407.

[83] Pedersen-bjergaard, J, Pedersen, M, Roulston, D, & Philip, P. Different genetic pathways in leukemogenesis for patients presenting with therapy-related myelodysplasia and therapy-related acute myeloid leukemia. Blood (1995). , 86(9), 3542-3552.

[84] Dissing, M, Le Beau, MM, & Pedersen-Bjergaard, J. . Inversion of chromosome 16 and uncommon rearrangements of the CBFB and MYH11 genes in therapy-related acute myeloid leukemia: rare events related to DNA-topoisomerase II inhibitors? Journal of clinical oncology (1998). , 16(5), 1890-1896.

[85] Smith, S. M, Le Beau, MM, Huo, D, Karrison, T, Sobecks, RM, Anastasi, J, Vardiman, JW, Rowley, JD, & Larson, RA. . Clinical-cytogenetic associations in 306 patients with therapy-related myelodysplasia and myeloid leukemia: the University of Chicago series. Blood (2003). , 102(1), 43-52.

[86] Ross, J. A, Potter, J. D, & Robison, L. L. Infant leukemia, topoisomerase II inhibitors, and the MLL gene. Journal of the National Cancer Institute (1994). , 86(22), 1678-1680.

[87] Nitiss, J. L. Targeting DNA topoisomerase II in cancer chemotherapy. Nature reviews Cancer (2009). , 9(5), 338-350.

[88] Allan, J. M, & Travis, L. B. Mechanisms of therapy-related carcinogenesis. Nature reviews Cancer (2005). , 5(12), 943-955.

[89] Joannides, M, & Grimwade, D. Molecular biology of therapy-related leukaemias. Clinical & translational oncology (2010). , 12(1), 8-14.

[90] Salzer, W. L, Devidas, M, Carroll, W. L, Winick, N, Pullen, J, Hunger, S. P, & Camitta, B. A. Long-term results of the pediatric oncology group studies for childhood acute lymphoblastic leukemia 1984-2001: a report from the children's oncology group. Leukemia (2010). , 24(2), 355-370.

[91] Pui, C. H, Ribeiro, R. C, Hancock, M. L, Rivera, G. K, Evans, W. E, Raimondi, S. C, Head, D. R, Behm, F. G, Mahmoud, M. H, Sandlund, J. T, et al. Acute myeloid leukemia in children treated with epipodophyllotoxins for acute lymphoblastic leukemia. The New England journal of medicine (1991). , 325(24), 1682-1687.

[92] Neglia, J. P, Meadows, A. T, Robison, L. L, Kim, T. H, Newton, W. A, Ruymann, F. B, Sather, H. N, & Hammond, G. D. Second neoplasms after acute lymphoblastic leukemia in childhood. The New England journal of medicine (1991). , 325(19), 1330-1336.

[93] Kreissman, S. G, Gelber, R. D, Cohen, H. J, Clavell, L. A, Leavitt, P, & Sallan, S. E. Incidence of secondary acute myelogenous leukemia after treatment of childhood acute lymphoblastic leukemia. Cancer (1992). , 70(8), 2208-2213.

[94] Jankovic, M, Fraschini, D, Amici, A, Aricò, M, Arrighini, A, Basso, G, & Colella, R. DiTullio MT, Haupt R, Macchia P, et al. Outcome after cessation of therapy in childhood acute lymphoblastic leukaemia. The Associazione Italiana Ematologia ed Oncologia Pediatrica (AIEOP). European journal of cancer (1993). A(13) 1839-1843.

[95] Winick, N. J, Mckenna, R. W, Shuster, J. J, Schneider, N. R, Borowitz, M. J, Bowman, W. P, Jacaruso, D, Kamen, B. A, & Buchanan, G. R. Secondary acute myeloid leukemia in children with acute lymphoblastic leukemia treated with etoposide. Journal of clinical oncology (1993). , 11(2), 209-217.

[96] Pagano, L, Annino, L, Ferrari, A, Camera, A, Martino, B, Montillo, M, Tosti, M. E, Mele, A, Pulsoni, A, Vegna, M. L, Leone, G, & Mandelli, F. Secondary haematological neoplasm after treatment of adult acute lymphoblastic leukemia: analysis of 1170 adult ALL patients enrolled in the GIMEMA trials. Gruppo Italiano Malattie Ematologiche Maligne dell'Adulto. British journal of haematology (1998). , 100(4), 669-676.

[97] Armstrong, S. A, Golub, T. R, & Korsmeyer, S. J. MLL-rearranged leukemias: insights from gene expression profiling. Seminars in hematology (2003). , 40(4), 268-273.

[98] Gewirtz, D. A. Does bulk damage to DNA explain the cytostatic and cytotoxic effects of topoisomerase II inhibitors? Biochemical pharmacology (1991). , 42(12), 2253-2258.

[99] Vanhees, K, De Bock, L, Godschalk, R. W, & Van Schooten, F. J. van Waalwijk van Doorn-Khosrovani SB. Prenatal exposure to flavonoids: implication for cancer risk. Toxicological sciences (2011). , 120(1), 59-67.

[100] Croft, K. D. The chemistry and biological effects of flavonoids and phenolic acids. Annals of the New York Academy of Sciences (1998).

[101] Stalikas, C. D. Extraction, separation, and detection methods for phenolic acids and flavonoids. Journal of separation science (2007). , 30(18), 3268-3295.

[102] Lanoue, L, Green, K. K, Kwik-uribe, C, & Keen, C. L. Dietary factors and the risk for acute infant leukemia: evaluating the effects of cocoa-derived flavanols on DNA topoisomerase activity. Experimental biology and medicine (2010). , 235(1), 77-89.

[103] Balzer, J, Rassaf, T, Heiss, C, Kleinbongard, P, Lauer, T, Merx, M, Heussen, N, Gross, H. B, Keen, C. L, Schroeter, H, & Kelm, M. Sustained benefits in vascular function through flavanol-containing cocoa in medicated diabetic patients a double-masked, randomized, controlled trial. Journal of the American College of Cardiology (2008). , 51(22), 2141-2149.

[104] Corder, R, Mullen, W, Khan, N. Q, Marks, S. C, Wood, E. G, Carrier, M. J, & Crozier, A. Oenology: red wine procyanidins and vascular health. Nature (2006).

[105] Duthie, G, & Crozier, A. Plant-derived phenolic antioxidants. Current opinion in clinical nutrition and metabolic care (2000). , 3(6), 447-451.

[106] Grassi, D, Aggio, A, Onori, L, Croce, G, Tiberti, S, Ferri, C, Ferri, L, & Desideri, G. Tea, flavonoids, and nitric oxide-mediated vascular reactivity. The Journal of nutrition (2008). S-1560S.

[107] Adlercreutz, H, Markkanen, H, & Watanabe, S. Plasma concentrations of phyto-oestrogens in Japanese men. Lancet (1993). , 342(8881), 1209-1210.

[108] Schröder-van der Elst JP van der Heide D, Rokos H, Morreale de Escobar G, Köhrle J. Synthetic flavonoids cross the placenta in the rat and are found in fetal brain. The American journal of physiology (1998). Pt 1) EE256., 253.

[109] Strick, R, Strissel, P. L, Borgers, S, Smith, S. L, & Rowley, J. D. Dietary bioflavonoids induce cleavage in the MLL gene and may contribute to infant leukemia. Proceedings of the National Academy of Sciences of the United States of America (2000). , 97(9), 4790-4795.

[110] Ross, J. A, Potter, J. D, Reaman, G. H, Pendergrass, T. W, & Robison, L. L. Maternal exposure to potential inhibitors of DNA topoisomerase II and infant leukemia (United States): a report from the Children's Cancer Group. Cancer Causes Control (1996). , 7(6), 581-590.

[111] Jensen, C. D, Block, G, Buffler, P, Ma, X, Selvin, S, & Month, S. Maternal dietary risk factors in childhood acute lymphoblastic leukemia (United States). Cancer Causes Control (2004). , 15(6), 559-570.

[112] Petridou, E, Ntouvelis, E, Dessypris, N, & Terzidis, A. Trichopoulos D; Childhood Hematology-Oncology Group. Maternal diet and acute lymphoblastic leukemia in young children. Cancer epidemiology, biomarkers & prevention (2005). , 14(8), 1935-1939.

[113] Kwan, M. L, Jensen, C. D, Block, G, Hudes, M. L, Chu, L. W, & Buffler, P. A. Public health reports (2009). , 124(4), 503-514.

[114] Sam, T. N, Kersey, J. H, Linabery, A. M, Johnson, K. J, Heerema, N. A, Hilden, J. M, Davies, S. M, Reaman, G. H, & Ross, J. A. MLL gene rearrangements in infant leukemia vary with age at diagnosis and selected demographic factors: a Children's Oncology Group (COG) study. Pediatric blood & cancer (2012). , 58(6), 836-839.

Chapter 8

Infection During the First Year of Life and Acute Leukemia: Epidemiological Evidence

Janet Flores-Lujano, Juan Carlos Núñez-Enríquez, Angélica Rangel-López, David Aldebarán-Duarte, Arturo Fajardo-Gutiérrez and Juan Manuel Mejía-Arangué

Additional information is available at the end of the chapter

http://dx.doi.org/10.5772/52717

1. Introduction

The role of infection in the etiology of leukemia was revealed for the first time more than ninety years ago through a series of cases reported by Gordon Ward in the year 1917. These cases included 1457 children with acute leukemia, but the results were inconclusive. Later, in another study by Poynton, Thursfield and Paterson, the authors reported that it was not possible to attribute the etiology of leukemia to a single infectious agent and emphasized the importance of host susceptibility in the acquirement of an infection and the development of acute leukemia.[1,2]

In 1937, in a study conducted in England by Kellet, it was mentioned that an infection could be the causative agent for acute leukemia when the infection is widely distributed but has low infectivity. This conclusion was supported by Cooke in 1942 in a study involving 33 pediatric care units in the United States, who found that the peak age of 2 to 5 years in children with acute leukemia correlated with the peak of increased incidence of diseases, such as measles and diphtheria. [3,4]

One of the most important scientific contributions in this regard was made by Kinlen et al., who found a relationship between high incidence rates of acute leukemia and Non-Hodgkin's lymphoma and infections in children living near rural areas. Kinlen's findings resulted in the emergence of a hypothesis proposing that leukemia could be caused by exposure to an infectious agent in a susceptible population and, in this case, a mixed population (rural-urban), causing an abnormal immune response that increases the risk of developing the disease. [5,7]

Moreover, Greaves et al. provided a new approach to the hypothesis that had been raised by Kellet, now basing it on biological and epidemiological data on acute leukemia. These authors suggested the hypothesis of late infection, which is explained by two stages: the first stage occurs with a mutation in utero at the same time that precursor B cells are developing and a second stage, during the postnatal period, in which the cell that undergoes a mutation is exposed to a common infection late in the first year of the child's life. [8-13]

2. Measuring exposure to infection with proxy variables

Over time, in epidemiological studies that have attempted to determine whether an association between early infections and the development of leukemia exists, some indicators have been used to quantify the exposure to infection. These indicators are designated as "proxies" and include socioeconomic status, surgical history, allergic diseases, immunizations, attendance at daycare, breastfeeding, neonatal infections, and prenatal history, among others. [14-25]

2.1. Socioeconomic status

In several epidemiological studies that have assessed infections during the first year of life in children, it was considered to be important to adjust for socioeconomic status because a high socioeconomic status is consistently associated with the development of leukemia and protection against infection. On the contrary, those who have a low socioeconomic status are at a higher risk for the presence of common infections. [26-30] It is important to note, however, that the methods used to measure this variable are not consistent. For example, Steensel-Moll et al. measured socioeconomic status in The Netherlands (1973-1980) according to the parents' education, while other authors have used, for example, the number of people per room, home ownership, and family income as indicators of socioeconomic status. [15-17,21,22,31-33]

2.2. Prenatal history

The study of prenatal history is interesting as a proxy because it assesses the association between infections and the development of leukemia before birth in an indirect manner, taking into account the fact that, being part of a binomial mother-fetus, the child may have been exposed to infection during the intrauterine period if the mother had an infection during pregnancy. For example, in a study by Fedrick and Alberman in 1972, a positive association was reported between influenza during pregnancy and the development of leukemia and lymphoma, where a RR of 9 ($p < 0.001$) was obtained. Other studies have used other variables associated with pregnancy for the same purpose. For example, whether antimicrobials and/or antiviral drugs were used if the mother had infections was considered. [34] Moreover, the authors of several studies considered a history of antibiotic and/or antiviral use by mothers during pregnancy to reflect the fact that they had been exposed to an infectious process. In this regard, Infante-Rivard et al. noted during 1989 to 1995 that the use of antimicrobials during pregnancy increased the risk of leukemia, with an OR of 1.5 (95% CI:1.02-2.21). When the data were fur-

http://dx.doi.org/10.5772/52717

ther adjusted for the child's age being <4 years at diagnosis, the OR was 1.78 (95% CI: 1.04-3.04). Furthermore, in 2010, these results were supported by the German study of Kaatsch et al., who reported an OR of 1.47 (95% CI: 1.06-2.04). [33,35] These findings, however, are inconsistent with those reported by other authors. [36-45]

2.3. Neonatal infections

While there are maternal protective barriers during pregnancy that help to prevent infections that may occur in the child at some point after birth, when these barriers cease to exist and the immune system is not well developed, the child is at greater risk for developing infections. Therefore, many epidemiological studies have considered the neonatal period to be a crucial step in the assessment of the relationship between infections and the development of acute leukemia. In 1999, McKinney et al. reported that the presence of neonatal infection was associated with a decreased risk of acute lymphoblastic leukemia (ALL) in Scottish children, with an OR of 0.49 (95% CI: 0.26 to 0.95) being more evident in cases of skin infections, such as omphalitis and/or infection in the skin around the umbilical cord, with an OR of 0.20 (95% CI: 0.05 to 0.87) for all leukemias and for acute lymphoblastic leukemia, regardless of birth type (vaginal or by cesarean section). [46]

2.4. Breastfeeding

Breast milk is considered to be the first vaccine that a child receives during the first months of life, and it protects against infections by stimulating the immune system. There are many mechanisms by which breast milk exerts its antimicrobial and immunological properties. Among the most important mechanisms are the immunoglobulins, interleukins, lactoferrin, mucin, various types of enzymes (e.g., lysozyme and lipases), opsonins, cytokines, prostaglandins and other small peptides. Also involved in these functions are T and B lymphocytes, which are present in breast milk. Thus, the study of breastfeeding as a protective factor against infections during the first year of life has generated scientific interest. [47-50] In most epidemiological studies, it has been documented that breastfeeding favorably influences both the response to infection and the modulation of the child's immune system. [21,33,51-64]

These factors require further investigation, as there is inconsistency among the epidemiological studies conducted thus far regarding whether a child's immune system will respond appropriately to an infectious agent after the child has been breastfed for the first six months of life. However, if the child has had recurrent common infections, his/her immune system will have an adequate response to a delayed infection.

2.5. Attendance at daycare

The child's attendance at daycare also represents a quantifiable index of infection during the first year of life in relation to the development of leukemia. For its implementation in epidemiological studies, investigators have used the age of entry to kindergarten, the hours spent in child care, the number of partners in the nursery, the presence of infection during their stay in the nursery, the social activities being undertaken by the child during the first year, the type of staff who attended to the child during their stay and the hours they remained at home, among others. There is evidence reported by some studies that there is a dose-response effect with respect to the number of hours that a child remains in a nursery and a lower risk of developing leukemia, and the more a child is in contact with other children, the risk is increased for common and recurring infections, thus favoring a better stimulation and maturation of the immune system. [17,65] In the UK, Gilham et al. also found child attendance at day care during the first year of life to have a protective effect, reporting an OR = 0.69 (95% CI: 0.51 to 0.93, p = 0.02), but this effect was more significant when the child attended during the first 3 months of age, with an OR = 0.52 (95% CI: 0.32 to 0.83, p = 0.007). [66]

2.6. Immunizations

Knowing the vaccination history of children is another important approach to understanding the role of infections in the modern-day development of childhood acute leukemia. This is based on the assumption that vaccines are infectious antigenic stimuli that enable the formation of antibodies and, therefore, a better performance of the immune system. Vaccines could also be the mechanism by which the development of acute leukemia is prevented. [67] Meanwhile, Schüz et al. conducted a study in Germany (1999) and reported that, in children older than 4 years of age, there was an increased risk of developing leukemia in those with a history of fewer than three vaccines, with an OR of 1.8 (95% CI: 1.2-2.7), and a low risk in children with a history of 4-6 shots, with an OR of 1.3 (95% CI:1.0-1.7), which supports the following dose-response relationship: as the number of vaccines given to children increases, the risk of developing acute leukemia decreases. [68] The role of immunization is still controversial, however, because, as mentioned above, while some authors conclude that immunizations provide protection, others have reported the opposite result. [67,69-74]

2.7. Allergic diseases

The role of allergic diseases (e.g., rhinitis, atopic dermatitis, asthma, and urticaria) as a protective factor for the development of leukemia has been controversial in epidemiological reports. Two hypotheses have been proposed to explain the causal relationship between allergic diseases and cancer, including acute leukemia.

The first hypothesis that we will mention is that of "immune surveillance", which postulates that the immune system can recognize the antigens of malignant cells as foreign and respond to remove them from the body, preventing the potential development of cancer in most cases. Therefore, it is believed that the presence of an allergic disease would increase the surveillance, providing better control and identifying and eliminating any malignant cells, resulting in an increased incidence of malignancy in people who are immunocompromised compared with those with an intact immune system. [75,76]

The second hypothesis refers to a "chronic stimulation of the immune system" that would be conferred by allergens that trigger the carcinogenic potential through both the proliferation of large numbers of immune cells and the increased likelihood of genetic errors caused by pro-oncogenic mutations, which could not be repaired in subsequent divisions. [77-78]

Linabery et al. conducted a meta-analysis to investigate the relationship between allergic diseases and the development of acute leukemia. Three studies reported a positive association in this regard, with an OR of 1.42 (95% CI: 0.60-3.35). Six studies examined whether there was an association between acute lymphoblastic leukemia (ALL) (OR = 0.69; 95% CI: 0.54 to 0.89) and acute myeloid leukemia (AML) (OR = 0.87; 95% CI: 0.62-1.22), but there was heterogeneity among the results. We also performed such a study in asthmatics, and inverse associations were observed between asthma (OR = 0.79; 95% CI: 0.61-1.02), eczema (OR = 0.74; 95% CI: 0.58-0.96) and hay fever (OR = 0.55, 95% CI: 0.46-0.66) and the development of ALL. [79]

2.8. Surgical history

The individual susceptibility of children who suffer from common diseases and recurrences has been considered to be the main factor leading to surgical interventions that are performed as part of the treatment of these infections. Some examples of these treatments are adenoidectomy, tonsillectomy, interventions for ear surgery, and appendectomy. It is worth noting that these anatomical structures are important parts of the lymphatic tissue and immune system, especially during the first two years of life. Thus, their removal would result in immune dysfunction and an increased risk of infections that occur especially during the first year of life, and this mechanism could be involved in the development of acute leukemia during that time. It is for this reason that epidemiological studies that examine infections as an exposure factor in the development of leukemia are controlled by this variable, but there is no epidemiological evidence that surgical interventions studied as a proxy are associated with the development of childhood acute leukemia. [68]

3. Epidemiological studies

Some types of infections that have been evaluated in most epidemiological studies are respiratory tract infections, gastroenteritis, and those caused by specific infectious agents, such as streptococcus and influenza virus. Other diseases that have been considered are exanthematous diseases, allergic diseases (e.g., asthma, acute rhinitis, and atopic dermatitis) and gastrointestinal diseases because these diseases are recurrent during the first year of life. This recurrence would result in the child's immune system performing better when mature, decreasing the risk of aberrant responses to infections that could result in the development of acute leukemia. [80,81] This finding was consistent with that of Perillat et al., who conducted a study in France in a sample of 280 children with acute leukemia (cases) and 288 healthy children (controls). The authors reported that if the child suffered from recurrent infections before 2 years of age, he/she would be protected from the development of acute leukemia, with an OR = 0.6 (95% CI: 0.4-1.0). These results were statistically significant and consistent with those reported by Neglia et al. [21,22,32,68]

However, Schüz et al. (1999) conducted a case-control study in Germany during 1992-1997. They studied 1184 families of children with acute leukemia (cases) and 2588 families of healthy children (controls) and found no association between common infections and an increased incidence of leukemia. It is notable, however, that they reported that when the children had a history of surgical procedures, such as appendectomy/tonsillectomy, at least once in their life, their risk of developing acute leukemia increased, with an OR of 1.4 (95% CI: 1.0-1.9). These authors also observed a significant association with pneumonia, with an OR of 1.7 (95% CI: 1.2-2.3), whereas bronchitis was not associated with the development of acute leukemia, with an OR of 1.1 (95% CI: 0.9-1.4). Moreover, they observed a moderate risk (OR = 1.3; 95% CI: 1.0-1.7) when the children were breastfed for no more than 1 month, specifically in children diagnosed with common ALL. [68]

Neglia et al. performed a case-control study in children under 15 years of age in the U.S. The cases of newly diagnosed ALL were ascertained from the Children's Cancer Group (CCG), and the controls were randomly selected using a random digit-dialing methodology and individually matched to the cases by age, race and telephone area code and exchange between January 1, 1989, and June 15, 1993. They observed a slight decrease in the risk of developing acute leukemia when the child had repeated ear infections during their first year of life, with ORs of 0.86 (95% CI: 0.61-1.22), 0.83 (95% CI: 0.63-1.09) and 0.71 (95% CI: 0.50-1.01) for 1 episode, 2-4 episodes and 5 or more episodes, respectively, and continuous infections were associated with an OR of 0.69 (95% CI: 0.35-1.37; p = 0.026), but these results were not statistically significant. Moreover, it should be noted that these results are similar to a dose-response gradient, as the risk of developing acute leukemia was decreased with an increasing number of infections in the child during the first year of life. This association was more evident in children aged 2 to 5 years with pre-B ALL who presented with ear infections (between 2 and 4 episodes), with an OR of 0.65 (95% CI: 0.43-1.00). No other factor studied was associated with the development of acute leukemia. Furthermore, no association was observed between day care and the development of common acute lymphoblastic leukemia (ALL), with an OR of 1.05 (95% CI: 0.80-1.37). [32]

Using a design similar to that of Perillat et al. (2002) and Neglia et al. (2000), Jourdan-Da et al. evaluated the role of childhood infections in the risk of developing acute leukemia in France. This study included 473 cases of acute leukemia and 567 population-based controls. They found a strong inverse association between gastrointestinal infections and the need to assist the child in day care, with an OR of 0.6 (95% CI: 0.4-0.8). Additionally, a history of asthma decreases the risk of developing leukemia (OR = 0.5; 95% CI: 0.3-0.9). Breastfeeding was not associated with the development of leukemia, but an increasing order of the child's birth increases the risk of developing acute lymphoblastic leukemia, with an OR of 2.0 (95% CI: 1.1-3.7). [15,16,32]

Meanwhile, Rudant et al., also in France, used a case-control design of a National Register (ESCALE) and included 765 incident cases of acute leukemia and 1,681 controls. They observed positive associations when the child presented with recurrent common infections, a history of asthma or a history of eczema, with ORs of 0.7 (95% CI: 0.6-0.9), 0.7 (95% CI: 0.4-1.0) and 0.7 (95% CI: 0.6 -0.9), respectively. Having regular contact with farm animals

http://dx.doi.org/10.5772/52717

(OR = 0.6; 95% CI: 0.5-0.8) and breastfeeding (OR = 0.7; 95% CI: 0.5-1.0) were found to be protective factors for this disease, as was also found in children who had visited farms often in their first year of life, with an OR of 0.4 (95% CI: 0.3-0.6). No significant association was found for assistance of the child in daycare before one year of age (OR = 0.8; 95% CI: 0.6-1.1). One can conclude that repeated infections, such as asthma, play an important role in the etiology of leukemia. [82]

Moreover, Urayama et al., in the USA, conducted two epidemiological studies, namely a case-control study and a meta-analysis. The first study showed that in non-Hispanic white children who attended day care before 6 months of age, the risk of developing leukemia was decreased (OR = 0.90; 95% CI: 0.82-1.00), but this association was not observed in the population of Hispanic children. However, Hispanic children who had ear infections were found to have a decreased risk of developing acute leukemia, with an OR of 0.45 (95% CI: 0.25 to 0.79). Did not report any associations for the other variables studied. In the second study (meta-analysis), these authors evaluated the association between daycare attendance during infancy and the risk of developing acute leukemia; specifically, they wanted to assess whether early exposure to infection protected children from the disease. They concluded that the risk of developing acute leukemia was decreased in children who were exposed to common infections in the first year of life (OR = 0.76; 95% CI: 0.67 to 0.87). [24,25] These findings are consistent with the findings of Perillat et al., Jourdan-Da et al., Dockerty et al., and Ma X et al. [15-19,21,22]

In New Zealand, Dockerty et al. conducted a case-control study that included 121 children diagnosed with acute leukemia and 303 controls (with ages less than 14 years in both groups). They found that exposure to the influenza virus is a risk factor for developing leukemia; that is, a child infected with the influenza virus during the first year of life has a 7-fold risk of developing acute leukemia compared with children who had influenza, with an OR of 6.8 (95% CI: 1.8-25.7). [15,32]

Cardwell et al., using a different epidemiological case-control nested design in a cohort, reported positive evidence of upper respiratory tract infections as a risk factor for the development of acute leukemia (OR = 1.56; 95% CI: 1.08-2.27) and acute lymphoblastic leukemia (OR = 1.59; 95% CI: 1.02-2.49). Similarly, in children presenting with an exanthematous disease, namely chicken pox, we obtained ORs of 2.41 (95% CI: 1.14-5.09) and 2.62 (95% CI: 1.12-6.13) for acute leukemia and acute lymphoblastic leukemia, respectively. [83]

MacArthur et al. conducted a study that included 399 cases and 399 controls who were matched for age and gender and lived in the same area. They evaluated the relationship between vaccination, infectious diseases and common infection and use of medications in children, but their results were not statistically significant, as they found no relationship between childhood diseases and acute leukemia.[84]

Chan et al. performed a population-based, case-control study in China and found that the incidence of roseola and/or fever rash in the first year of life is a protective factor for the development of acute leukemia, with an OR of 0.33 (95% CI: 0.16 to 0.68); however, the risk of developing acute leukemia was increased if the child had a history of tonsillitis in the period 3-12 months before the reference date (OR = 2.56; 95% CI: 1.22-5.38). No association was found between acute leukemia incidence and daycare attendance. In a study similar to that of Chan et al., Roman et al. found that exposure to fungal infections during the first year of life increases the risk of developing acute leukemia, with an OR of 1.4 (95% CI: 1.0-1.9).[14,85]

4. Infections during the first year of life and development of acute leukemia in children with Down syndrome

In the literature, there are few epidemiological studies that have evaluated the effect of early infections and breastfeeding on the development of acute leukemia in children with Down syndrome; however, the results obtained are very interesting. One such study was conducted by Canfield et al. in a population of children diagnosed with acute leukemia between January 1997 and October 2002 (data were obtained from the records of the Children's Oncology Group). The sample group consisted of 158 children with Down syndrome and leukemia, and the control group consisted of 173 children with Down syndrome, all of whom were randomly selected. The results of this study were that children with Down syndrome who had infections during the first 2 years of life had a lower risk of developing acute leukemia, with an OR of 0.55 (95% CI: 0.33 to 0.92), compared with children with Down syndrome who had not been infected. [86,87]

In another study that was conducted in children with Down syndrome in Mexico City, however, this association could not be verified. That study sought to assess whether breastfeeding and infections during the first year of life were associated with the development of acute leukemia. In that study, both breastfeeding and the development of infections during the first year of life in children with Down syndrome were protective factors for the development of leukemia, with ORs of 0.84 (95% CI: 0.43-1.61) and 1.70 (95% CI: 0.82-3.52), respectively, but the results were not statistically significant. Infections requiring hospitalization were also evaluated, and it was found that children >6 years of age had a higher risk of developing acute leukemia, with an OR of 3.57 (95% CI: 1.59-8.05). Thus, these results do not support those of the previously mentioned study or the hypothesis proposed by Greaves that infections are a protective factor for developing acute leukemia. [88]

Author, Year (Country)	Van Steensel et al., 1986 (The Netherlands)	Schüz et al., 1999 (Germany)	Dockerty et al., 1999 (New Zealand)
Design of study	Case-control study (1973-1980)	Two-part case-control study (1980-1994)	Case-control study (1991-1995)
Size of sample	492 cases, 480 controls; Age: 0-14 years	1184 cases, 2588 controls; Age: 0-14 years	121 cases, 303 controls; Age: 0-14 years
Data collection	Mailed questionnaire; addressed to the diagnosed	Telephone interviews with the parents	Mothers interviewed at the home; standardized

			questionnaires and serological tests were conducted
Variables	Breastfeeding; birth order; family size; social class; number of rooms in the household; infections; hospitalization or consultation for infections; primary infections (measles, chicken pox, mumps, or rubella); periods of fever	First-born child; duration of breastfeeding; deficit in social contacts; routine immunizations; infections; tonsillectomy or appendectomy; allergies of the child; allergies of the mother	Social class; marital status; ethnic group; educational level of the parent; home ownership; length of gestation; age of the mother at the child's birth; weight of the child at birth; exposure of the mother to X-rays during the first trimester; exposure of the child to X-rays or radiotherapy before onset of the illness; tobacco smoking by the mother in the first trimester or before the pregnancy
Odds ratios and relevant results	Common colds (RR: 0.8, 95% CI: 0.6-1.0); periods of fever (RR: 0.9; 95% CI: 0.7-1.2); and primary infections (RR: 0.8; 95% CI: 0.4-2.0). These variables were adjusted for birth order, family size, social class, and residential space. Infectious diseases requiring hospitalization (RR: 0.6; 95% IC: 0.4-1.0).	Routine immunizations between 0-3 years of age and having had a tonsillectomy or appendectomy increased the child's risk of developing leukemia (OR: 3.2; 95% CI: 2.3-4.6 and OR: 1.4; 95% CI: 1.1-1.9, respectively), whereas allergies showed a protective effect (OR: 0.6; 95% IC: 0.5-0.8).	A positive association was found between infection caused by influenza during the first year of life and the risk of developing leukemia (OR: 6.8; 95% CI: 1.8-25.7). No other variable was related to acute leukemia.
Author, Year (Country)	Neglia et al., 2000 (USA)	Infante et al., 2000 (Canada)	Rosenbaum et al., 2000 (USA)
Design of study	Case-control study (January 1, 1989-June 15,1993)	Case-control study (1989-1995)	Case-control study (1980-1991)
Size of sample	1842 cases, 1986 controls; Age: <15 years	491 cases, 491 controls; Age: 0-9 years	255 cases, 760 controls; Age: 0-14 years; 31 county regions (cases)
Data collection	Structured interview	Structured questionnaire administered to the mothers by telephone	Standardized questionnaires mailed to the parents
Variables	Interview of the mother; gender; age; race; educational level of the mother; educational level of the father; family income; immunophenotype class.	Educational level of the mother; family income at the time of the child's diagnosis; mother's age; father's age; tobacco use by the mother; infections during the pregnancy; child's birth order; attendance at day care or a nursery; principal feeding method (breast or bottle); length of breastfeeding; history of recurrent infections of the mother; use of antibiotics during pregnancy	Gender; race; educational level of the mother; birth order; feeding status at birth (breast, bottle); age at the diagnosis; day care or preschool program; family outcome; maternal employment during the pregnancy
Odds ratios and relevant results	Neither attendance at nor time remaining in daycare was associated with the risk of developing leukemia. For children with 1-4 episodes of ear infections or sustained infections, the association between infections and	Early attendance at daycare or at a nursery and breastfeeding were protective factors against the development of acute leukemia (OR: 0.49; 95% CI: 0.31-0.77 and OR: 0.68; 95% CI: 0.49-0.95, respectively).	Children who attended day care for >36 months had a lower risk of developing leukemia (OR: 1.32, 95% CI: 0.70-2.52) than those who attended day care for 1-18 months (OR: 1.74; 95% CI:

	the development of acute leukemia was not statistically significant.		0.89-3.42) or for 19-36 months (OR: 1.32; 95% CI: 0.64-2.71).
Author, Year (Country)	Perillat et al., 2002 (France)	Chan et al., 2002 (China)	Jourdan-Da et al., 2004 (France)
Design of study	Case-control study	Population-based, case-control study (November 1994-December 1997)	Case-control study (1995-1998)
Size of sample	280 incident cases, 288 hospital controls	116 cases, 788 controls; Age: 2-14 years; the Hong Kong Pediatric Hematology and Oncology Study Group	473 cases, 567 population-based controls
Data collection	Standardized, face-to-face interviews of the mothers	Standardized, face-to-face interviews	Questionnaire
Variables	Diagnosed categories (acute leukemia classification and immunophenotype); gender; age; ethnic origin; hospital where the case was identified; educational level of the mother; occupation of the mother at the time of the interview; socio-professional categories; place of residence; birth order; number of siblings; daycare attendance; age at the start of daycare; repeated infections before the age of 2 years; incidence of surgical operation for early ear-nose-throat infections before the age of 2 years; breastfeeding	Medical history (infectious illnesses) in the first year of life; breastfeeding; daycare/social contacts of the index patient and siblings; household environment; community environment	Gender; age at the time of diagnosis; region of the residence at the time of diagnosis; socio-professional categories; educational level of the mother; educational level of the father; birth weight; term of pregnancy; birth order; mother's age at birth; Down syndrome; breastfeeding; infections in the first year of life
Odds ratios and relevant results	An inverse association was found between the development of acute leukemia and attendance at daycare (OR: 0.6; 95% CI: 0.4-1.0), repeated (≥4 per year) early common infections before the age of 2 years (OR: 0.6; 95% CI: 0.4-1.0), and surgery for infection of the nose, ear, or throat before the age of 2 years (OR: 0.5; 95% CI: 0.2-1.0). A statistically significant interaction was found between attendance at daycare and repeated common infections.	If the child had rubella and/or fever during the first year of life, the risk was lowered (OR: 0.33; 95% CI: 0.16-0.68). A change of residence during the first year of life presented a lower risk of the child developing leukemia (OR: 0.47; 95% CI: 0.23-0.98), whereas with such a change during the second year, the risk increased (OR: 3.92; 95% CI: 1.47-10.46).	A strong association was found between childhood gastrointestinal illnesses and attendance at daycare and a lowered risk of developing leukemia (OR: 0.6; 95% CI: 0.4-0.8); however, no association was found for breastfeeding. Birth order (4th or later) showed a significant association with an increased risk of acute lymphoblastic leukemia (OR: 2.0; 95% CI: 1.1-3.7), while prior episodes of asthma were associated with a lower risk of developing acute lymphoblastic leukemia (OR: 0.5; 95% CI: 0.3-0.9).
Author, Year (Country)	Rosenbaum et al., 2005 (USA)	Ma et al., 2005 (USA)	Roman et al., 2007 (United Kingdom)
Design of study	Population-based, case-control study (1980-1991)		Population-based, case-control study (1991-1996)

http://dx.doi.org/10.5772/52717

Size of sample	255 cases, 760 controls; Age: 0-14 years	294 incident cases, 376 controls; Age: 0-14 years	455 cases, 1031 controls; Age: 0-14 years
Data collection	Questionnaire	Personal interview of the parents	Interview of the parents
Variables	Gender; race; birth year; mother's educational level; family income; maternal smoking status; infant feeding at birth; birth order; attendance at daycare before 25 months of age; year of diagnosis of leukemia; age at diagnosis of leukemia; allergies; history of allergies; common infections (e.g., colds, otitis media, influenza, croup, bronchiolitis, pneumonia, vomiting, diarrhea)	Age; gender; household income; mother's educational level; mother's age at birth; birth weight; birth order; duration of breastfeeding; day care attendance; infections during infancy	Gender; age; diagnosis of an infectious disease
Odds ratios and relevant results	The results showed that infection late in the first year of the child's life was associated with an increase in the risk of developing leukemia.	Attendance at daycare and infections during infancy were associated with a decrease in the risk of developing acute lymphoblastic leukemia within the white, Hispanic population (OR: 0.42; 95% CI: 0.18-0.99 and OR: 0.32; 95% CI: 0.14-0.74, respectively); corresponding data for the Hispanic population, even for those living in the same area, did not agree.	The cases had more episodes of infection than did the controls, which was more notable in the neonatal period (≤1 month): 18% of the controls and 24% of the cases with leukemia were diagnosed with an average of <1 infection (OR: 1.4; 95% CI: 1.1-1.9; $p < 0.05$). The cases with ≥1 episodes of infection in the neonatal period tended to be diagnosed with acute lymphoblastic leukemia at a relatively young age.
Author, Year (Country)	MacArthur et al., 2007 (Canada)	Cardwell et al., 2008 (United Kingdom)	Urayama et al., 2010 (USA)
Design of study	Population-based, case-control study (January 1,1990 - December 31,1994)	Nested case-control (cohort) study	Case-control study (1995-1999)
Size of sample	399 cases, 399 controls; Age: 0-14 years	62 cases, 2215 matched controls	669 cases, 977 controls; Age: 1-14 years
Data collection	Standardized personal interviews in the child's home	Data-based	
Variables	Gender; age; mother's age; father's age; numbers of live births; annual household income; mother's education; father's education; ethnicity; vaccinations; illness and infections; breastfeeding; allergies; immunosuppressant medication for the child; vitamins; antibiotics for the child	Gender; age; consultations; number of consultations; antibiotic prescriptions; common infections	Gender; mother's age at the child's birth; mother's educational level; annual household income; birth weight; breastfeeding; mother's tobacco use; daycare attendance; history of common infections in the child; ethnicity
Odds ratio and relevant results	No association was found between early infections and acute leukemia; however, vitamin use was associated with a risk of developing acute leukemia (OR; 1.66; (95% CI: 1.18-2.33); the use of	One or more infections in the first year of life reduced the risk of leukemia (OR: 10.5; 95% CI: 0.69-1.59;	When variables were evaluated separately, both attendance at daycare at 6 months of age and birth order reduced the risk of leukemia (OR: 0.90; 95% CI:

	immunosuppressants by the child decreased the risk of leukemia (OR: 0.37; 95% CI: 0.16-0.84); breastfeeding for >6 months had a protective effect against the development of leukemia ($p < 0.05$).	$p = 0.83$) and of acute lymphoblastic leukemia (OR: 1.05; 95% CI: 0.64-1.74; $p = 0.84$).	0.82-1.00 and OR: 0.68; 95% CI: 0.50-0.92, respectively) in a white, non-Hispanic population, but not in a Hispanic population; however, if these children had ear infections, the risk of developing acute leukemia was reduced (OR: 0.45, 95% CI: 0.25-0.79).

Author, Year (Country)	Rudant J et al., 2010 (France)	Urayama et al., 2011 (USA)
Design of study	National registry-based, case-control study ESCALE (2003-2004)	Observational studies (1993-2008)
Size of sample	765 incident cases, 1,681 controls.	14 case-control study
Data collection	Questionnaire, interviews by telephone	Searches of the PubMed database and bibliographies of the publications
Variables	Mother's educational level; parental professional category; place of residence at the time of diagnosis; mother's age at the child's birth; number of children age <15 years in the household; birth order; breastfeeding; duration of breastfeeding; early common infections; surgical operation for ear, nose, or throat infections; history of allergies; contact with animals; farm visits before the age of 2 years	N/A
Odds ratios and relevant results	Negative associations were found for children with repeated common infections (OR: 0.7; 95% CI: 0.6-0.9); with a history of asthma or eczema (OR: 0.7; 95% CI: 0.4-1.0 and OR: 0.7; 95% CI: 0.6-0.9, respectively); with attendance at daycare before 1 year of age (OR: 0.8; 95% CI: 0.6-1.1); and with prolonged breastfeeding (OR: 0.7; 95% CI: 0.5-1.0).	Attendance at daycare is associated with a reduced risk of acute lymphoblastic leukemia (OR: 0.76; 95% CI: 0.67-0.87).

Table 1. Summary of reviewed articles concerning the epidemiology of early infection and acute childhood leukemia.

5. Conclusions

The vast majority of the epidemiological studies conducted thus far on the association between infection during the first year of life and the development of acute leukemia in children have corresponding case-control designs. Additionally, the results of these studies appear to suggest a lower risk of developing acute leukemia among children who were ex-

http://dx.doi.org/10.5772/52717

posed to early infections compared with those who were not exposed. No such association, however, has been reported by other authors; therefore, infections that occur during the first year of life are still considered to be a controversial exposure factor. To achieve better epidemiological evidence, the consistent study of proxy variables in different studies should be performed to enable a better quantification of exposure.

Acknowledgements

This work was funded by the Consejo Nacional de la Ciencia y la Tecnología (CONACYT) through its program, Fondo Sectorial de Investigación en Salud y Seguridad Social (SALUD 2007-1-71223/FIS/IMSS/PROT/592); the Fondo Sectorial de Investigación para la Educación (CB-2007-1-83949/FIS/IMSS/PROT/616) and by Instituto Mexicano del Seguro Social (FIS/IMSS/PROT/G10/846).

Author details

Janet Flores-Lujano, Juan Carlos Núñez-Enríquez, Angélica Rangel-López, David Aldebarán-Duarte, Arturo Fajardo-Gutiérrez and Juan Manuel Mejía-Aranguré*

*Address all correspondence to: arangurejm@hotmail.com

Research Unit in Clinical Epidemiology, Hospital of Pediatrics, National Medical Center 21st Century, Mexican Institute of Social Insurance (IMSS), Mexico City, Mexico

References

[1] Ward, G. The infective theory of acute leukemia. British Journal of Children's Diseases 1917; 14 10-20

[2] Poynton, F.; Thursfield, H. & Paterson, D. The Severe Blood Diseases of Childhood, London XIX. British Journal of Children's Diseases. 1922,128

[3] Kellet, C. Acute myeloid leukemia in one of identical twins. Archives of disease in childhood 1937;12(70) 239-252

[4] Cooke, J. V. The incidence of acute leukemia in children. The Journal of the American Medical Association 1942; 119 547-550

[5] Kinlen, L. Epidemiological evidence for an infective basis in childhood leukaemia. British Journal of Cancer 1995;71(1) 1-5

[6] Kinlen, L.; Dickson, M. & Stiller, C. Childhood leukemia and non-Hodgkin's lymphoma near large rural construction sites, with a comparison with Sellafield nuclear site. British Journal of Cancer 1995;310 763-768

[7] Kinlen, L. Evidence for an infective cause of childhood leukaemia: comparison of a Scottish new town with nuclear reprocessing sites in Britain. Lancet 1998;2(8624) 1323-1327

[8] Greaves, M. Speculations on the cause of childhood acute lymphoblastic leukemia. Leukemia 1988;2(2) 120-125

[9] Greaves, MF & Alexander, FE. An infectious etiology for common acute lymphoblastic leukemia in childhood? Leukemia 1993;7(3) 349-360

[10] Greaves, M.; Colman, S.; Beard, M.; Bradstock, K.; Cabrera, M.; Chen, PM.; Jacobs, P.; Lam-Po-Tan, P.; MacDougall, L. & Williams, C. Geographical distribution of acute lymphoblastic leukemia subtypes: second report of the collaborative group study. Leukemia 1993;7(1) 27-34

[11] Greaves, M. & Alexander, F. Epidemiological characteristics of childhood acute lymphocytic leukemia. Leukemia 1994;8(10) 1793-1794, ISSN 0887-6924

[12] Greaves, M. Science, Medical and the future: Childhood leukaemia. British Medical Journal 2002;2(324) 283-287

[13] Greaves, M. Infection, immune responses and the aetiology of childhood leukemia. Nature Reviews Cancer 2006;6(3) 93-203

[14] Chan, L.; Lam, T.; Li, C.; Lau, Y.; Li, C.; Yuen, H.; Lee, C.; Ha, S.; Yuen, P.; Leung, N.; Patheal, S.; Greaves, M. & Alexander, F. Is the timing of exposure to infection a major determinant of acute lymphoblastic leukaemia in Hong Kong?.Paediatric and Perinatal Epidemiology 2002;16(2) 154-165

[15] Dockerty, J.; Skegg, D.; Elwood, J.; Herbison, G.; Becroft, D. & Lewis, M. Infections, vaccinations, and the risk of childhood leukaemia. British Journal of Cancer, 1999; 80(9) 1483-1489

[16] Jourdan-Da, S.; Perel, Y.; Méchinaud, F.; Plouvier, E.; Gandemer, V.; Lutz, P.; Vannier, J.; Lamagnére, J.; Margueritte, G.; Boutard, P.; Robert, A.; Armari, C.; Munzer, M.; Millot, F.; De Lumley, L.; Berthou, C.; Rialland, X.; Pautard, B.; Hémon, D. &Clavel, J. Infectious diseases in the first year of life, perinatal characteristics and childhood acute leukaemia. British Journal of Cancer 2004; 90(1) 139-145

[17] Ma, X.; Buffler, P.; Wiemels, J.; Selvin, S.; Metayer, C.; Loh, M.; Does, M. &Wiencke, J. Ethnic difference in daycare attendance, early infections, and risk of childhood acute lymphoblastic leukemia. Cancer Epidemiology, Biomarkers & Prevention 2005;14(8) 1928-1934

[18] Ma, X.; Metayer, C.; Does, M. &Buffler, P. Maternal pregnancy loss, birth characteristics, and childhood leukemia (United States). Cancer Causes & Control 2005;16(9) 1075-1083

[19] Ma, X.; Urayama, K.; Chang, J.; Wiemels, J. &Buffler, P. Infection and pediatric acute lymphoblastic leukemia. Blood Cells, Molecules & Diseases 2009;42(2) 117-120

[20] Roman, E.; Simpson, J.; Ansell, P.; Lightfoot, T. & Smith, A. Infectious proxies and childhood leukemia: Findings from the United Kingdom Childhood Cancer Study (UKCCS). Blood Cells, Molecules and Diseases 2009;42(2) 126–128

[21] Perillat, F.; Clavel, J.; Jaussent, I.; Baruchel, A.; Leverger, G.; Nelken, B.; Philippe, N.; Schaison, G.; Sommelet, D.; Vilmer, E. &Hemon, D. Breast-feeding, fetal loss and childhood acute leukemia. European Journal of Pediatrics 2002;161(4) 235-237

[22] Perrillat, F.; Clavel, J.; Auclerc, M.; Baruchel, A.; Leverger, G.; Nelken, B.; Philippe, N.; Schaison, G.; Sommelet, D.; Vilmer, E. &Hémon, D. Day-care, early common infections and childhood acute leukaemia: a multicentre French case-control study. British Journal of Cancer 2002;8(86) 1064-1069

[23] Rosenbaum, P.; Buck, G. &Brecher, M. Early child-care and preschool experiences and the risk of childhood acute lymphoblastic leukemia. American Journal of Epidemiology 2000;152(12) 1136-1144

[24] Urayama, K.; Buffler, P.; Gallagher, E.; Ayoob, J. & Ma, X. A meta-analysis of the association between day-care attendance and childhood acute lymphoblastic leukaemia. International Journal of Epidemiology 2010;39(3) 718–732

[25] Urayama, K.; Ma, X.; Selvin, S.; Metayer, C.; Chokkalingam, A.; Wiemels, J.; Does, M.; Chang, J.; Wong, A.; Trachtenberg, E. &Buffler, P. Early life exposure to infections and risk of childhood acute lymphoblastic leukemia. International Journal of Cancer 2011;128(7) 632-643

[26] Githens, J.; Elliot, F. & Saunders, L. The relation of socioeconomic factors to incidence of childhood leukemia. Public Health Reports 1965;80 573–578

[27] Alexander, F.; Cartwright, R.; McKinney, P. & Ricketts, T. Leukaemia incidence, social class and estuaries: an ecological analysis. Journal of Public Health Medicine, 1990;12(2) 109–117

[28] Draper, GJ. The Geographical Epidemiology of Childhood Leukaemia and Non-Hodgkin Lymphomas in Great Britain, 1966–83, OPCS Studies on Medical and Population Subjects No. 53 1991. London: OPCS; (ed).

[29] Stiller, C. & Boyle, P. Effect of population mixing and socioeconomic status in England and Wales, 1979–85, on lymphoblastic leukaemia in children. British Medical Journal 1996;313 1297–1300

[30] Borugian, M.; Spinelli, J.; Mezei, G.; Wilkins, R.; Abanto, Z. & McBride, M. Childhood leukemia and socioeconomic status in Canada. Epidemiology 2005;16(4) 526–531

[31] Van Steensel, H.; Valkenburg; H. & van Zanen G. Childhood leukemia and infectious diseases in the first year of life: a register-based case-control study. American Journal of Epidemiology 1986;124(4) 590-594

[32] Neglia, J.; Linet, M.; Shu, X.; Severson, R.; Potter, J.; Mertens, A.; Wen, W.; Kersey, J. & Robison, L. Patterns of infection and day care utilization and risk of childhood acute lymphoblastic leukaemia. British Journal of Cancer 2000;82(1) 234-240

[33] Infante, C.; Fortier, I. & Olson E. Markers of infection, breast-feeding and childhood acute leukemia. British Journal of Cancer 2000;83,(11) 1559-1564

[34] Fedrick, J &Alberman, ED. Reported influenza in pregnancy and subsequent cancer in the child. British Medical Journal, 1972;27(2) 485-488

[35] Kaatsch P, Scheidemann-Wesp U, Schüz J. Maternal use of antibiotics and cancer in the offspring: results of a case-control study in Germany. Cancer Causes Control 2010 21(8) 1335-1345.

[36] Van Steensel-Moll, H.; Valkenburg, H.; Vandenbroucke, J. & van Zanen, G. Are maternal fertility problems related to childhood leukaemia? International Journal of Epidemiology 1985;14(4) 555-559

[37] Thapa, P.; Whitlock, J.; Brockman-Worrell, K.; Gideon, P.; Mitchel, E Jr.; Roberson, P.; Pais, R. & Ray, W. Prenatal Exposure to Metronidazole and Risk of Childhood Cancer A Retrospective Cohort Study of Children Younger than 5 Years. Cancer 1998;83(7), 1461-1468

[38] Gilman, E.; Wilson, L.; Kneale, G. & Waterhouse, J. Childhood cancers and their association with pregnancy drugs and illnesses. Paediatric and Perinatal Epidemiology 1989;3(1) 66-94

[39] Rodvall, Y.; Pershagen, G.; Hrubec, Z.; Ahlbom, A.; Pedersen, N. &Boice, J. Prenatal X-ray exposure and childhood cancer in Swedish twins. International Journal of Cancer 1990;46(3) 362-365

[40] vanDuijn, C.; van Steensel-Moll, H.; Coebergh, J. & van Zanen, G. Risk factors for childhood acute non-lymphocytic leukemia: An association with maternal alcohol consumption during pregnancy? Cancer Epidemiology, Biomarkers & Prevention 1994;3(6) 457-460

[41] Roman, E.; Ansell, P. & Bull, D. Leukaemia and non-Hodgkin's lymphoma in children and young adults: are prenatal and neonatal factors important determinants of disease? British Journal of Cancer 1997;76(3) 406–415

[42] Naumburg, E.; Bellocco, R.; Cnattingius. S.; Jonzon, A. &Ekbom, A. Perinatal exposure to infection and risk of childhood leukemia. Medical and Pediatric Oncology 2002;38(6) 391-397

[43] Wen, W.; Shu, X.; Potter, J.; Severson, R.; Buckley, J.; Reaman, G. & Robison, L. Parental medication use and risk of childhood acute lymphoblastic leukemia. Cancer 2002;95(8) 1786-1794

[44] Alexander, F.; Patheal, S.; Biondi A.; Brandalise, S.; Cabrera, M.; Chan, L.; Chen, Z.; Cimino, G.; Cordoba, J.; Gu, L.; Hussein, H.; Ishii, E.; Kamel, AM.; Labra, S.; Magalhães, I.; Mizutani, S.; Petridou, E.; de Oliveira, M.; Yuen, P.; Wiemels, J. & Greaves, M. Transplacental chemical exposure and risk of infant leukemia with MLL gene fusion. The Journal of Cancer Research 2001;61(6) 2542-6

[45] Shaw, A.; Infante-Rivard, C. & Morrison, H. Use of medication during pregnancy and risk of childhood leukemia (Canada). Cancer Causes Control 2004;15(9) 931-937

[46] McKinney, P.; Juszczak E.; Findlay E.; Smith K. & Thomson, C. Pre- and perinatal risk factors for childhood leukaemia and other malignancies: a Scottish case control study. British Journal of Cancer 1999;80(11) 1844-51

[47] Field, C. The immunological components of human milk and their effect on immune development in infants. The Journal of Nutrition 2005;13(1) 1-4

[48] Macías, S.; Rodríguez, S.; &Ronayne, P. Leche materna: composición y factores condicionantes de la lactancia. ArchivosArgentinos de Pediatría 2006;104(5) 423-430

[49] Parker, L. Breast-feeding and cancer prevention. European Journal of Cancer 2001;37(2) 55-8

[50] Riveron, R. Valor inmunológico de la leche materna. Revista Cubana de Pediatría1995;67(2) 1-16

[51] Altinkaynak, S.; Selimoglu, M.; Turgut, A.; Kilicaslan, B. &Ertekin, V. Breast-feeding duration and childhood acute leukemia and lymphomas in a sample of Turkish children. Journal of Pediatric Gastroenterology and Nutrition 2006;42(5) 568-572

[52] Bener, A.; Denic, S. &Galadari, S. Longer Breast-feeding and protection against childhood leukaemia and lymphomas. European Journal of Cancer 2001;37(2) 234-238

[53] Beral, V.; Fear, N.; Alexander, F. & Appleby, P. Breastfeeding and childhood cancer. UK Childhood Cancer Study Investigators. British Journal of Cancer 2001;85(11) 1685-1694

[54] [54] Davis, K. Review of the evidence for an association between infant feeding and childhood cancer. International Journal of Cancer supplement 1998;11 29-33

[55] Guise, J.; Austin, D. & Morris C. Review of case-control studies related to breastfeeding and reduced risk of childhood leukemia. Pediatrics 2005;116(5) 724-731

[56] Ip, S.; Chung, M.; Raman, G.; Chew, P.; Magula, N.; DeVine, D.; Trikalinos, T. & Lau, J. Breastfeeding and maternal and infant health outcomes in developed countries. Evidence Report/Technology Assessment 2007;153 1-186

[57] Kwan, L.; Buffler, P.; Abrams, B. &Kiley, V. Breastfeeding and the risk of childhood leukemia: a meta-analysis. Public Health Reports 2004;119(6) 521-535

[58] Kwan, M.; Buffler, P.; Wiemels, J.; Metayer, C.; Selvin, S.; Ducore, J. & Block, G. Breastfeeding patterns and risk of childhood acute lymphoblastic leukaemia. British Journal of Cancer 2005;93(3) 379-384

[59] Shu, X.; Clemens, J.; Zheng, W.; Ying, D.; Ji, B. & Jin, F. Infant breastfeeding and the risk of childhood lymphoma and leukaemia. International Journal of Epidemiology 1995;24(1) 27-32

[60] Shu, X.; Linet, M.; Steinbuch, M.; Wen, W.; Buckley, J.; Neglia, J.; Potter, J.; Reaman, G. & Robison, L. Breast-feeding and risk of childhood acute leukemia. Journal National Cancer Institute 1999;91(20) 1765-1772

[61] Stuebe, A. The risks of not breastfeeding for mothers and infants. Reviews in Obstetrics and Gynecology 2009;2(4) 222-231

[62] Cushing, A.; Samet, J.; Lambert, W.; Skipper, B.; Hunt, W.; Young, S. & McLaren, L. Breastfeeding reduces risk of respiratory illness in infants. American Journal of Epidemiology 1998;147(9) 863-870

[63] Lancashire, R.; Sorahan, T. & OSCC. Breastfeeding and childhood cancer risks: OSCC data. British Journal of Cancer 2003;88(7) 1035-1037

[64] Paricio, J.; Lizán, M.; Otero, A.; Benlloch, M.; Beseler, B.; Sánchez, M.; Santos, L. & Rivera, L. Full breastfeeding and hospitalization as a result of infections in the first year of life. Pediatrics 2006;118(1) e92-e99

[65] Menegaux, F.; Olshan, A.; Neglia, J.; Pollock, B. &Bondy, M. Day care, childhood infections and risk of neuroblastoma. American Journal of Epidemiology 2004;159(9) 843-851

[66] Gilham, C.; Peto, J,; Simpson J, Roman E, Eden TO, Greaves MF, Alexander FE; UKCCS Investigators. Day care in infancy and risk of childhood acute lymphoblastic leukaemia: findings from UK case-control study. British Medical Journal 2005;330(7503) 1294

[67] Kneale, G.; Stewart, A. & Wilson, L. Immunizations against infectious diseases and childhood cancers. Cancer immunology, immunotherapy 1986;21(2) 129–132

[68] Schüz, J.; Kaletsch, U.; Meinert, R.; Kaatsch, P. &Michaelis, J. Association of childhood leukaemia with factors related to the immune system. British Journal of Cancer 1999;80(3-4) 585-90

[69] Haro, AS. The effect of BCG-vaccination and tuberculosis on the risk of leukemia. Developments in biological standardization, (Part A), 1986;58 433-449

[70] Hartley, A.; Birch, J.; McKinney, P.; Blair, V.; Teare, M.; Carrette, J.; Mann, J.; Stiller, C.; Draper, G. & Johnston, H. The Inter-Regional Epidemiological Study of Childhood Cancer (IRESCC): past medical history in children with cancer. Journal of Epidemiology and Community Health 1988;42(3) 235–242

[71] Nishi, M. & Miyake, H. A case-control study of non-T cell acute lymphoblastic leukaemia of children in Hokkaido, Japan. Journal of Epidemiology & Community Health 1989;43(4) 352–355

[72] Buckley, J.; Buckley, C.; Ruccione, K.; Sather, H.; Waskerwitz, M.; Woods, W. & Robison, L. Epidemiological characteristics of childhood acute lymphocytic leukemia. Analysis by immunophenotype. The Children's Cancer Group. Leukemia 1994;8 856–864

[73] Petridou, E; Trichopoulos, D; Kalapothaki, V; Pourtsidis, A; Kogevinas, M; Kalmanti, M; Koliouskas, D; Kosmidis, H; Panagiotou, J; Piperopoulou, F. &Tzortzatou, F. The risk profile of childhood leukemia in Greece: a nationwide case-control study. British Journal of Cancer 1997;76(9) 1241–1247

[74] Petridou, E.; Dalamaga, M.; Mentis, A.; Skalkidou, A.; Moustaki, M.; Karpathios, T; Trichopoulos, D. & Childhood Haematologists-Oncologists Group. Evidence on the infectious etiology of childhood leukemia: the role of low herd immunity (Greece). Cancer Causes & Control 2001;12(7) 645-52

[75] Markiewicz MA, Gajewski TF. The immune system as anti-tumor sentinel: molecular requirements for an anti-tumor immune response. Critical Reviews in Oncogenesis. 1999;10(3):247-260

[76] Rosenbaum, P.; Buck, G. &Brecher, M. Allergy and infectious disease histories and the risk of childhood acute lymphoblastic leukaemia. Paediatric and Perinatal Epidemiology 2005;19(2) 152-164

[77] Eriksson, N.; Mikoczy, Z, &Hagmar, L. Cancer incidence in 13811 patients skin tested for allergy. Journal of Investigational Allergology& Clinical Immunology 2005;15(3) 161-166

[78] Turner, M.; Chen, Y.; Krewski, D. &Ghadirian, P. International journal of cancer. Journal international du cancer. International Journal of Cancer 2006;118(12) 3124-32

[79] Linabery, A.; Jurek, A.; Duval, S. & Ross, J. The association between atopy and childhood/adolescent leukemia: a meta-analysis. American Journal of Epidemiology 2010;171(7) 749-64

[80] McNally, R. & Eden, T. An infectious aetiology for childhood acute leukaemia: a review of the evidence. British Journal of Haematology 2004;127(3) pp.243-263,

[81] McNally, R.; Cairns, D.; Eden, O.; Alexander, F.; Taylor, G.; Kelsey, A. & Birch, J. (2002). An infectious aetiology for childhood brain tumours?. Evidence from space-time clustering and seasonality analyses. British Journal of Cancer 2002;86(7) 1070-1077

[82] Rudant, J.; Orsi, L.; Menegaux, F.; Petit, A.; Baruchel, A.; Bertrand, Y.; Lambilliotte, A.; Robert, A.; Michel, G.; Margueritte, G.; Tandonnet, J.; Mechinaud, F.; Bordigoni, P.; Hémon, D. &Clavel, J. (2010). Childhood acute leukemia, early common infections, and allergy: The ESCALE Study. American Journal of Epidemiology 2010;172(9) 1015-1027

[83] Cardwell, C.; McKinney, P.; Patterson, C. & Murray, L. Infections in early life and childhood leukaemia risk: a UK case-control study of general practitioner records. British Journal of Cancer 2008;99(9) 1529-33

[84] MacArthur, A.; McBride, M.; Spinelli, J.; Tamaro, S.; Gallagher, R. &Theriault, G. (2008). Risk of childhood leukemia associated with vaccination, infection, and medication use in childhood: the Cross-Canada Childhood Leukemia Study. American Journal of Epidemiology 2008;167(5) 598-606

[85] Roman, E.; Simpson, J.; Ansell, P.; Kinsey, S.; Mitchell, C.; McKinney, P.; Birch, J.; Greaves, M.; Eden, T. & United Kingdom Childhood Cancer Study Investigators. Childhood acute lymphoblastic leukaemia and infections in the first year of life: A report from the United Kingdom Childhood Cancer Study. American Journal of Epidemiology 2007;165(5) 496–504

[86] Canfield, K.; Spector, L.; Robison, L.; Lazovich, D.; Roesler, M.; Olshan, A.; Smith, F.; Heerema, N.; Barnard, D.; Blair, C. & Ross, J. Childhood and maternal infections and risk of acute leukaemia in children with Down syndrome: a report from the Children's Oncology Group. British Journal of Cancer 2004;91(11) 1866-18872

[87] Ross, J.; Spector, L.; Robison, L. &Olshon, A. Epidemiology of leukemia in children with Down syndrome. Pediatric Blood & Cancer 2005;44(1) 8-12

[88] Flores, J.; Pérez, M.; Fuentes, E.; Gorodezky, C.; Bernaldez, R.; Del Campo, M.; Martínez, A.; Medina, A.; Paredes, R.; De Diego, J.; Bolea, V.; Rodríguez, M.; Rivera, R.; Palomo, M.; Romero, L.; Pérez, P.; Alvarado, M.; Salamanca, F.; Fajardo, A. &Mejía, J. Breastfeeding and early infection in the aetiology of childhood leukaemia in Down syndrome. British Journal of Cancer 2009;101(5) 860-864

Section 4

Prognostic of ALL

Chapter 9

Genetic Markers in the Prognosis of Childhood Acute Lymphoblastic Leukemia

M.R. Juárez-Velázquez, C. Salas-Labadía,
A. Reyes-León, M.P. Navarrete-Meneses,
E.M. Fuentes-Panana and P. Pérez-Vera

Additional information is available at the end of the chapter

http://dx.doi.org/10.5772/54288

1. Introduction

Acute leukemia is a broad term used to identify several malignancies of immature hematopoietic cells. Although, variable incidences have been reported between countries, ranging from 46 to 57 cases by million children, it is considered the most common childhood cancer worldwide [1]. Acute lymphoblastic leukemia (ALL) is the most frequent subtype (75%-80% of cases; with the remaining 20-25% being of myeloid origin, AML). In ALL, B cell origin is the most frequently diagnosed (B cell ALL) representing 83%, and T cell ALL comprises 15% [2]. The total of ALL cases represents 30-40% of all types of pediatric cancer[3].

One of the major achievements in cancer therapy has been the increased cure rates for ALL, from 10% in the 60s to 76-86% today, although these favorable numbers are mainly valid for developed countries[4,5]. The improvement in ALL cure rates can be in part attributed to the assessment of conventional prognostic factors and identification of molecular markers associated with a better response to therapy. Suitable risk stratification has permitted a more personalized treatment, selecting patients for receiving standard or intensified therapy, alone or in combination with drugs against ALL specific targets, and together with an enhanced supportive care have contributed to the increase in the event-free survival (EFS) rates[4]. Conventional childhood ALL stratification is based on prognostic factors related to characteristics of the patient (age at diagnosis) and the disease itself white blood cell (WBC) count at diagnosis, immunophenotype of the leukemic cells, presence of known genetic fusions, numerical abnormalities or abnormal gene expression, and early response to therapy (evaluated by morphological methods or using a more accurate measurement such as minimal residual disease (MRD) analysis) [4–6].

From a genetic point of view, ALL is one of the best characterized malignancies. Numerical and structural chromosomal abnormalities have been described by cytogenetic methods, fluorescence *in situ* hybridization (FISH), polymerase chain reaction (PCR), and more recently, by next generation sequencing. Chromosomal abnormalities are clonal markers of the ALL blast, since the cytogenetic and molecular analyses have revealed that approximately 75% of ALL-children present these genetic lesions [7,8]. To date, more than 200 genes have been found participating downstream of common ALL translocations [9]; interestingly, a handful of these genes are consistently affected in many subtypes of the disease paving the way to better understand homeostatic lymphopoiesis and the leukemogenic process [10].

2. Signaling and transcription factors important in lymphopoiesis and leukemogenesis

Generation of lymphoid cells is a highly ordered multi-step process that in adult mammals starts in bone marrow with the differentiation of multipotent hematopoietic stem cells (HSC) (Figure 1A). HSCs start a differentiation pathway in which the capacity to form multiple lineages is gradually lost coinciding with a gain of lineage specific functions. Thus, HSCs yield multipotent progenitor cells (MPPs) still with myeloid and lymphoid potential, which eventually give rise to lymphoid-primed multipotent progenitor (LMPP) and early lymphoid progenitor (ELP) populations, with a progressive more restrictive lymphoid program. Similarly, ELPs generate early T lineage progenitors (ETP) and common lymphoid progenitors (CLP), and these populations, although still exhibit high plasticity, preferentially give rise *in vivo* to T and B cells, respectively [11,12]. Intrinsic signaling and transcriptional programs shape this differentiation pathway guiding lineage decisions. When these developmental programs are abnormally activated or repressed, can induce the leukemogenic process.

B and T cells are characterized by their potential to express receptors with a highly diverse repertoire of specificities: the B and T cell receptors (BCR and TCR). This diverse specificity is given by a recombination process termed VDJ recombination and it is the sequential assembly and testing of the BCR and TCR what defines the B/T development pathway. The first stages (pro and pre) are characterized by recombination of the antigen binding variable sequences (heavy and light chains for the BCR, and the β, α, γ or δ chains for the TCR) (Figure 1B). The subsequent stages require elimination of auto-reactive clones, and only clones selected against self-recognition become functional mature cells. Genetic and biochemical studies have shown that all forms of the BCR and TCR are required for progression through several defined developmental checkpoints [13,14]. This is an important concept, since it illustrates that different signaling and transcription programs are operating through all developmental stages, and therefore, if an aberrant program is established, development is unable to proceed. As we will see in the following sections, the leukemic gene fusions and other genetic abnormalities produce aberrant signaling pathways or abnormal transcriptional activities, leading to a developmental arrest in specific stages, events that seem to be required and characterize B and T cell ALL.

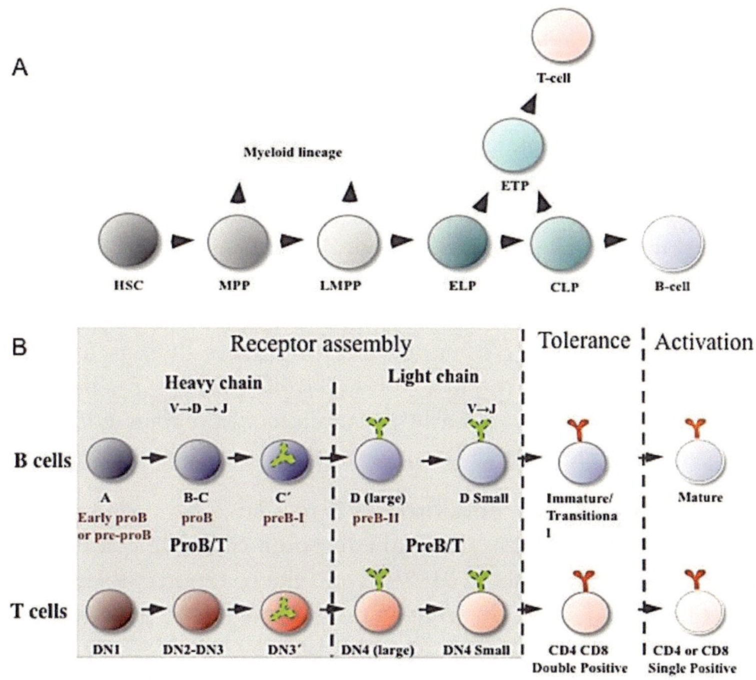

Figure 1. Schematic drawing of the early hematopoietic development. A) HSCs (hematopoietic stem cells), MPPs (multipotent progenitors), LMPPs (lymphoid-primed MPPs), ELPs (early lymphoid progenitors), CLPs (common lymphoid progenitors), ETPs (early T lineage progenitors). Important branch points during lineage decisions are shown with arrows. B) All B- and T-cell stages can be divided according to the main processes guiding development: receptor assembly, tolerance, and activation. Receptor assembly stages (light gray box) in B and T cells are differentiated by the process of VDJ recombination in the heavy (IgH) and light (IgL) chains, which are recombined in the pro-B and pre-B stages, respectively (b and a rearrangement in DN1-3 and DN4 abT cells). B cells only rearrange heavy and light chains, while T cells can follow two different pathways of TCR chains, ab and gd. Intimate contact between immature B /DP T cells and the stromal cells of the bone marrow and thymus allows those receptors capable of recognizing self-antigens to be identified and eliminated through a variety of mechanisms collectively termed "tolerance". Non-self-reactive cells transit to the mature stage where they become functional cells that could be activated and respond to foreign antigens. The nomenclature of each sub-stage in the mouse model is shown in black letters, e.g. A-D for B cells and DN1–4 for T cells; the most common human nomenclature is shown in red letters. The dashed lines separating all stages indicate checkpoints at which signaling from the pre-BCR/TCR and BCR/TCR is required for positive selection and progression along the maturation pathway. The preBCR, preTCR, and mature receptors are also illustrated in their respective stages. B cell development occurs in bone marrow and T cell development in the thymus.

Early developmental stages are the ones generally found compromised in human pediatric B and T cell ALL. These stages in B cell ALL are early proB or pre-proB (before heavy-chain recombination), preB-I (after heavy-chain recombination), and preB-II (before light-chain rearrangement) (Figure 1B). These stages are also recognized by the expression of stage specific markers, a characteristic that has helped to classify the different types of pediatric ALL. B cells are recognized by the expression of CD19 and CD10, common B cell ALL by the expression of the BCR (IgM) either in cytoplasm (preB-I) or membrane (preB-II), and preB-I can also be differentiated from preB-II cells by expression of the enzyme terminal deoxynucleotidyl transferase (TdT) [10].

T cells are recognized by the expression of CD3, CD5 and CD7. Early T cells lack expression of CD4 and CD8 (double negative or DN stages). Contrary to B cell ALL, T cell ALL clones often express markers of more advanced stages of development (for instance double positive stages). However, these clones also show a lack of expression or cytoplasmic TCRβ, indicating that transformation happened before rearrangement of this TCR component or just after, and thus arguing that transformation targeted ETP/DN1 or DN3′cells [15]. The acquisition of markers of more mature cells is probably due to marker aberrant expression or leukemia-induced developmental progression in absence of the TCR signal. Although, postnatal B cell early maturation only happens in bone marrow, T cells mature in thymus. LMPP, ELP, CLP and ETP cells are all able to leave bone marrow in response to environmental signals and complete the T cell maturation program in thymus. Therefore, ETP/DN1 cells are normal residents of bone marrow, while double positive T cells are only found in thymus. T cell transformation of very early populations also agrees with the predominant presence of the T cell leukemic clone in bone marrow [15].

Limitation of lineage choice during development is regulated by a combination of signaling pathways and transcription factors. The main receptor controlling the proB stage is the IL-7R, which is composed of an α chain (IL-7Rα) and the common cytokine receptor G chain (GC) [16,17]. Deletion of IL-7Rα or GC leads to developmental arrest at the early proB stage [18–21]. IL-7 activates three major signaling pathways: 1) JAK–STAT, 2) phosphatidylinositol 3-kinase (PI3K)–Akt and 3) Ras-Raf-Erk [22]. STAT5 (signal transducer and activator of transcription 5) is the predominant STAT protein activated by IL-7 [22,23] and STAT5 loss also arrest B cells at the early proB stage. Once the preBCR is expressed, it can take over many of the functions performed by the IL-7 receptor, since the preBCR also activates the PI3K-Akt and Ras-Raf-Erk pathways [24,25].

Downstream of IL-7 two transcription factors have been documented as the most important for cell entry into the B cell lineage: E2A/TCF3 (immunoglobulin enhancer binding factors E12/E47/transcription factor 3) and EBF1 (Early B cell Factor 1) [26–28]. On the other hand, PAX5 (Paired box 5) is the more important transcription factor for B cell commitment. Loss of E2A and EBF1 blocks entry into the B cell lineage, and loss of PAX5 redirects B cells into other lineages [28–30]. One of the main molecular functions of PAX5 (acting together with E2A, EBF1 and STAT5) is to allow VDJ recombination [31,32]. Ectopic expression of PAX5 and E2A allows VDJ recombination in non-B cells [45, 46]. Also, E2A, PAX5, IKZF1 and RUNX1, among other transcription factors, are responsible for expression of the VDJ recombinase (RAG) [33,34].

The most important cells that give rise to T cells are ELPs and CLPs. Although, both B and T cells are mainly originated from them, an important genetic difference between cells prone to the B lineage is the expression of EBF1 and PAX5, while for T cells is NOTCH1 signaling. NOTCH1 directs progenitors into the thymus and it is the master orchestrator of T cell lineage entry and development [35,36]. NOTCH contains multiple epidermal growth factor (EGF)-like repeats through which it binds its ligands DLL-1, -2, -4 (Delta-like ligand), and Jagged-1 and -2 expressed by bone marrow and thymus stromal cells. Upon ligand binding NOTCH1 initiates a series of proteolytic cleavage events, the first one catalyzed by the

http://dx.doi.org/10.5772/54288

ADAM family of metalloproteinases and the second by the γ–secretase complex. This cleavage activates NOTCH1 removing the extracellular portion and translocating to the nucleus its intracellular region (ICN), where it becomes part of a large transcriptional activation complex together with CSL and histone acetylase p300. Also, ICN has a C-terminal PEST domain involved in regulation of NOTCH1 ubiquitylation and proteasome-mediated degradation, therefore controlling protein turnover [35–38].

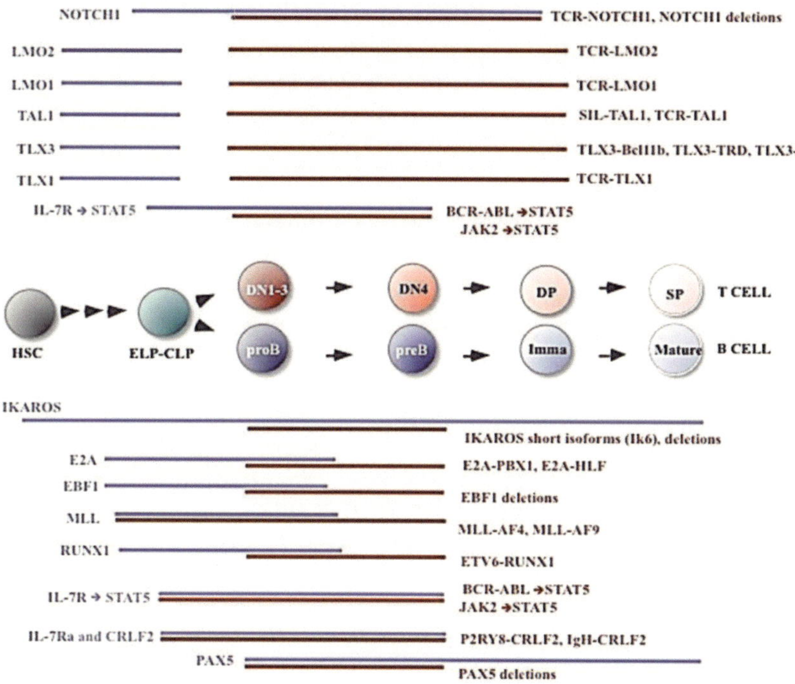

Figure 2. Schematic drawing of homeostatic and leukemic expression of acute leukemia inducing genes. Normal (in blue) and leukemic (in red) expression of receptors, signaling proteins and transcription factors is shown along the B and T cell development pathways. Homeostatic factors are shown to the left of the figure and their most common modified forms in ALL are shown to the right; the upper part showing the ones compromised in T cells and the bottom part in B cells. Developmental stages are indicated starting with the hematopoietic stem cell (HSC) and then with the early lymphoid progenitor (ELP) and the common lymphoid progenitor (CLP) and further into the T and B cell pathways. Of note, the proB and preB stages are the ones usually compromised in B cell ALL; in T cell ALL, marker expression is indicative of double positive stages but TCR recombination status shows that leukemic stages most probably belong to double negative stages. Therefore, the red line representing abnormal leukemic expression extends from DN to DP stages in T cell development. Also, several of the transcription factors compromised in T cell ALL are not normally expressed in these stages but ectopically expressed through the inducing genomic lesion.

NOTCH1 expression is importantly regulated by E2A [39], and is essential for activation of genes necessary for T cell entry and early development. Indeed, NOTCH1 expression is turned off in late stages of T cell development, forced expression of NOTCH1 in multipotent progenitor cells direct them to the T cell lineage and controls the expression of several transcription factors important for T cell early development, e.g. *HES1, Bcl11b, GATA3, TCF1, Pu1* and *RUNX1*, among many more [38]. Many of these genes are required to turn off transcriptional programs of multipotent progenitor cells or other hematopoietic lineages, or for T cell specific functions such as recombinase expression or TCR recombination.

Some of the transcription factors drivers of T cell ALL are normally expressed in non-malignant thymocytes since they are essential regulators of T-cell ontogeny, while others are not expressed in normal ones, but they are rather ectopically expressed by transformed cells (Figure 2). This is contrary to B cells, in which most of the transcription factors associated with transformation fulfill an important regulatory function (Figure 2). This observation supports different mechanisms for the origin of B and T cell ALL. In agreement, *TLX1, TLX3, TAL1, LMO1* and *LMO2* gene loci remain open during TCR recombination, increasing the probability of aberrant rearrangements [39,40]. The identification of the signaling proteins and transcription factors compromised in B and T cell ALL has helped us to understand normal B and T cell development and its oncogenic counterpart, and as we will emphasize in the following sections, they have also provided an important tool to classify patients with specific genetic characteristics into risk groups matching disease prognosis.

3. Criteria for ALL risk stratification

The clinical and laboratory criteria supporting risk stratification vary among institutions, with most groups considering as high risk the following characteristics: age ≥ 10 or <1 years at presentation, WBC ≥ 50,000/μl, presence of extramedullary disease, T cell immunophenotype, presence of adverse genetic abnormalities such as t(9;22) (*BCR-ABL1*), *MLL* gene rearrangements, hypodiploidy <44 chromosomes and near haploidy. Finally, a poor response to therapy resulting in ≥ 5% bone marrow blasts at days 15, 19, 29, 35 or 43 post-treatment is also considered of bad prognosis [6].

All the above-mentioned prognostic factors are used to classify patients into two risk groups, high and standard risk. For instance, it is known that increased WBC count confers poor prognosis for B cell ALL patients and in T cell ALL, a leukocyte count greater than 100,000/μl is associated with high risk of relapse in the central nervous system. Also, patients with hyperleukocytosis, greater than 400,000/μl, are at high risk of central nervous system hemorrhage and pulmonary and neurological events due to leukostasis. However, most of these risk criteria are better understood for B cell and they are not as clear for T cell ALL patients [3]. Recently, evaluation of early response to therapy has been demonstrated being an important parameter for treatment efficacy and disease prognosis. Based on the latter criteria, it is possible to identify the group of patients that require augmented therapy to improve their outcome.

3.1. Prognostic significance of treatment response

The frequency of bone marrow or circulating lymphoblasts after one week of chemotherapy is associated with risk for relapse [41] and nowadays, this constitutes one of the most useful prognostic factors in childhood ALL. An efficient early response to treatment is determined by evaluating clearance rates of leukemic cells after the induction phase of treatment [42].

This pharmacological response depends on numerous variables, including drug sensitivity / resistance of the leukemic cells, the dosage and the ability of individual patients to metabolize and eliminate anti-leukemic drugs [43,44].

The Berlin-Frankfurt Munster (BFM) group has traditionally employed the response to prednisone for 7 days and one dose of intrathecal methotrexate to stratify patients. Peripheral blood blast count of 1,000/µl after prednisone treatment is used as a threshold to assign patients into two groups, prednisone good responders (GR) and poor responders (PR). The ALL-BMF Group demonstrated in large series of infant patients treated with effective risk-based ALL therapy that prednisone response is a strong prognostic parameter for outcome; 75% of infants were good responders (GR) and achieved an EFS of 53% at 6 years using conventional therapy, whereas poor responder infants had an EFS of 15% [41]. The Tokyo Cancer Children´s Leukemia Group also showed that B and T cell ALL patients with high blast counts at day 8, had a 4 years EFS of 74%; in contrast, patients without blasts presented an EFS of 89% for B and 95% for T cell ALL [43]. Thus, it is well accepted that early response to prednisone treatment is a strong indicator of EFS [41]. However, this assessment is limited by the low sensitivity (5-10% blasts) of microscopy-based methods of blast quantification [45]. The morphological analysis of blasts by conventional methods easily underestimates the presence and frequency of residual cells. PCR or flow cytometry- based methods for detecting MRD are at least 100 times more sensitive.

The common principle for all MRD assessments is that leukemogenic process results in molecular and cellular changes, which distinguish leukemic cells from their normal counterparts [46]. In patients with ALL, MRD can be monitored by flow cytometry, PCR amplification of gene fusion transcripts, and PCR amplification of the B and T cell antigen receptors (BCR/TCR specific VDJ recombinants). Combining information about cell size, granularity and expression of surface and intracellular molecules, it is possible to identify by flow cytometry a phenotypic signature characteristic of leukemic cells. Flow cytometry-based identification of cell immunophenotypes allows the detection of one leukemic cell among 10,000 normal cells (0.01%) [47,48]; however, these assays require high expertise for quality results, previous knowledge of immunophenotypic profiles of normal and leukemic cells and experience to select the best markers useful for each patient [49]. Other option to distinguish leukemic from normal cells is the PCR screening of gene fusion transcripts, produced by specific chromosomal translocations, among the most common of them are: *BCR-ABL1, MLL-AF4, E2A-PBX1* and *ETV6-RUNX1* [50]. These genetic abnormalities can be detected by PCR with high sensitivities ranging from 0.1- 0.001% [51]. Clonal rearrangements of the BCR and TCR genes are also useful tools for detecting MRD. Specific VDJ rearrangements result in unique molecular signatures that can be detected by real-time quantitative PCR, with a sensitivity of 0.01-0.001% [52]. The applicability of this latter method is useful in 90% of cases, however, a leukemic blast can be associated with more than one VDJ rearrangement during disease progression; for this reason, it is recommended to use at least two different rearrangements as a target for each patient [53].

MRD studies revealed that many patients who achieve remission by traditional methods harbored residual disease predisposing them to relapse [46,48]. The most immediate application of MRD testing is the identification of patients who are candidates for treatment intensification, since levels of MRD are proportional to the risk of relapse [51]. The most appropriate time for evaluation of MRD vary between different groups, for the ALL-BMF 95 protocol in Austria, MRD quantification by flow cytometry of bone marrow samples must be estimated on days 33 and 78 post-treatment. In the experience of St. Jude Children's Research Hospital, the presence of 0.01% residual cells on days 19, 46, or subsequent time points during treatment, is strongly associated with a high risk of relapse [54,55]. The Children's Oncology Group quantifies MRD in bone marrow on day 29 post-treatment, and ≥ 0.01% of MRD is associated with poor outcome [56]. The Dana-Farber Cancer Institute ALL Consortium, considers MRD cut-off values of 0.1% for prediction of 5-year relapse hazard [57]. Recently, the Italian cooperative group AIEOP identified 3 risk groups based on MRD values by flow cytometry of bone marrow samples on day 15 of treatment. Those risk groups are: standard (<0.01% MRD) with a 5-years cumulative incidence of relapse (CIR) of 7.5%, intermediate (0.01% - <10% MRD) with CIR of 17.5%, and high (>10% MRD) with CIR of 47.2% [58]. MRD is also useful as an independent predictor of second relapse in patients with ALL who had a previous relapse and achieved a second remission [59,60]. Notably, the time of first relapse and MRD are the only 2 significant predictors of outcome in a multivariate analysis [60].

3.2. Genetic abnormalities in ALL as prognostic factors

From a genetic point of view, ALL is one of the best characterized malignancies. Numerical and structural chromosomal abnormalities have been described by cytogenetic methods, FISH, PCR, and more recently, by next generation sequencing. Chromosomal abnormalities are clonal markers of the ALL blast, since the cytogenetic and molecular analyses have revealed that approximately 75% of ALL-children present these genetic lesions [7]. To date, more than 200 genes have been found participating, downstream of common ALL translocations. Interestingly, a handful of these genes are affected by more than one translocation, thus supporting specific mechanisms of leukemogenesis [9].

The genetic abnormalities found in ALL are basically of two types: 1) gains or losses of one or several chromosomes (numerical abnormalities) and 2) translocations generating gene fusions that encode proteins with novel functions (chimeric proteins), or that re-locate a gene close to a strong transcriptional promoter causing gene overexpression. These translocations are produced by double-strand breaks (DSB) in different chromosomes or different regions of one chromosome, that are then recombined through non-homologous end-joining mechanisms [9,61]. These events of illegitimate recombination result in juxtaposition of normally separated regions, relocating a gene or producing a chimeric fusion gene [3].

Several studies have demonstrated that the first genetic lesion in childhood ALL often occurs in uterus. Screening of many of the genetic lesions that characterize the ALL blast in blood samples from Guthrie cards supports their prenatal origin. These studies have shown the presence of the same gene fusion in blood samples collected at birth and in the leukemic blasts at diagnosis. Thus, an intrauterine origin of *MLL-AF4* has been observed in 100% of the studied cases, *ETV6-RUNX1* in 75% of cases, *E2A-PBX1* in 10% of cases and a numerical

http://dx.doi.org/10.5772/54288

abnormality, hyperdiploidy, in 100% of patients in one study [9]. However, it is accepted that for all mentioned cases this first oncogenic hit is not sufficient, and additional postnatal mutational events are required for disease initiation [62].

The known ALL genetic abnormalities have been relevant for the identification of genes involved in cancer and therefore for the insights in the biology of the leukemogenic process. Importantly, these genetic abnormalities are a disease signature that has been an invaluable tool for the precise disease diagnosis, prognosis and stratification into risk groups, guiding patient management and treatment choice [63]. The Third International Workshop on Chromosomes in Leukemia was the first major study demonstrating the independent prognostic significance of cytogenetic findings in ALL, providing data on clinical relevance of chromosomal recurrent aberrations, and elucidating its molecular basis and biologic consequences [64]. Given their importance, it is the main goal of this chapter to describe in detail the most important genetic abnormalities in the stratification of ALL patients, highlighting aspects of their oncogenic mechanisms, incidence and prognosis.

4. Molecular and cytogenetic subgroups in pediatric B cell ALL

As it was previously mentioned, several genetic abnormalities are characteristic of ALL and have been relevant for the identification of genes involved in cancer and therefore have given insights into the biology of the leukemogenic process, plus they have been an invaluable tool for the precise disease diagnosis, prognosis and stratification into risk groups. Several of them will be discussed in the coming sections.

4.1. *BCR-ABL1* fusion

The *BCR-ABL1* fusion is generated by a reciprocal translocation between sequences of the *BCR* (Breakpoint cluster region; do not confuse with the B cell receptor) gene located at 22q11.23, and the *ABL1* (Abelson tyrosine-protein kinase 1) gene located at 9q34.1. This translocation generates a derivative chromosome 22 known as the Philadelphia (Ph) chromosome, and was first observed in adult patients with chronic myeloid leukemia (CML), but later also in approximately 3-5% of pediatric ALL patients. The *BCR* gene contains 23 exons and encodes a 160 kD phosphoprotein of still unclear function. However, its first exon, which is normally present in the BCR-ABL1 protein, contains a serine/threonine kinase activity and SH2 binding sites [65]. On the other hand, *ABL1* is a proto-oncogene that encodes a cytoplasmic and nuclear protein tyrosine kinase implicated in cell differentiation, cell division, cell adhesion, and stress response [66,67]. The *BCR-ABL1* fusion produces a chimeric protein with cytoplasmic localization and oncogenic potential because retains the catalytic domain of ABL1 fused to the BCR domain, which mediates constitutive oligomerization of the fusion protein in the absence of physiologic activating signals, thereby promoting aberrant tyrosine kinase constitutive activity, inducing aberrant signaling and activating multiple cellular pathways [3,68–70]. Among the signaling pathways activated contributing to leukemogenesis are JAK2 kinase/STAT5, MAP kinases and PI3K/Akt, which includes several members of the Bcl-2 family of anti-apoptotic proteins.

The Ph chromosome detected in CML varies from the one in ALL, with different *BCR* breakpoints between diseases. Two chimeric proteins with different leukemogenic potential are encoded, one of 210 kDa prevalent in CML and other of 190 kDa prevalent in childhood ALL [70,71]. *In vitro* studies showed that the 190kDa BCR-ABL exhibits a greater tyrosine kinase activity than the 210kDa form. Thus, this fusion defines one of the subgroups of ALL with the worst clinical prognosis, mainly because it leads to genetic instability through the reduction in DNA repair fidelity and by generation of reactive oxygen species, that enhance spontaneous DNA damage in tumor cells that can yield the accumulation of additional genetic mutations [72,73].

Ph positive childhood ALL is associated with older age at presentation, high leukocyte count, French-American-British (FAB) L2 morphology, and high incidence of central nervous system. Age at ALL presentation influences the prognosis of this genetic rearrangement; patients with ages ranging from one to nine years have a better prognosis than adolescents and young adults [70,74]. Thus, Ph positive is associated with a very high risk and poor prognosis. Although more than 95% of patients achieve an adequate response to induction therapy, these remissions are shallow and short-lived [6]; additionally, these patients frequently present high levels of MRD at the end of the induction therapy [75]. Ph positive ALL incidence varies among different cohorts (Table 1), ranging between 2-3% for Western European countries (Germany, Italy, Austria, Britain, Switzerland) [76–78], 1-4% for American countries (USA and Mexico) [4,79] and 7-15% for Eastern countries (China, Taiwan, Malaysia-Singapore) [63].

Intensive research efforts were done to demonstrate the BCR-ABL1 transforming activity *in vitro* and *in vivo*, as well as to describe the downstream signaling pathways and transcriptional programs affected by this translocation. These studies led to the development of successful targeted therapy with small-molecule tyrosine kinase inhibitors (TKI), such as STI571 (Imatinib mesylate, Gleevec®, Novartis Pharmaceuticals, Basel, Switzerland). This TKI has successfully been used for treatment of Ph positive CML patients [69,87] and has also permitted a better management of ALL patients. Remissions have been achieved when Imatinib has been used either as single agent or as part of combination regimens. In accordance with COG ALLL0031 trial (2002-2006), patients who received a regimen that included Imatinib achieved a 3-year EFS of 80%, which was more than the double of the EFS rate of patients treated without this agent. Although the number of treated patients was small in this study, it supported that the addition of Imatinib to intensive chemotherapy can improve the outcome of Ph positive ALL children [74,87]. Genomic studies have identified a subtype of pediatric B cell ALL Ph negative patients with a gene-expression profile similar to *BCR-ABL1* positive ones, it is thought that these "*BCR-ABL1* like" disease harbors mutations that deregulate cytokine receptor and tyrosine kinase signaling, this subset of B cell ALL patients might also be benefited by the TKI therapy [87]. "*BCR-ABL1* like" group will be mentioned in a following section.

Genetic abnormalities	Frequency in different populations (%)									Clinical implication
	Europe		America				Asia			
	UK Medical Research Council ALL97/99 [77]	ALL-BFM90 [78,80]	UKCCG [81]	StJChRH [82]	Hispanics [83]	Mexico [84]	India [4]	China [85]	Malaysia-Singapore [86]	
Numerical changes										
Hyperdiploidy >50 chromosomes	38	-	31	25	41	31	-	24	-	Excellent prognosis with anti-metabolite treatment
Hypodiploidy <44 chromosomes	-	-	-	1-2	<1	-	-	-	-	Poor prognosis
Structural changes										
t(1;19)(q23;p13) *E2A-PBX1*	4	2	-	5	5 *E2A-PBX1* or *E2A-HLF*	5	7	5	4	Improved prognosis with high-dose methotrexate treatment
11q23 rearrangements *MLL*	2	3	2	8	2	9	0	3	5	Poor prognosis
t(9;22) (q34;q11.2) *BCR-ABL1*	3	2	2	2	1	4	5	17	7	Improved early treatment outcome with imatinib
t(12;21) (p13;q22) *ETV6-RUNX1*	25	22	21	25	13	9	7	19	13	Excellent prognosis with asparaginase

-, non described

Table 1. Frequency of numerical and structural changes among B-ALL patients of different cohorts

4.2. *E2A-PBX1* fusion

The *E2A-PBX1* fusion results from the balanced translocation t(1;19)(q23;p13) or the unbalanced derivative der(19)t(1;19), that involve *E2A* (previously described as the Immunoglobulin enhancer binding factors E12/E47, also named *TCF3*) and *PBX1* (Pre-B cell leukemia transcription factor 1) genes. *E2A* encodes two basic helix-loop-helix (bHLH) transcription factors, E12 and E47, through alternative splicing. Both transcription factors are immunoglobulin enhancer binding proteins involved in the regulation of immunoglobulin gene expression [34] and in the initiation and specification of the B cell lineage [29]. *PBX1* also encodes a transcription factor (Leukemia Homeobox 1), a member of the three amino acid loop extension (TALE) family of homeodomain proteins. PBX1 forms heterodimers with HOX family homeodomain proteins and together with them cooperatively regulates transcription of several target genes according to the HOX partner [88,89]. PBX1 regulates the self-renewal potential of HSC by maintaining their quiescence state; additionally, it modulates early stages of B-cell development. PBX1 is also important for the multi-linage potential of human embryonic stem cells (hESC) [90].

E2A-PBX1 fusion results in chimeric proteins that contain the transcriptional activation domain of E2A linked to the DNA-binding domain and HOX heterodimerization domain of PBX1. The resulting oncogenic transcription factor inappropriately activates the expression of genes normally regulated by the PBX1-HOX heterodimers [3,91]. Among the transcriptional targets of E2A-PBX1 are *WNT16* and *MerTK*. Since the WTN family is widely recognized to be involved in oncogenesis, it is possible that *E2A-PBX1* initiates the leukemogenic process through its potent expression of WNT16 [10,92]. MerTK is a receptor with a coupled tyrosine kinase activity that regulates self-renewal of bone marrow precursor cells, and although MerTK is not normally expressed in committed lymphocytes, high level expression is detected in B and T cell ALL and mantle cell lymphomas [93,94].

According to studies in different populations (Table 1), *E2A-PBX1* translocation is present in approximately 2-6% of pediatric ALL cases; however its incidence among the specific pre-B ALL subtype (the one with cytoplasmic or membrane IgM) is approximately 25% [64,95,96]. The Total Therapy Study XIIIB at St Jude Children's Research Hospital reported an incidence of 4.7%, with 5-year EFS of 80-90% [4,97]. On the other hand, the reported incidences for European countries, such as Great Britain, Germany, Italy, Austria and Switzerland, is between 2.1 and 4%, while the reported incidences for Eastern countries (Malaysia, Singapore and China) range from 4.12 to 5.37%. *E2A-PBX1* has barely been detected in Guthrie cards of B cell ALL patients, which suggests that in most cases emerges postnatally [9]. Also, the molecular breakpoints of the *E2A-PBX1* fusion in IgM positive or IgM negative cases are generally dissimilar suggesting different origins of the disease [3,98].

Clinical features of pre-B ALL positive for *E2A-PBX1*, include 5 year age at presentation, WBC count of 21-28,000/μl and pseudodiploid karyotypes [64,87,99]. Risk stratification for *E2A/PBX1* patients is controversial. It is considered of poor prognosis in adult cases, while in children it has been reported either relatively favorable or of poor prognosis. This could be explained in part by treatment differences; although it was initially considered of an unfavorable outcome, rate cures have been improved with the use of more effective therapies, such as dosage intensification with methotrexate [64,82]. Future treatment improvements could be achieved based on the discovery of pathways for treatment resistance of *E2A-PBX1* positive cells. It has been shown that *MerTK* is activated by GAS6 (Growth arrest specific 6) produced in bone marrow by mesenchymal cells, which are part of the HSC supporting

http://dx.doi.org/10.5772/54288

stroma. One of the important functions regulated by GAS6 is HSC self-renewal and it is possible that the leukemic blast becomes resistant to conventional chemotherapy due to GAS6 induced quiescence. Similar to BCR-ABL1 targeted therapy, GAS6-MerTK interaction might be an important target for directed therapy [94].

Another translocation involving the *E2A* gene in ALL is t(17;19)(q22;p13), present in 1% of children, which produces the fusion of *E2A* to *HLF* (Hepatic leukemia factor). *HLF* is a member of the bZIP family of transcription factors and the E2A-HLF fusion protein contains the transcriptional activation domain of E2A linked to the DNA-binding and protein-protein interaction motifs of HLF. The resulting chimeric protein most probably activates the transcription of genes normally regulated by HLF. It is suggested that E2A-HLF inhibits apoptosis through the aberrant up-regulation of SLUG and LMO2, which are anti-apoptotic factors in normal hematopoietic progenitor cells [10,100].

4.3. *MLL* translocations

Myeloid/lymphoid or Mixed lineage leukemia gene (*MLL, MLL1, ALL1, TRX,* and *HTRX*) is the human homologue of the *Drosophila melanogaster* trithorax gene; it is located at 11q23 and consists of 36 exons. It encodes a 430 kDa DNA binding protein that positively regulates *HOX* gene expression through methylation of lysine 4 of histone 3 (H3K4) [101]. MLL is a large multi-domain protein, the N-terminus contains three short AT-hook motifs (ATH 1–3), which are thought to mediate DNA binding. There are two speckled nuclear localization sites (SNL1 and SNL2) immediately C-terminal to the ATH motifs that are followed by a transcriptional repression domain consisting of two functional subunits, RD1 and RD2. RD1 contains a DNA methyltransferase (DMT) homology domain with a CxxC zinc-finger motif that might recruit transcriptional repressors. RD2 recruits histone deacetylases HDAC1 and HDAC2. There is also a plant homology domain (PHD) zinc-finger motif that might mediate protein-protein interactions and a C-terminal SET (Su(var)3-9, enchancer-of-zeste, trithorax) domain that possesses histone H3 lysine 4 (H3K4) methyltransferase activity [95]. Despite RD1 and RD2, MLL is thought to be primarily a transcriptional activator due to its methyltransferase activity and to the transcriptional activation domain, which recruits the transcriptional co-activator CBP (CREB-binding protein). MLL is thought to be a master gene for epigenetic transcriptional memory regulation.

MLL in its mature form consists of two non-covalently associated subunits, an N-terminal 320 kDa fragment (MLL_N) and a C-terminal 180 kDa moiety (MLL_C), which are both core components of the MLL complex and result from the cleavage of nascent MLL by an aspartic protease named taspase 1. The MLL_N fragment is thought to bind DNA regulatory regions of clustered *HOX* genes as part of a multi-subunit complex that includes components of the basal transcription machinery and mediate transcriptional repression of *HOX* genes. However, in the presence of MLL_C, the MLL_N complex can lead to transcriptional activation. The MLL_C subunit contains the SET motif and associates with at least four proteins that modify chromatin for efficient transcription through methylation, acetylation and nucleosome remodeling processes [101,102]. *MLL* gene is ubiquitously expressed in haematopoietic cells including stem and progenitor populations, and *HOX* genes are direct targets of MLL during development [7,95,102]. Also, MLL is a key constituent of the mammalian DNA damage response pathway, and it is reported that deregulation of the S-phase checkpoint mediated by *MLL* aberrations contributes to the pathogenesis of human *MLL* positive leukemias [103].

Most *MLL* translocations initiate within a well-characterized 8.3 kb breakpoint cluster region that encompasses exons 5-11. This region is AT-rich, contains Alu, LINE, and MER repetitive sequences, putative DNA topoisomerase-II cleavage recognition sites, as well as a scaffold and matrix attachment region (SAR/MAR); these elements have been proposed to play a direct or indirect role in promoting 11q23 rearrangements [104]. The proposed mechanisms that yield *MLL* translocations include recombination of Alu elements, recombination mediated by topoisomerase-II poisons, and an error prone non-homologous end joining (NHEJ) of DSB [101,104]. *MLL* fusions are diverse, since it has been found in more than 70 different translocations with numerous partner genes. The most frequent are *AF4, AF9, ENL, AF10, ELL* and *AF6*. *MLL-AF4* results from the translocation t(4;11)(q21;q23) that is commonly found in patients younger than one year of age (infant ALL), while *MLL-AF9* is generated by the translocation t(9;11)(p22;q23) that is more frequently seen in secondary, therapy-induced malignancies. Although infrequent, other type of rearrangement involving *MLL* is the partial tandem amplification [7].

All *MLL* fusions encode proteins that share a common transcriptional regulator function capable of regulating HOX genes expression. Some of the *MLL* fusion partners are themselves chromatin modifiers that function in histone acetylation, whereas other fusion partners can recruit histone methyl-transferases, such as DOT1; methylation at lysine 79 of histone H3 catalyzed by DOT1 has been recognized as a hallmark of chromatin activated by MLL fusion proteins [7,102,104]. MLL fusion proteins efficiently transform hematopoietic cells into leukemic cells with stem cell-like self-renewal properties [7].

MLL translocations define subgroups of high risk ALL with specific clinical and biological characteristics associated to adverse prognosis. These subgroups include infant acute leukemia (IAL), therapy-related leukemia (a subtype of leukemia developed by patients previously treated with etoposide after a cancer episode) and T cell ALL [102]. *MLL* translocations are found in approximately 10% of all human leukemias including ALL, AML and biphenotypic (mixed lineage) leukaemia, this latter one is characterized by the expression of both myeloid and lymphoid antigens such as CD14 and CD19 in the leukemic blast [7,102]. *MLL* translocations are particularly frequent (70-80%) in high risk IAL.

MLL-AF4 is one of the leukemia-inducing genetic rearrangements documented to emerge *in utero* during fetal hematopoiesis. Concordant *MLL-AF4* positive leukemia studies in identical monozygotic twins demonstrated that both siblings share the same breakpoints, although the disease usually presents at different times in each twin [105]. Moreover, *MLL-AF4* can be detected in archived neonatal blood from Guthrie cards in IAL or in ALL patients. This evidence coupled with the short period of latency observed in patients that develop IAL, strongly suggests that some leukemia-driving gene fusions can be acquired prenatally [9,62,95]. These observations have raised the question if *in utero* exposition to specific environmental mutagens can induce *MLL* breakage and anomalous recombination events. *In vitro* and *in vivo* assays have identified bioflavonoids, hormones and insecticides

http://dx.doi.org/10.5772/54288

as potential inductors of *MLL* aberrations [80,106–110]. Additionally, the best-known inductor of *MLL* aberrations is etoposide, which is a DNA topoisomerase-II inhibitor commonly used as a chemotherapeutic agent. Etoposide induced genetic aberrations might be due to increased concentrations of DNA topoisomerase-II DNA cleavage complex. 11q23 rearrangements, particularly those that generate *MLL-AF9* fusions, are found in 5-15% of secondary therapy-related leukemias [104,107,111–113].

As mentioned before, the frequency of *MLL* rearrangements in IAL, particularly the *MLL-AF4* fusion, is approximately 80%; however, this frequency diminishes in older children with ALL. *MLL* rearrangements incidences reported from American countries ranged from 2.2-3.3%, while for European countries (Germany, Italy, Austria, UK and Switzerland) was between 2.1-6%. The incidence of *MLL* rearrangements in Eastern countries (China, Taiwan, Malaysia and Singapore) also ranged from 2.1-4.9%. The estimated 5-year EFS for patients with *MLL* translocations ranged between 30-40% [4] and therefore it is considered of very bad prognosis.

4.4. *ETV6-RUNX1* fusion

RUNX1 (Runt-related transcription factor 1 and also known as *AML1* or *CBFα2*) is a gene that maps in 21q22.3. *RUNX1* encodes a transcription factor that contains a Runt domain essential for interaction with transcription factor CBFβ and for DNA binding [114]. The RUNX1-CBFβ heterodimer is a master regulator of early hematopoietic genes transcription. *ETV6* (E-Twenty-Six, also named *TEL*), is localized in 12p13.1, belongs to the *ets* transcription factor family, and contains two major domains: ETS and helix-loop-helix (HLH). ETV6 participates in fetal hematopoiesis of all lineages [115,116]. A substantial proportion (7-25% of children and 2% of adults, Table 1) of ALL patients present the *ETV6/RUNX1* fusion as a result of the translocation t(12;21)(p13;q21). The chimeric protein from this fusion contains the N-terminal region of ETV6 fused to almost all RUNX1, including the Runt domain. The ETV6 fragment losses the DNA binding domain but retains the protein binding domain that interacts with cellular proteins with transcriptional repression activity, N-CoR and mSin3a, producing stable repression complexes at the promoters of RUNX1 target genes. mSin3a transcriptional repressor function is due to a histone deacetylase activity(HDAC) [10] but the ETV6-RUNX1 fusion has additional repressor functions through sequestration of transcriptional complexes and competitive inhibition of the wild-type ETV6 activity [10,116].

Several abnormalities secondary to *ETV6-RUNX1* fusion have been detected, such as *ETV6* loss, *ETV6/RUNX1* duplication and extra copies of *RUNX1* originated by trisomy 21. Recently, it has been described that *ETV6* loss occurs postnatally in more mature cells than the *ETV6-RUNX1* fusion. Analysis of this deletion revealed an unexpected similarity with SINE and LINE retrotransposons, suggesting their participation in this loss of heterozygosity-like mechanism of ETV6 loss. These findings are consistent with Greaves′ double hit model of leukemogenesis for this subtype of ALL [117].

ETV6/RUNX1 positive patients have been defined as a group with excellent outcome at 5 years follow-up, which cannot be identified by standard prognostic features [118,119]. In several studies based on different populations, this subgroup represented about 25% of cases with B cell precursor immunophenotype [120]; and this genetic marker could also be found in T cell ALL [81]. Other studies support different incidence rates for *ETV6/RUNX1* fusions depending on ethnicity and geographic origin [83,85,121,122] (Table 1). In particular, the lowest frequencies have been described for Hispanic [83,121] and Oriental patients [85,123], compared to patients from West Europe and the United States. Given this difference, further studies should be conducted looking for environmental and genetic etiologic factors, including exposure to leukemogenic agents, analysis of predisposition genes associated to ALL and genetic ancestry in different populations.

Several studies have supported that *ETV6-RUNX1* positive patients have an excellent outcome in clinical trials after treatment with corticosteroids, vincristine, and asparaginase [82]. Nevertheless, *ETV6/RUNX1* has been considered as a non-significant prognostic factor in other studies, since this fusion has been found in relapsed patients [124,125]. In spite of their excellent initial treatment response, and favorable short-term outcome, up to 24% of patients relapse [124], and this usually occurs in patients out of treatment, often several years after cessation of treatment and occasionally as long as 10 to 20 years later [125]. Efforts have been made for obtaining a better understanding about the origin of relapses in this group of ALL patients. Analyses of copy number abnormalities (CNAs) have provided evidence that *ETV6-RUNX1* positive patients have an average of 6 CNAs at diagnosis, with increasing abundance of these CNAs at relapse, and the genes involved in CNAs usually include cell cycle regulator genes [125,126].

The clonal origin of relapse has been investigated comparing CNA profiles from matched *ETV6/RUNX1* positive patients at diagnosis and relapse. Genes associated with cell cycle control (cyclin-dependent kinase inhibitors *CDKN2A, CDKN2B, CCNC)* were found deleted in relapsed patients. As a novel finding, trisomy 16 was observed as a recurrent abnormality, although its significance is presently unknown [125]. A model of abnormalities acquisition from diagnosis to relapse has been proposed; mutations detected recurrently or known to be involved in a leukemogenic pathway were classified as driver mutations, while mutations defined as non-recurrent or without a known function in leukemogenesis were considered passenger mutations. Four genetic profiles have been proposed with this analysis: 1) diagnosis and relapse clones with the same abnormalities; 2) relapse clones with acquired extra driver mutations; 3) relapse clones with losses and gains of driver mutations and 4) relapse clones without all original CNAs but with a novel profile of genetic alterations [125]. At least 3 of these groups support that clones present at diagnosis are responsible for relapses occurring months or years after treatment cessation. In one patient with a remission lasting 119 months a backtracking FISH analysis was performed, and a low number of leukemic subclone was identified at presentation whose genotype matched that observed in the relapse clone. This patient showed clonal diversity at diagnosis and the relapse subclone probably remained due to active mechanisms of chemotherapy resistance and quiescence. The authors suggested that this case of relapse represents an effect of a dormant clone with low proliferative capacity and associated drug insensitivity rather than a mutation-induced resistance effect [125]. This patient might exemplify the genetic variation sometimes observed between initiating and relapse clones. Thus, this study argues that evolutionary genetic changes between the leukemic blast at presentation and relapse most probably are due to the frequency and intrinsic genetic characteristics of the relapsed clone.

More recently, it has been shown that genes associated with glucocorticoid mediated apoptosis could be deleted in *ETV6/RUNX1* relapsed patients. One of the most altered genes is the Bcl2 modifying factor (BMF), whose deletion is often detected at diagnosis and relapse. The glucocorticoid receptor NR3C1, and genes of the mismatch repair pathways are also deleted, but this was only observed at relapse. All these genes participate in apoptosis induced by gluococorticoids, supporting that a drug resistance mechanism could contribute to the episode of leukemia relapse, e.g. *BMF* deletions leading to survival of a specific leukemic clone after gluococorticoid treatment [126]. This information is relevant for future evaluation of *ETV6/RUNX1* patients and perhaps this genetic lesion should be diagnosed in ALLs together with BMF, NR3C1 and other CNAs as a guide for novel treatment approaches.

4.5. Hyperdiploidy

Hyperdiploidy with 51-65 chromosomes is also a frequent abnormality, 25-41% of ALL patients present this numerical aberration [10,83,85] and are generally associated with a favorable outcome (Table 1). This includes age 3-5 years and relative low WBC count at presentation, B cell precursor immunophenotype [127] and a 5-year EFS estimate of 85-95% when patients are treated with anti-metabolite based therapy [4,127]. Leukemic lymphoblasts in this subgroup have a high propensity to undergo apoptosis *in vitro* and *in vivo*, and accumulate greater quantities of methotrexate and its active polyglutamate metabolites than other ALL subgroups. These features are probably very important for the associated good prognosis of this subtype of ALL.

High hyperdiploidy can be detected by cytogenetic analysis or flow cytometry. This latter technique measures the DNA content of the leukemic blasts in comparison to the normal cell pool and DNA content of 1.16 is considered as a prognostic indicator of favorable outcome. However, it is recommended to perform additional cytogenetic studies to detect specific chromosome gains, and discard the presence of additional genetic rearrangements, which could also influence disease outcome. About 50% of hyperdiploid cases present additional abnormalities as duplications of 1q or isochromosome 17q, this last abnormality confers adverse prognosis [128]. High hyperdiploidy is often characterized cytogenetically by massive aneuploidy, originating a non-random gain of specific chromosomes, including some or all of +X, +4, +6, +10, +14, +17, +18, and +21; trisomies and tetrasomies of other chromosomes are also present in this group of patients [127].

In spite of the excellent prognosis associated to this genetic subtype, about 25% of the patients develop adverse events, indicating outcome differences and genetic subgroups between high hyperdiploid patients. For this reason, diverse studies have been performed trying to identify prognostic characteristics in these ALL patients. Based on cytogenetic studies and survival analyses, specific trisomies have been found associated to prognosis. Results from univariate analyses informed that gain of individual chromosomes 6, 4, 10 and 18 improves prognosis, in contrast, trisomy 5 confers worse prognosis

[129–131]. Currently, the Children's Cancer Group (CCG) and the Pediatric Oncology Group (POG) consider the presence of simultaneous trisomies of chromosomes 4, 10, and 17 as a favorable prognostic factor [132].

Analysis by SNP array of high hyperdiploid patients have been performed and revealed that 80% presented CNAs, which are not detected by traditional cytogenetic methods. An association between duplication of 1q and +5 has often been observed, and also uniparental isodisomies of chromosomes 9 and 11, gains of chromosomes 17q and 21q, deletions and microdeletions of *ETV6*, cyclin-dependent kinase inhibitor 2A (*CKDN2A*), *PAX5* and PAN3 poly(A) specific ribonuclease subunit homolog (*PAN3*). Interestingly, partial deletions of AT rich interactive domain 5B (*ARID5B*) were also detected [127] and polymorphisms of this gene were recently associated to susceptibility for developing ALL, particularly associated with the high hyperdiploid subtype [133].

ALL cases with 47-50 chromosomes have an intermediate prognosis [71], near-triploidy (69 to 81 chromosomes) [134] have a response to therapy similar to that of non-hyperdiploid, and ALL cases with near tetraploidy (82 to 94 chromosomes) have a high frequency of T cell immunophenotype (see T cell ALL section) and frequently harbors a cryptic ETV6-RUNX1 fusion [135]. These tetraploid leukemias, although significantly less common, have a worse prognosis than the ones with 51-65 chromosomes. The genetic reason for this differential prognosis is presently unclear.

4.6. Hypodiploidy

The hypodiploid ALL is defined as leukemic blasts with less that 46 chromosomes and it is present in 6-7% of patients with childhood ALL. Three different subgroups have been defined according to the number of chromosomes, which are also important for disease outcome: near-haploid ALL (less than 30 chromosomes), low hypodiploid ALL (33-39 chromosomes) and high hypodiploid ALL (42-45 chromosomes). Near-haploidy is observed approximately in 0.5% of ALL cases and it is most frequently associated with females, and together with low hypodiploidy is related with the worst prognosis. Also, children with near-haploidy tend to be younger than those with low hypodiploidy [134,136]. Most of the hypodiploid ALL patients belong to the high hypodiploid group.

The pattern of chromosome loss in near-haploidy is not random as there is preferential retention of two copies of chromosomes 6, 8, 10, 14, 18, 21, and the sex chromosomes. In rare cases, an apparent hyperdiploid genome is observed but the number of chromosomes results from doubling haploid or near-haploid chromosome content. In these cases, although there is an increased in the total number of chromosomes, this ALL is still characterized by losses of specific chromosomes. This ALL is frequently wrongly diagnosed without a careful cytogenetic and DNA content analysis [136], and an appropriate diagnosis is important as near-haploidy defines a rare type of ALL associated with short remission duration and poor prognosis. Therefore, a clear diagnosis of the total chromosome number is essential to stratify patients into the appropriate risk group.

http://dx.doi.org/10.5772/54288

5. Molecular and cytogenetic subgroups in pediatric T-cell ALL

T cell ALL is a neoplastic disorder characterized by malignant transformation of early thymocytes [37]. It accounts for approximately 10-15% of pediatric ALL cases [2,37,137–139] and tends to present clinically with high circulating blast cell counts, mediastinal masses, and often central nervous system involvement [37,140]. Therefore, it is a high risk ALL with a relapse rate of about 30% within the first 2 years following diagnosis [15,139]. T cell ALL is caused by genetic alterations leading to a variety of changes that can affect cell cycle control, unlimited self-renewal capacity, impaired differentiation and loss of sensitivity to death signals [37]. As previously described, T cell ALL shares some chromosome rearrangements with B cell ALL; however, about 50% of T-ALL patients have recurrent chromosomal translocations specific of this subtype. The most common chromosome abnormalities include rearrangements affecting the *TCR* regulatory elements: juxtaposing promoter and enhancer elements from the *TCRA/D* locus (T-cell receptor α/δ, 14q11) and *TCRB* (T-cell receptor β, 7q34) to developmentally important transcription factor genes such as homeobox genes (*TLX1, TLX3*); helix-loop-helix genes (*TAL1/SCL, TAL2, LYL1*) or LIM-domain genes (*LMO1, LMO2*) (Table 2) [15,37,139–142]. Other important genetic abnormalities frequently targeted during malignant transformation of T cells are interstitial deletion on *TAL1/SCL* and *NOTCH1* point mutations (Table 2). Translocations not involving *TCR* loci have also been described, relevant examples are the gene fusion *CALM-AF10* and the episomal recombination between *NUP214* and *ABL1* genes (Table 2) [35,141].

Genetic abnormalities	Frequency (%)	Function	Outcome	References
TCR-mediated translocations in T-ALL				
t(10;14)(q24;q11) TLX1-TCR α/δ t(7;10)(q35;q24) TCR β-TLX1	4-10	Homeodomain transcription factor Spleen development	Good	[37,38,143]
t(1;14)(p32;q11) TAL1-TCR α/δ	3	bHLH transcription factor HSC survival	Undefined	[15,37]
t(7;9)(q34;q34.3) TCR β-NOTCH1	<1	Transmembrane receptor T-cell development	Poor	[35–38]
Non-TCR-mediated translocations and mutations in T-ALL				
t(5;14)(q35;q32) TLX3-BCL11b	20	Homeodomain transcription factor Neural development	Poor	[37,38,137]
1p32 deletion SIL-TAL1	17	bHLH transcription factor	Undefined	[15,37]
NOTCH1 mutations	>50	Transmembrane receptor T-cell development	Poor	[35–38]

HSC, Hematopoietic Stem Cell

Table 2. Translocations and mutations in T-ALL

5.1. Impaired differentiation caused by defects in transcription factors expression/function

5.1.1. Deregulation of TLX1 and TLX3 Homeobox genes

Homeobox genes (*HOX*) are divided into two classes: class I *HOX* genes (*HOXA-D*) and class two *HOX* genes (*TLX1* and *TLX3*). Class II *HOX* genes have been extensively studied In T cell ALL and from them *TLX1* has been found activated in 4-10% of childhood T cell ALL, most frequently by t(10;14)(q24;q11) and t(7;10)(q35;q24) chromosomal translocations [36,37,40,137,143–145]. Both rearrangements lead to the transcriptional activation of *TLX1* gene by re-location of *TLX1* coding sequences under the transcriptional control of the TCR regulatory sequences (Table 2) [36,37,40,137]. *TLX1* is not normally expressed in healthy T cells. Interestingly, overexpression of TLX1 has also been observed in absence of known translocations, suggesting that other mechanisms of up-regulation are involved. Epigenetic changes mediated by promoter demethylation can also lead to *TLX1* aberrant expression [36,137,145]. *TLX1*+ T cells are virtually all arrested at a developmental stage phenotypically similar to the early cortical (CD1+) CD4+CD8+ "double-positive" stage of thymocyte development (early cortical thymocytes) [40]. However, these leukemic T cells lack preTCR expression suggesting that the oncogenic event occurred very early in development (probably to ETP/DN1 cells) and *TLX1* aberrant expression helped the cell to bypass the first developmental checkpoints until the cells were finally arrested at the double positive stage [139]. The favorable clinical outcome of patients with this phenotype might support the arrest in the double positive stage, since it is characterized by lack of expression of anti-apoptotic genes because of the tolerance and negative selection mechanisms that are at work to eliminate self-reactive T cell clones [35–37,143–145].

The cryptic chromosomal translocation t(5;14)(q35;q32) juxtaposes *TLX3* to the distal region of *BCL11B* producing a strong expression of *TLX3*, a genetic lesion present in approximately 20% of childhood T cell ALL (Table 2) [15,35–37,137,141]. Like *TLX1*, *TLX3* is not expressed during normal T cell development [36]. Rare variants of t(5;14) have also been reported: t(5;14)(q32;q11) involving *TRA/TRD* and t(5;7)(q35;q21) involving *CDK6* [35–37]. Some studies indicated that *TLX3* confers a bad response to treatment, but this is controversial since variation has been found between different populations [139]. It is possible that the prognostic meaning of *TLX3* overexpression might be influenced by the presence of additional altered oncogenes such *NUP214-ABL1* or *NOTCH1* [15,37].

5.1.2. Deregulation of TAL1, a basic Helix-Loop-Helix (bHLH) gene

Two different models have explained the oncogenic potential and transformation mechanism of *TAL1*: 1) inappropriate activation of *TAL1* target genes and 2) through a dominant-negative mechanism in which *TAL1* binds to and inhibits the normal activity of the E2A (E47)/HEB transcription factor complex. The second mechanism suggests that E2A proteins may directly regulate cell cycle in thymocyte precursors [35,37,146]. *TAL1* maps on chromosome 1p32 and abnormal function of this gene is one of the most common transcriptional defects in childhood T cell ALL (Table 2); in 17% of patients *TAL1* activation is a consequence of a cryptic interstitial deletion that generates a *SIL-TAL1* fusion, and in 3% of patients, t(1;14)(p32;q11) juxtaposes *TAL1* to TCR transcriptional regulatory elements causing its ectopic expression [37]. Ectopic *TAL1* expression is associated with a maturation arrest of thymocytes. TAL1 protein could also induce overexpression of BCL2A1, resulting in anti-apoptotic activities in the stage of T cell development arrest and a poor response to therapy, particularly in young children [35,37,147,148].

It is documented that *TLX3* expression confers a poor response to treatment, whereas *TLX1* activation is significantly associated with a better prognosis in T cell ALL. A high percentage of cryptic abnormalities of *TLX1*, *TLX3* and *TAL1* genes (both translocations and deletions), are mostly detected only using FISH with specific probes for each type of alteration [35]. Recently, quantitative RT-PCR and expression microarrays have permitted a better and technically simpler T cell ALL classification based on the differential oncogene expression pattern [35]. Most probably, these new methodologies will positively impact the outcome of T cell ALL patients, allowing for a better disease sub-typing and assignment of treatments with better therapeutic responses.

A novel subgroup of early T cell precursor leukemia has been reported, characterized by simultaneous expression of T cell/ stem-cell/myeloid markers and very poor prognosis when treated with standard intensive chemotherapy. Interestingly, this subgroup includes a part of those patients with *LYL1* and *LMO1* overexpression [2].

5.2. Activation of the NOTCH1 signaling pathway

The first alteration described affecting *NOTCH1* in T cell ALL was t(7;9)(q34;q34.3), which couples the coding sequences of the *NOTCH1* ICN to the *TCR β* locus. This alteration is present in <1% of T cell ALL patients [36,38,138]. Currently, gain-of-function mutations in *NOTCH1* are reported in >50% of all T cell leukemia patients. *NOTCH1* mutations are mainly observed in the HD and PEST domains. Mutations in HD result in NOTCH1 constitutive activation and cell transformation. These HD NOTCH1 mutants are observed in an average of 44% of T cell ALL patients. The deletion of the PEST domain enhances NOTCH1 intracellular signaling and is present in 30% of patients. Both, HD and PEST mutations together are found in 17% of cases, and have a synergistic effect on NOTCH1 activation [35,38,138]. *NOTCH1* mutations are found in all developmental subtypes of T cell ALL, supporting that these mutations might occur very early in T cell progenitors [35], and in general, they represent a marker of poor prognosis in patients with T cell ALL (Table 2) [138]. Zhu and cols reported that the outcome of patients with *NOTCH1* mutations varies according to the concomitant expression of *TLX1* and/or *TLX3*. Patients additionally positive for *TLX3* expression, have worse prognosis than those with *TLX1* expression since the latter ones tent to show prolonged survival [138].

Glucocorticoids are normally used to treat T cell ALL patients and glucocorticoid resistance have been mapped to NOTCH1 aberrant expression. Recently, a combination therapy with glucocorticoids and GSIs in a mouse model of resistant to treatment T cell ALL show promising results, arguing that NOTCH1 inhibitors in combination with traditional anti-leukemic drugs might improve disease prognosis in patients with NOTCH1 mutations [149].

6. New prognostic markers detected by genomic variation assays and gene expression evaluation in childhood ALL

The previously described genetic abnormalities in ALL influence the aggressive behavior of leukemic cells and the response to treatment in an important manner. Unfortunately, those abnormalities are not 100% predictive of disease outcome. More recently, genome wide analysis has identified genes associated with risk to relapse in patients with primary gene fusions and hyperdiploidy. These studies have also found novel gene abnormalities probably leading to altered signaling pathways and gene expression patterns in the leukemic blast. Nowadays, many novel cryptic translocations, mutations, deletions, and abnormal expression profiles are considered useful outcome markers in children with ALL and several of these more common markers will be further detailed in this section.

6.1. *CASP8AP2*

The Caspase-8-Associated Protein 2 gene, also known as FLICE associated Huge Protein (*CASP8AP2* or *FLASH*), is located at 6q15. *CASP8AP2* encodes a protein with multiple functions; although it has been traditionally recognized as a key mediator of apoptosis, several studies have demonstrated that also participates in cell division [150], NF-kappaB signaling [151,152], c-Myb activation [153,154], S phase progression [155], histone transcription and 3′-end maturation of histone mRNAs [155–157]. CASP8AP2 interacts with the death-effector domain (DED) of caspase 8 and hence it plays an important regulatory role in Fas-mediated apoptosis.

The clinical significance of *CASP8AP2* was first reported in Flotho and cols study [158], in which differences in expression levels were associated with *in vivo* responses to multiagent chemotherapy. *CASP8AP2* expression was analyzed in 99 patients enrolled in St Jude Total Therapy Study XIII and patients were divided into 3 groups according to expression. Patients with high expression levels had significantly better EFS rates and lower cumulative incidences of relapse than those with intermediate or low *CASP8AP2* expression. The pro-apoptotic function of CASP8AP2 and its low expression in leukemic blasts from patients with persistent MRD, suggest that this gene could be a powerful predictor of treatment response in childhood ALL. Furthermore, Flotho and cols [159] identified a signature of 14 genes associated with MRD, and *CASP8AP2* was among the signature genes with a low level expression. Other genes down regulated in these high risk patients were the H2A histone family member Z (*H2AFZ*), budding uninhibited by benzimidazoles 3 homolog (*BUB3*) and CDC28 protein kinase regulatory subunit 1B (*CKS1B*). All these patients showed suboptimal responses to remission induction therapy and they eventually relapsed [159].

Analyses of *CASP8AP2* as a prognostic marker used for risk stratification have been made in leukemic patients from different populations. In a cohort of 39 newly diagnosed ALL patients enrolled in Beijing Children`s Hospital (BCH)-ALL 2003 protocol, the bone marrow expression of *CASP8AP2* at diagnosis was an useful indicator for relapse. In the same study, 106 patients enrolled in Chinese Children´s Leukemia Group (CCLG)-ALL 2008 protocol were also analyzed, and patients with low *CASP8AP2* expression presented higher relapse rates, lower relapse free survival and lower overall survival, in comparison to the high-expression group [160].

Biologic basis of the variation of *CASP8AP2* expression could be deletions at band 6q15-16.1, which are often detected in patients with T cell ALL. This abnormality results in down regulation of *CASP8AP2* expression and poor response to early treatment. In 73 T cell ALL samples obtained from patients enrolled in the multicenter ALL-BFM 1990, ALL-BFM 1995 and ALL-BFM 2000 protocols, deletion 6q15-16.1 was associated with unfavorable MRD levels. Although deletion 6q15-16.1 involves several genes, *CASP8AP2* was the single gene with a better association between the deletion and the less efficient induction of apoptosis by chemotherapy [161].

The usefulness of *CASP8AP2* expression as a potential marker of early response to treatment and relapse is still controversial. Yang et. al. [157] failed to show prognostic significance for this gene expression in a group of 78 B cell ALL and 12 T cell ALL newly diagnosed patients enrolled in the Taiwan Pediatric Oncology Group (TPOG). Further studies should be performed in ALL children from different populations and measuring different treatment protocols in order to clarify the prognostic significance of *CASP8AP2*.

6.2. *IKZF1*

The *IKZF1* or *LyF1* gene encodes Ikaros, a transcription factor located on chromosome 7p12, whose largest transcript comprises 6 zinc finger domains in 7 exons; four of these fingers are required for DNA binding and the other 2 for homo and heterodimeric associations with other Ikaros family members, for example Helios and Aiolos [162].

IKZF1 encodes 11 isoforms through a mechanism of alternative splicing, each isoform containing a different set of zinc finger domains dictating differential DNA binding capabilities. Five of these isoforms (Ik-1, Ik-2, Ik-2A, Ik-3 and Ik-3A,) are considered as "long" and functional, because they conserve at least 3 N-terminal DNA binding domains, which permit them entering to the nucleus and presenting high transcriptional activity. The remaining isoforms are referred as "short" (Ik-4, Ik-4A, Ik-5, Ik-6, Ik-7 and Ik-8) and have 2 or less N-terminal DNA binding domains. They are unable to bind DNA with high affinity, do not enter the nucleus, therefore neither activate transcription, but retain the protein binding domains and then the ability to form homo and heterodimers. This group might act as non-DNA-binding dominant-negative isoforms, reducing Ikaros activity. In particular, Ik-6 is not efficiently translocated to the nucleus, resulting in null transcriptional activity [162,163].

Ikaros plays an essential role in development and differentiation of lymphoid and myeloid lineages. It acts as a tumor suppressor and as a regulator of gene expression through a chromatin remodeling function. In normal cells, long Ik-1 and Ik-2 isoforms are more expressed than the predominantly dominant-negative isoforms, Ik-3, Ik-4, Ik-5 and Ik-6 [162,163]. During alternative splicing Ikaros is susceptible to loss the amino-terminal DNA-binding domain, leading to increased expression of specific isoforms, in particular Ik-6, which is strongly associated with B and T cell ALL [164–166].

On the other hand, SNP array analysis of B cell ALL children has revealed deletions of complete *IKZF1* locus; there were also deletions of coding exons 3 through 6, resulting in Ik-6 expression in B-ALL patients. It has also detected point mutations (R111, L117fs, G158S, H224fs, S402fs and E504fs); in particular G158 attenuates the DNA-binding activity and might act as a dominant-negative Ikaros allele. [167]. Approximately 28% of high risk B cell ALL patients, and 9% of unselected risk patients show *IKZF1* deletions [167,168]. Deletions in *IKZF1* in unselected B cell ALL Asian patients are present in 10-15%; this incidence is similar to the one previously seen in Caucasian countries [85,157].

"Short" and "long" isoforms can be expressed in leukemic cells from both B and T cell ALL patients, however, the frequency and expression levels seem to vary between specific immunophenotype and genetic subgroups [169,170]. For instance, Ph positive B cell ALL patients tend to have higher levels of Ik-6 in contrast to Ik-1 and Ik-2 [170]. Interestingly, one study found that *IKZF1* is deleted in 84% of Ph positive B cell ALL patients, supporting its important role in the pathogenesis of this genetic subtype [168]. Ik-6 has also been found overexpressed in patients with the *MLL-AF4* fusion [171].

Regarding prognosis, there is a strong correlation between mutations, deletions in *IKZF1* or presence of non-functional Ikaros isoforms, and poor outcome in both B and T cell ALL patients. Nevertheless, this association is independent of the presence of the *BCR-ABL1* fusion, since both Ph positive and negative patients have poor outcome when *IKZF1* is altered [167,168]. Furthermore, approximately 35% of ALL relapsed cases, this condition also contributes to chemotherapy resistance [172,173]. Events of relapse have been predicted in 79% of non-high risk ALL patients based in both MRD and *IKZF1* deletions [174]. Recently, a novel high risk ALL subgroup called "*BCR-ABL1* like" has been identified, 39% of them presented *IKZF1* deletions or mutations and they had a highly unfavorable prognosis as that found in the Ph positive B cell ALL group. About 20% of the total of B cell ALL patients belong to this "*BCR-ABL1* like" subgroup [175].

6.3. *JAK2*

The *JAK2* gene is located on 9p24 and encodes a kinase that belongs to the JAK family of protein tyrosine kinases (JAK1, JAK2, JAK3 and TYK2). All members of the JAK family are activated by tyrosine phosphorylation and participate in proliferation, differentiation, and cellular migration processes after activation. Additionally, JAK2 regulates apoptosis during hematopoiesis. After JAK2 is activated, this tyrosine phosphorylates STAT5 leading to its dimerization, nuclear translocation and regulation of its target genes. The JAK/STAT pathway is the main signaling mechanism for numerous cytokines and growth factors. Mutations in different members of the JAK family are associated with inflammatory disease, erythrocytosis and childhood ALL [176,177].

Recently, it has been shown that the mutation R683, within the JAK2 pseudokinase domain, is present in approximately 3-4% of childhood ALL patients [178]. About 10% of high risk B cell ALL patients are R683+, however, the incidence is increased in patients with Down syndrome (18-28%) [179–181]. The incidence of *JAK2* mutations is about 10% in the high-risk "*BCR-ABL1* like" group [182]. *JAK2* mutations have also been observed in cell lines MHH-

http://dx.doi.org/10.5772/54288

CALL4 and MUTZ5, derived from B cell ALL patients without Down syndrome [183]. *JAK2* mutations in ALL are significantly associated with poor outcome and the prognosis is worse when are associated with *IKZF1* deletions; this is an important observation since it has been estimated that 87% of high risk ALL cases harbor *JAK2* mutations together with *IKZF1* deletions [182].

6.4. *CRLF2*

The *Cytokine receptor-like factor 2* or *CRLF2* gene also termed thymic stromal lymphopoietin receptor *(TSLPR)*, encodes a type I cytokine receptor. This gene is located in the pseudoautosomal region 1 (PAR1) at both sex chromosomes, X (Xp22.3) and Y (Yp11.3). CRLF2 forms a heterodimeric receptor with IL7Rα which binds the thymic stromal lymphopoietin (TSLP) ligand. CRLF2 plays an important role during T cell and dendritic cell development, promotes B cell survival and proliferation, and is involved in inflammation, allergic responses and malignant transformation [183,184].

Approximately 40% of children with B cell ALL have *CRLF2* cryptic genetic alterations, which induce abnormal signaling during B cell development [178]. *CRLF2* is involved in 2 types of genomic rearrangements: 1) an interstitial deletion within the PAR1 region of chromosome X or Y that places the *CRLF2* gene under the transcriptional control of the *P2RY8* promoter (*P2RY8-CRLF2*), and 2) two cryptic chromosomal translocations t(X;14)(p22; q32) and t(Y;14)(p11;q32), both involving the locus of the B cell antigen receptor heavy chain (fusion *IGH-CRLF2*) [183,185,186]. PAR1 deletions seem to be more frequent than *IGH-CRLF2* translocation, however some groups report that translocation is the most frequent; these observations are still controversial. *CRLF2* rearrangements are associated with aberrant overexpression of *CRLF2* in B cell ALL patients and might contribute to the pathogenesis of the disease [187–190]. Approximately 50% of patients with high *CRLF2* expression present a *CRLF2* rearrangement. However, in a few studies, low *CRLF2* expression has been detected in ALL with the *P2RY8-CRLF2* rearrangement. This low expression could result from a low frequency of the leukemic clone with the *P2RY8-CRLF2* lesion within the heterogeneous pool of leukemic blasts, further studies will be necessary to clarify it [85,187,190].

About 5-7% of Caucasian non-selected B cell ALL patients present *CRLF2* rearrangements and overexpression. This frequency increased to 16-19% in high risk B cell ALL patients; for this reason *CRLF2* abnormalities have been associated with adverse prognosis [85,178,183,186,189–191]. Occurrence of *CRLF2* abnormalities differs among ALL populations, this is probably influenced by the ethnic origin. Harvey and colleagues found that 35.3% of Hispanic/Latin high risk B cell ALL patients have *CRLF2* rearrangements and high expression of its protein [188], this fact could explain in part the poor response to treatment observed in this group [178,187–190]. *CRLF2* analysis by different groups have demonstrated that rearrangements in this gene do not coexist with other non-random ALL chromosomal abnormalities [186,189,190]; except for a couple of *BCR-ABL1* positive patients that showed a high *CRLF2* expression, but not genomic alterations of the gene [187].

Rearrangements and overexpression of *CRLF2* and *JAK2* mutations are particularly abundant in B cell ALL children with Down syndrome, coexistence of both lesions have been found in up to 45-60% [178,186]. For this group of patients, *CRLF2* rearrangements are more frequent than other ALL aberrations as high hyperdiploid, *ETV6-RUNX1, E2A-PBX1* and *MLL-AF4*. A point mutation in *CRLF2* (F232C) has been identified in 9% of Down syndrome cases leading to *CRLF2* overexpression [191]; it has been proposed that this alteration could be the first leukemogenic event in these children [178,183].

A strong interaction among *IKZF1* deletion, *CRLF2* overexpression and *JAK2* mutations has been described in B cell ALL. Recent studies support that 100% of B cell ALL patients with *JAK2* mutations have *CRLF2* overexpression, however, the opposite is not true. Analyses of different children ALL populations have identified coexistence of these abnormalities: 81% of Hispanic/Latin patients present *CRLF2* overexpression and *IKZF1* deletions, and 69% of them have *JAK2* mutations [188]; in 40% of Caucasian patients with *CRLF2* overexpression *IKZF1* deletions have been found [189]; 95% of Chinese patients with *JAK2* mutations also present high *CRLF2* expression [85]. In Dutch children with Down syndrome, deletions of *IKZF1* were found in 35%, *JAK2* mutations in 15% and *CRLF2* overexpression in 62% of cases [192].

According to these observations, it has been speculated that *IKZF1* deletion, *CRLF2* overexpression and *JAK2* mutations collaborate during B lymphoid transformation perturbing the normal lymphoid development. Furthermore, cooperative mutations could contribute to increase the risk of relapse and promoting therapy resistance and treatment failure. Particularly, *CRLF2* alterations might be the first step in carcinogenic signaling, given that its overexpression is associated with activation of the STAT5 pathway through tyrosine phosphorylation in primary B-cell progenitors [183,189,193].

7. Conclusions

Progress in risk adapted treatment of childhood ALL can currently cure up to 80% of patients. Prognostic factors including patient and disease characteristics as well as response to treatment, play a key role in stratification. Through exhaustive genetic characterization of ALL, gene fusions, point mutations, deletions and gross losses or gains of genetic material have been associated to prognosis. Recently, gene expression and comparative genomic hybridization microarrays have identified new potential genetic markers for predicting outcome. These markers have been evaluated in order to recognize patients prone to relapse, even when they present low risk characteristics by conventional parameters of risk stratification. Based on those studies, gene signatures, mutations and signaling pathways no previously associated to ALL have been identified. Detected abnormalities are involved in diverse cellular processes, as cell cycle progression, cell death, and regulation of gene expression. These activities directly influence how the leukemic blast responds to treatment, and have an important role in the relapse process. Novel genetic alterations that have been associated with poor outcome in ALL patients are rearrangements/mutations that trigger *CRLF2* overexpression; *JAK2* mutations; *IKZF1* deletions and mutations, and down expression of *CASP8AP2*. Genomic analysis of relapse leukemic clones has also been useful detect-

http://dx.doi.org/10.5772/54288

ing novel genetic abnormalities that influence the aggressive behavior of leukemic cells and in consequence the response to treatment. Recently, new mutations have been found in patients with high hyperdiploidy or with *ETV6-RUNX1* fusion. These recent findings are important in the stratification of these subgroups of patients. ALL is one of the best characterized malignancies at the genetic level, and the increased survival of ALL patients in recent years is without a doubt due to the knowledge of the genes involved in ALL etiology. Next generation technologies and discovery of new genetic markers will keep providing a better understanding of the disease and a more comprehensive biological frame to stratify patients into more reliable risk groups. This knowledge will also reveal potential therapeutic targets that could yield personalized treatments, increasing the number of cured ALL children with less adverse sequelae.

Acknowledgements

To CONACyT FONSEC SSA/IMSS/ISSSTE//44402. (PPV) and CONACyT PhD grant 165427 (RJV).

Author details

M.R. Juárez-Velázquez[1], C. Salas-Labadía[1], A. Reyes-León[1], M.P. Navarrete-Meneses[1], E.M. Fuentes-Pananá[2] and P. Pérez-Vera[1]

1 Tissue Culture Laboratory, Department of Research in Human Genetics, National Pediatrics Institute, Secretariat of Health, Mexico City, Mexico

2 Unit of Medical Research in Infectious and Parasitic Diseases, High Specialty Medical Care Unit of the Pediatric Hospital, National Medical Center XXI Century, Mexican Institute of Social Security, Mexico City, Mexico

References

[1] Pérez-Saldivar ML, Fajardo-Gutiérrez A, Bernáldez-Ríos R, Martínez-Avalos A, Medina-Sanson A, Espinosa-Hernández L, et al. Childhood acute leukemias are frequent in Mexico City: descriptive epidemiology. BMC Cancer. 2011;11:355.

[2] Coustan-Smith E, Mullighan CG, Onciu M, Behm FG, Raimondi SC, Pei D, et al. Early T-cell precursor leukaemia: a subtype of very high-risk acute lymphoblastic leukaemia. Lancet Oncol. 2009 Feb;10(2):147–56.

[3] Pui C-H, Campana D. Childhood Leukemia. In Abeloff's Clinical Oncology. (ed.) Elsevier Inc: Churchill Livingstone; 2008. p. 2139–69.

[4] Pui C-H, Carroll WL, Meshinchi S, Arceci RJ. Biology, risk stratification, and therapy of pediatric acute leukemias: an update. J. Clin. Oncol. 2011 Feb 10;29(5):551–65.

[5] Neale GAM, Campana D, Pui C-H. Minimal residual disease detection in acute lymphoblastic leukemia: real improvement with the real-time quantitative PCR method? J. Pediatr. Hematol. Oncol. 2003 Feb;25(2):100–2.

[6] Bhojwani D, Howard SC, Pui C-H. High-risk childhood acute lymphoblastic leukemia. Clin Lymphoma Myeloma. 2009;9 Suppl 3:S222–230.

[7] Krivtsov AV, Armstrong SA. MLL translocations, histone modifications and leukaemia stem-cell development. Nat. Rev. Cancer. 2007 Nov;7(11):823–33.

[8] Pui CH, Crist WM, Look AT. Biology and clinical significance of cytogenetic abnormalities in childhood acute lymphoblastic leukemia. Blood. 1990 Oct 15;76(8):1449–63.

[9] Greaves MF, Wiemels J. Origins of chromosome translocations in childhood leukaemia. Nat. Rev. Cancer. 2003 Sep;3(9):639–49.

[10] Pérez-Vera P, Reyes-León A, Fuentes-Pananá EM. Signaling proteins and transcription factors in normal and malignant early B cell development. Bone Marrow Res. 2011;2011:502751.

[11] Richie Ehrlich LI, Serwold T, Weissman IL. In vitro assays misrepresent in vivo lineage potentials of murine lymphoid progenitors. Blood. 2011 Mar 3;117(9):2618–24.

[12] Schlenner SM, Madan V, Busch K, Tietz A, Läufle C, Costa C, et al. Fate mapping reveals separate origins of T cells and myeloid lineages in the thymus. Immunity. 2010 Mar 26;32(3):426–36.

[13] Fuentes-Pananá EM, Bannish G, Karnell FG, Treml JF, Monroe JG. Analysis of the individual contributions of Igalpha (CD79a)- and Igbeta (CD79b)-mediated tonic signaling for bone marrow B cell development and peripheral B cell maturation. J. Immunol. 2006 Dec 1;177(11):7913–22.

[14] Fuentes-Pananá EM, Bannish G, Monroe JG. Basal B-cell receptor signaling in B lymphocytes: mechanisms of regulation and role in positive selection, differentiation, and peripheral survival. Immunol. Rev. 2004 Feb;197:26–40.

[15] van Grotel M, Meijerink JPP, Beverloo HB, Langerak AW, Buys-Gladdines JGCAM, Schneider P, et al. The outcome of molecular-cytogenetic subgroups in pediatric T-cell acute lymphoblastic leukemia: a retrospective study of patients treated according to DCOG or COALL protocols. Haematologica. 2006 Sep;91(9):1212–21.

[16] Noguchi M, Nakamura Y, Russell SM, Ziegler SF, Tsang M, Cao X, et al. Interleukin-2 receptor gamma chain: a functional component of the interleukin-7 receptor. Science. 1993 Dec 17;262(5141):1877–80.

[17] Milne CD, Paige CJ. IL-7: a key regulator of B lymphopoiesis. Semin. Immunol. 2006 Feb;18(1):20–30.

[18] Peschon JJ, Morrissey PJ, Grabstein KH, Ramsdell FJ, Maraskovsky E, Gliniak BC, et al. Early lymphocyte expansion is severely impaired in interleukin 7 receptor-deficient mice. J. Exp. Med. 1994 Nov 1;180(5):1955–60.

[19] von Freeden-Jeffry U, Vieira P, Lucian LA, McNeil T, Burdach SE, Murray R. Lymphopenia in interleukin (IL)-7 gene-deleted mice identifies IL-7 as a nonredundant cytokine. J. Exp. Med. 1995 Apr 1;181(4):1519–26.

[20] Cao X, Shores EW, Hu-Li J, Anver MR, Kelsall BL, Russell SM, et al. Defective lymphoid development in mice lacking expression of the common cytokine receptor gamma chain. Immunity. 1995 Mar;2(3):223–38.

[21] DiSanto JP, Müller W, Guy-Grand D, Fischer A, Rajewsky K. Lymphoid development in mice with a targeted deletion of the interleukin 2 receptor gamma chain. Proc. Natl. Acad. Sci. U.S.A. 1995 Jan 17;92(2):377–81.

[22] Kovanen PE, Leonard WJ. Cytokines and immunodeficiency diseases: critical roles of the gamma(c)-dependent cytokines interleukins 2, 4, 7, 9, 15, and 21, and their signaling pathways. Immunol. Rev. 2004 Dec;202:67–83.

[23] Hennighausen L, Robinson GW. Interpretation of cytokine signaling through the transcription factors STAT5A and STAT5B. Genes Dev. 2008 Mar 15;22(6):711–21.

[24] Ramadani F, Bolland DJ, Garcon F, Emery JL, Vanhaesebroeck B, Corcoran AE, et al. The PI3K isoforms p110alpha and p110delta are essential for pre-B cell receptor signaling and B cell development. Sci Signal. 2010;3(134):ra60.

[25] Marshall AJ, Fleming HE, Wu GE, Paige CJ. Modulation of the IL-7 dose-response threshold during pro-B cell differentiation is dependent on pre-B cell receptor expression. J. Immunol. 1998 Dec 1;161(11):6038–45.

[26] Cobaleda C, Schebesta A, Delogu A, Busslinger M. Pax5: the guardian of B cell identity and function. Nat. Immunol. 2007 May;8(5):463–70.

[27] Nutt SL, Kee BL. The transcriptional regulation of B cell lineage commitment. Immunity. 2007 Jun;26(6):715–25.

[28] Nutt SL, Heavey B, Rolink AG, Busslinger M. Commitment to the B-lymphoid lineage depends on the transcription factor Pax5. Nature. 1999 Oct 7;401(6753):556–62.

[29] Smith E, Sigvardsson M. The roles of transcription factors in B lymphocyte commitment, development, and transformation. J. Leukoc. Biol. 2004 Jun;75(6):973–81.

[30] O'Riordan M, Grosschedl R. Coordinate regulation of B cell differentiation by the transcription factors EBF and E2A. Immunity. 1999 Jul;11(1):21–31.

[31] Sato H, Saito-Ohara F, Inazawa J, Kudo A. Pax-5 is essential for kappa sterile transcription during Ig kappa chain gene rearrangement. J. Immunol. 2004 Apr 15;172(8): 4858–65.

[32] Fuxa M, Skok J, Souabni A, Salvagiotto G, Roldan E, Busslinger M. Pax5 induces V-to-DJ rearrangements and locus contraction of the immunoglobulin heavy-chain gene. Genes Dev. 2004 Feb 15;18(4):411–22.

[33] Kuo TC, Schlissel MS. Mechanisms controlling expression of the RAG locus during lymphocyte development. Curr. Opin. Immunol. 2009 Apr;21(2):173–8.

[34] Bain G, Maandag EC, Izon DJ, Amsen D, Kruisbeek AM, Weintraub BC, et al. E2A proteins are required for proper B cell development and initiation of immunoglobulin gene rearrangements. Cell. 1994 Dec 2;79(5):885–92.

[35] Graux C, Cools J, Michaux L, Vandenberghe P, Hagemeijer A. Cytogenetics and molecular genetics of T-cell acute lymphoblastic leukemia: from thymocyte to lymphoblast. Leukemia. 2006 Sep;20(9):1496–510.

[36] Van Vlierberghe P, Pieters R, Beverloo HB, Meijerink JPP. Molecular-genetic insights in paediatric T-cell acute lymphoblastic leukaemia. Br. J. Haematol. 2008 Oct;143(2): 153–68.

[37] De Keersmaecker K, Marynen P, Cools J. Genetic insights in the pathogenesis of T-cell acute lymphoblastic leukemia. Haematologica. 2005 Aug;90(8):1116–27.

[38] Koch U, Radtke F. Mechanisms of T cell development and transformation. Annu. Rev. Cell Dev. Biol. 2011 Nov 10;27:539–62.

[39] Ikawa T, Hirose S, Masuda K, Kakugawa K, Satoh R, Shibano-Satoh A, et al. An essential developmental checkpoint for production of the T cell lineage. Science. 2010 Jul 2;329(5987):93–6.

[40] Riz I, Hawley TS, Johnston H, Hawley RG. Role of TLX1 in T-cell acute lymphoblastic leukaemia pathogenesis. Br. J. Haematol. 2009 Apr;145(1):140–3.

[41] Dördelmann M, Reiter A, Borkhardt A, Ludwig WD, Götz N, Viehmann S, et al. Prednisone response is the strongest predictor of treatment outcome in infant acute lymphoblastic leukemia. Blood. 1999 Aug 15;94(4):1209–17.

[42] Pui C-H. Recent research advances in childhood acute lymphoblastic leukemia. J. Formos. Med. Assoc. 2010 Nov;109(11):777–87.

[43] Manabe A, Ohara A, Hasegawa D, Koh K, Saito T, Kiyokawa N, et al. Significance of the complete clearance of peripheral blasts after 7 days of prednisolone treatment in children with acute lymphoblastic leukemia: the Tokyo Children's Cancer Study Group Study L99-15. Haematologica. 2008 Aug;93(8):1155–60.

[44] Pui CH, Campana D, Evans WE. Childhood acute lymphoblastic leukaemia--current status and future perspectives. Lancet Oncol. 2001 Oct;2(10):597–607.

[45] Aricò M, Valsecchi MG, Conter V, Rizzari C, Pession A, Messina C, et al. Improved outcome in high-risk childhood acute lymphoblastic leukemia defined by prednisone-poor response treated with double Berlin-Frankfurt-Muenster protocol II. Blood. 2002 Jul 15;100(2):420–6.

[46] Szczepański T, Orfão A, van der Velden VH, San Miguel JF, van Dongen JJ. Minimal residual disease in leukaemia patients. Lancet Oncol. 2001 Jul;2(7):409–17.

[47] Campana D. Status of minimal residual disease testing in childhood haematological malignancies. Br. J. Haematol. 2008 Nov;143(4):481–9.

[48] Campana D. Determination of minimal residual disease in leukaemia patients. Br. J. Haematol. 2003 Jun;121(6):823–38.

[49] Campana D, Coustan-Smith E. Detection of minimal residual disease in acute leukemia by flow cytometry. Cytometry. 1999 Aug 15;38(4):139–52.

[50] Gabert J, Beillard E, van der Velden VHJ, Bi W, Grimwade D, Pallisgaard N, et al. Standardization and quality control studies of "real-time" quantitative reverse transcriptase polymerase chain reaction of fusion gene transcripts for residual disease detection in leukemia - a Europe Against Cancer program. Leukemia. 2003 Dec;17(12): 2318–57.

[51] Campana D. Minimal residual disease in acute lymphoblastic leukemia. Semin. Hematol. 2009 Jan;46(1):100–6.

[52] van der Velden VHJ, Hochhaus A, Cazzaniga G, Szczepanski T, Gabert J, van Dongen JJM. Detection of minimal residual disease in hematologic malignancies by real-time quantitative PCR: principles, approaches, and laboratory aspects. Leukemia. 2003 Jun;17(6):1013–34.

[53] Flohr T, Schrauder A, Cazzaniga G, Panzer-Grümayer R, van der Velden V, Fischer S, et al. Minimal residual disease-directed risk stratification using real-time quantitative PCR analysis of immunoglobulin and T-cell receptor gene rearrangements in the international multicenter trial AIEOP-BFM ALL 2000 for childhood acute lymphoblastic leukemia. Leukemia. 2008 Apr;22(4):771–82.

[54] Coustan-Smith E, Sancho J, Hancock ML, Boyett JM, Behm FG, Raimondi SC, et al. Clinical importance of minimal residual disease in childhood acute lymphoblastic leukemia. Blood. 2000 Oct 15;96(8):2691–6.

[55] Coustan-Smith E, Behm FG, Sanchez J, Boyett JM, Hancock ML, Raimondi SC, et al. Immunological detection of minimalresidual disease in children with acute lymphoblastic leukaemia. Lancet. 1998 Feb 21;351(9102):550–4.

[56] Borowitz MJ, Devidas M, Hunger SP, Bowman WP, Carroll AJ, Carroll WL, et al. Clinical significance of minimal residual disease in childhood acute lymphoblastic leukemia and its relationship to other prognostic factors: a Children's Oncology Group study. Blood. 2008 Jun 15;111(12):5477–85.

[57] Zhou J, Goldwasser MA, Li A, Dahlberg SE, Neuberg D, Wang H, et al. Quantitative analysis of minimal residual disease predicts relapse in children with B-lineage acute lymphoblastic leukemia in DFCI ALL Consortium Protocol 95-01. Blood. 2007 Sep 1;110(5):1607–11.

[58] Basso G, Veltroni M, Valsecchi MG, Dworzak MN, Ratei R, Silvestri D, et al. Risk of relapse of childhood acute lymphoblastic leukemia is predicted by flow cytometric measurement of residual disease on day 15 bone marrow. J. Clin. Oncol. 2009 Nov 1;27(31):5168–74.

[59] Eckert C, Biondi A, Seeger K, Cazzaniga G, Hartmann R, Beyermann B, et al. Prognostic value of minimal residual disease in relapsed childhood acute lymphoblastic leukaemia. Lancet. 2001 Oct 13;358(9289):1239–41.

[60] Coustan-Smith E, Gajjar A, Hijiya N, Razzouk BI, Ribeiro RC, Rivera GK, et al. Clinical significance of minimal residual disease in childhood acute lymphoblastic leukemia after first relapse. Leukemia. 2004 Mar;18(3):499–504.

[61] Pfeiffer P, Goedecke W, Obe G. Mechanisms of DNA double-strand break repair and their potential to induce chromosomal aberrations. Mutagenesis. 2000 Jul;15(4):289–302.

[62] Greaves M. In utero origins of childhood leukaemia. Early Hum. Dev. 2005 Jan;81(1): 123–9.

[63] Chen Z, Sandberg AA. Molecular cytogenetic aspects of hematological malignancies: clinical implications. Am. J. Med. Genet. 2002 Oct 30;115(3):130–41.

[64] Mrózek K, Harper DP, Aplan PD. Cytogenetics and molecular genetics of acute lymphoblastic leukemia. Hematol. Oncol. Clin. North Am. 2009 Oct;23(5):991–1010.

[65] Heisterkamp N, Stam K, Groffen J, de Klein A, Grosveld G. Structural organization of the bcr gene and its role in the Ph′ translocation. Nature. 1985 Jul 27;315(6022):758–61.

[66] Barilá D, Superti-Furga G. An intramolecular SH3-domain interaction regulates c-Abl activity. Nat. Genet. 1998 Mar;18(3):280–2.

[67] Chissoe SL, Bodenteich A, Wang YF, Wang YP, Burian D, Clifton SW, et al. Sequence and analysis of the human ABL gene, the BCR gene, and regions involved in the Philadelphia chromosomal translocation. Genomics. 1995 May 1;27(1):67–82.

[68] Fröhling S, Döhner H. Chromosomal abnormalities in cancer. N. Engl. J. Med. 2008 Aug 14;359(7):722–34.

[69] Chalandon Y, Schwaller J. Targeting mutated protein tyrosine kinases and their signaling pathways in hematologic malignancies. Haematologica. 2005 Jul;90(7):949–68.

[70] van Dongen JJ, Macintyre EA, Gabert JA, Delabesse E, Rossi V, Saglio G, et al. Standardized RT-PCR analysis of fusion gene transcripts from chromosome aberrations in acute leukemia for detection of minimal residual disease. Report of the BIOMED-1 Concerted Action: investigation of minimal residual disease in acute leukemia. Leukemia. 1999 Dec;13(12):1901–28.

[71] Raimondi SC, Roberson PK, Pui CH, Behm FG, Rivera GK. Hyperdiploid (47-50) acute lymphoblastic leukemia in children. Blood. 1992 Jun 15;79(12):3245–52.

[72] Nahar R, Ramezani-Rad P, Mossner M, Duy C, Cerchietti L, Geng H, et al. Pre-B cell receptor-mediated activation of BCL6 induces pre-B cell quiescence through transcriptional repression of MYC. Blood. 2011 Oct 13;118(15):4174–8.

[73] Skorski T. Genomic instability: The cause and effect of BCR/ABL tyrosine kinase. Curr Hematol Malig Rep. 2007 May;2(2):69–74.

[74] Pui C-H, Evans WE. Treatment of acute lymphoblastic leukemia. N. Engl. J. Med. 2006 Jan 12;354(2):166–78.

[75] Pieters R, Carroll WL. Biology and treatment of acute lymphoblastic leukemia. Hematol. Oncol. Clin. North Am. 2010 Feb;24(1):1–18.

[76] Szczepański T, Harrison CJ, van Dongen JJM. Genetic aberrations in paediatric acute leukaemias and implications for management of patients. Lancet Oncol. 2010 Sep; 11(9):880–9.

[77] Moorman AV, Ensor HM, Richards SM, Chilton L, Schwab C, Kinsey SE, et al. Prognostic effect of chromosomal abnormalities in childhood B-cell precursor acute lymphoblastic leukaemia: results from the UK Medical Research Council ALL97/99 randomised trial. Lancet Oncol. 2010 May;11(5):429–38.

[78] Schrappe M, Reiter A, Ludwig WD, Harbott J, Zimmermann M, Hiddemann W, et al. Improved outcome in childhood acute lymphoblastic leukemia despite reduced use of anthracyclines and cranial radiotherapy: results of trial ALL-BFM 90. German-Austrian-Swiss ALL-BFM Study Group. Blood. 2000 Jun 1;95(11):3310–22.

[79] Jiménez-Morales S, Miranda-Peralta E, Saldaña-Alvarez Y, Perez-Vera P, Paredes-Aguilera R, Rivera-Luna R, et al. BCR-ABL, ETV6-RUNX1 and E2A-PBX1: prevalence of the most common acute lymphoblastic leukemia fusion genes in Mexican patients. Leuk. Res. 2008 Oct;32(10):1518–22.

[80] Borkhardt A, Cazzaniga G, Viehmann S, Valsecchi MG, Ludwig WD, Burci L, et al. Incidence and clinical relevance of TEL/AML1 fusion genes in children with acute lymphoblastic leukemia enrolled in the German and Italian multicenter therapy trials. Associazione Italiana Ematologia Oncologia Pediatrica and the Berlin-Frankfurt-Münster Study Group. Blood. 1997 Jul 15;90(2):571–7.

[81] Harrison CJ, Moorman AV, Barber KE, Broadfield ZJ, Cheung KL, Harris RL, et al. Interphase molecular cytogenetic screening for chromosomal abnormalities of prognostic significance in childhood acute lymphoblastic leukaemia: a UK Cancer Cytogenetics Group Study. Br. J. Haematol. 2005 May;129(4):520–30.

[82] Pui C-H, Robison LL, Look AT. Acute lymphoblastic leukaemia. Lancet. 2008 Mar 22;371(9617):1030–43.

[83] Aldrich MC, Zhang L, Wiemels JL, Ma X, Loh ML, Metayer C, et al. Cytogenetics of Hispanic and White children with acute lymphoblastic leukemia in California. Cancer Epidemiol. Biomarkers Prev. 2006 Mar;15(3):578–81.

[84] Pérez-Vera P, Salas C, Montero-Ruiz O, Frías S, Dehesa G, Jarquín B, et al. Analysis of gene rearrangements using a fluorescence in situ hybridization method in Mexican patients with acute lymphoblastic leukemia: experience at a single institution. Cancer Genet. Cytogenet. 2008 Jul 15;184(2):94–8.

[85] Chen B, Wang Y-Y, Shen Y, Zhang W-N, He H-Y, Zhu Y-M, et al. Newly diagnosed acute lymphoblastic leukemia in China (I): abnormal genetic patterns in 1346 childhood and adult cases and their comparison with the reports from Western countries. Leukemia. 2012 Jul;26(7):1608–16.

[86] Ariffin H, Chen S-P, Kwok CS, Quah T-C, Lin H-P, Yeoh AEJ. Ethnic differences in the frequency of subtypes of childhood acute lymphoblastic leukemia: results of the Malaysia-Singapore Leukemia Study Group. J. Pediatr. Hematol. Oncol. 2007 Jan; 29(1):27–31.

[87] Hunger SP. Tyrosine kinase inhibitor use in pediatric Philadelphia chromosome-positive acute lymphoblastic anemia. Hematology Am Soc Hematol Educ Program. 2011;2011:361–5.

[88] Nourse J, Mellentin JD, Galili N, Wilkinson J, Stanbridge E, Smith SD, et al. Chromosomal translocation t(1;19) results in synthesis of a homeobox fusion mRNA that codes for a potential chimeric transcription factor. Cell. 1990 Feb 23;60(4):535–45.

[89] Biondi A, Masera G. Molecular pathogenesis of childhood acute lymphoblastic leukemia. Haematologica. 1998 Jul;83(7):651–9.

[90] Chan KK-K, Zhang J, Chia N-Y, Chan Y-S, Sim HS, Tan KS, et al. KLF4 and PBX1 directly regulate NANOG expression in human embryonic stem cells. Stem Cells. 2009 Sep;27(9):2114–25.

[91] LeBrun DP. E2A basic helix-loop-helix transcription factors in human leukemia. Front. Biosci. 2003 May 1;8:s206–222.

[92] Look AT. Oncogenic transcription factors in the human acute leukemias. Science. 1997 Nov 7;278(5340):1059–64.

[93] Graham DK, Salzberg DB, Kurtzberg J, Sather S, Matsushima GK, Keating AK, et al. Ectopic expression of the proto-oncogene Mer in pediatric T-cell acute lymphoblastic leukemia. Clin. Cancer Res. 2006 May 1;12(9):2662–9.

[94] Shiozawa Y, Pedersen EA, Taichman RS. GAS6/Mer axis regulates the homing and survival of the E2A/PBX1-positive B-cell precursor acute lymphoblastic leukemia in the bone marrow niche. Exp. Hematol. 2010 Feb;38(2):132–40.

[95] Armstrong SA, Look AT. Molecular genetics of acute lymphoblastic leukemia. J. Clin. Oncol. 2005 Sep 10;23(26):6306–15.

[96] Iacobucci I, Papayannidis C, Lonetti A, Ferrari A, Baccarani M, Martinelli G. Cytogenetic and molecular predictors of outcome in acute lymphocytic leukemia: recent developments. Curr Hematol Malig Rep. 2012 Jun;7(2):133–43.

[97] Pui C-H, Sandlund JT, Pei D, Campana D, Rivera GK, Ribeiro RC, et al. Improved outcome for children with acute lymphoblastic leukemia: results of Total Therapy Study XIIIB at St Jude Children's Research Hospital. Blood. 2004 Nov 1;104(9):2690–6.

[98] Privitera E, Kamps MP, Hayashi Y, Inaba T, Shapiro LH, Raimondi SC, et al. Different molecular consequences of the 1;19 chromosomal translocation in childhood B-cell precursor acute lymphoblastic leukemia. Blood. 1992 Apr 1;79(7):1781–8.

[99] Crist WM, Carroll AJ, Shuster JJ, Behm FG, Whitehead M, Vietti TJ, et al. Poor prognosis of children with pre-B acute lymphoblastic leukemia is associated with the t(1;19)(q23;p13): a Pediatric Oncology Group study. Blood. 1990 Jul 1;76(1):117–22.

[100] Inaba T, Inukai T, Yoshihara T, Seyschab H, Ashmun RA, Canman CE, et al. Reversal of apoptosis by the leukaemia-associated E2A-HLF chimaeric transcription factor. Nature. 1996 Aug 8;382(6591):541–4.

[101] Harper DP, Aplan PD. Chromosomal rearrangements leading to MLL gene fusions: clinical and biological aspects. Cancer Res. 2008 Dec 15;68(24):10024–7.

[102] Slany RK. The molecular biology of mixed lineage leukemia. Haematologica. 2009 Jul;94(7):984–93.

[103] Liu H, Takeda S, Kumar R, Westergard TD, Brown EJ, Pandita TK, et al. Phosphorylation of MLL by ATR is required for execution of mammalian S-phase checkpoint. Nature. 2010 Sep 16;467(7313):343–6.

[104] Sung PA, Libura J, Richardson C. Etoposide and illegitimate DNA double-strand break repair in the generation of MLL translocations: new insights and new questions. DNA Repair (Amst.). 2006 Sep 8;5(9-10):1109–18.

[105] Chuk MK, McIntyre E, Small D, Brown P. Discordance of MLL-rearranged (MLL-R) infant acute lymphoblastic leukemia in monozygotic twins with spontaneous clearance of preleukemic clone in unaffected twin. Blood. 2009 Jun 25;113(26):6691–4.

[106] Alexander FE, Patheal SL, Biondi A, Brandalise S, Cabrera ME, Chan LC, et al. Transplacental chemical exposure and risk of infant leukemia with MLL gene fusion. Cancer Res. 2001 Mar 15;61(6):2542–6.

[107] Bueno C, Catalina P, Melen GJ, Montes R, Sánchez L, Ligero G, et al. Etoposide induces MLL rearrangements and other chromosomal abnormalities in human embryonic stem cells. Carcinogenesis. 2009 Sep;30(9):1628–37.

[108] Schnyder S, Du NT, Le HB, Singh S, Loredo GA, Vaughan AT. Estrogen treatment induces MLL aberrations in human lymphoblastoid cells. Leuk. Res. 2009 Oct;33(10):1400–4.

[109] Blanco JG, Edick MJ, Relling MV. Etoposide induces chimeric Mll gene fusions. FASEB J. 2004 Jan;18(1):173–5.

[110] Barjesteh van Waalwijk van Doorn-Khosrovani S, Janssen J, Maas LM, Godschalk RWL, Nijhuis JG, van Schooten FJ. Dietary flavonoids induce MLL translocations in primary human CD34+ cells. Carcinogenesis. 2007 Aug;28(8):1703–9.

[111] Rojas E, Mussali P, Tovar E, Valverde M. DNA-AP sites generation by etoposide in whole blood cells. BMC Cancer. 2009;9:398.

[112] Moneypenny CG, Shao J, Song Y, Gallagher EP. MLL rearrangements are induced by low doses of etoposide in human fetal hematopoietic stem cells. Carcinogenesis. 2006 Apr;27(4):874–81.

[113] Brassesco MS, Montaldi AP, Gras DE, Camparoto ML, Martinez-Rossi NM, Scrideli CA, et al. Cytogenetic and molecular analysis of MLL rearrangements in acute lymphoblastic leukaemia survivors. Mutagenesis. 2009 Mar;24(2):153–60.

[114] Montero-Ruíz O, Alcántara-Ortigoza MA, Betancourt M, Juárez-Velázquez R, González-Márquez H, Pérez-Vera P. Expression of RUNX1 isoforms and its target gene BLK in childhood acute lymphoblastic leukemia. Leuk. Res. 2012 Sep;36(9):1105–11.

[115] Roudaia L, Cheney MD, Manuylova E, Chen W, Morrow M, Park S, et al. CBFbeta is critical for AML1-ETO and TEL-AML1 activity. Blood. 2009 Mar 26;113(13):3070–9.

[116] De Braekeleer E, Douet-Guilbert N, Morel F, Le Bris M-J, Basinko A, De Braekeleer M. ETV6 fusion genes in hematological malignancies: A review. Leuk. Res. 2012 Aug; 36(8):945–61.

[117] Wiemels JL, Hofmann J, Kang M, Selzer R, Green R, Zhou M, et al. Chromosome 12p deletions in TEL-AML1 childhood acute lymphoblastic leukemia are associated with retrotransposon elements and occur postnatally. Cancer Res. 2008 Dec 1;68(23):9935–44.

[118] Shurtleff SA, Buijs A, Behm FG, Rubnitz JE, Raimondi SC, Hancock ML, et al. TEL/AML1 fusion resulting from a cryptic t(12;21) is the most common genetic lesion in pediatric ALL and defines a subgroup of patients with an excellent prognosis. Leukemia. 1995 Dec;9(12):1985–9.

[119] Loh ML, Goldwasser MA, Silverman LB, Poon W-M, Vattikuti S, Cardoso A, et al. Prospective analysis of TEL/AML1-positive patients treated on Dana-Farber Cancer Institute Consortium Protocol 95-01. Blood. 2006 Jun 1;107(11):4508–13.

[120] Rubnitz JE, Downing JR, Pui CH, Shurtleff SA, Raimondi SC, Evans WE, et al. TEL gene rearrangement in acute lymphoblastic leukemia: a new genetic marker with prognostic significance. J. Clin. Oncol. 1997 Mar;15(3):1150–7.

[121] Pérez-Vera P, Montero-Ruiz O, Frías S, Ulloa-Avilés V, Cárdenas-Cardós R, Paredes-Aguilera R, et al. Detection of ETV6 and RUNX1 gene rearrangements using fluorescence in situ hybridization in Mexican patients with acute lymphoblastic leukemia: experience at a single institution. Cancer Genet. Cytogenet. 2005 Oct 15;162(2):140–5.

[122] Siraj AK, Kamat S, Gutiérrez MI, Banavali S, Timpson G, Sazawal S, et al. Frequencies of the major subgroups of precursor B-cell acute lymphoblastic leukemia in Indian children differ from the West. Leukemia. 2003 Jun;17(6):1192–3.

[123] Liang D-C, Shih L-Y, Yang C-P, Hung I-J, Liu H-C, Jaing T-H, et al. Frequencies of ETV6-RUNX1 fusion and hyperdiploidy in pediatric acute lymphoblastic leukemia are lower in far east than west. Pediatr Blood Cancer. 2010 Sep;55(3):430–3.

[124] Seeger K, Adams HP, Buchwald D, Beyermann B, Kremens B, Niemeyer C, et al. TEL-AML1 fusion transcript in relapsed childhood acute lymphoblastic leukemia. The Berlin-Frankfurt-Münster Study Group. Blood. 1998 Mar 1;91(5):1716–22.

[125] van Delft FW, Horsley S, Colman S, Anderson K, Bateman C, Kempski H, et al. Clonal origins of relapse in ETV6-RUNX1 acute lymphoblastic leukemia. Blood. 2011 Jun 9;117(23):6247–54.

[126] Kuster L, Grausenburger R, Fuka G, Kaindl U, Krapf G, Inthal A, et al. ETV6/RUNX1-positive relapses evolve from an ancestral clone and frequently acquire deletions of genes implicated in glucocorticoid signaling. Blood. 2011 Mar 3;117(9):2658–67.

[127] Paulsson K, Forestier E, Lilljebjörn H, Heldrup J, Behrendtz M, Young BD, et al. Genetic landscape of high hyperdiploid childhood acute lymphoblastic leukemia. Proc. Natl. Acad. Sci. U.S.A. 2010 Dec 14;107(50):21719–24.

[128] Pui CH, Raimondi SC, Williams DL. Isochromosome 17q in childhood acute lymphoblastic leukemia: an adverse cytogenetic feature in association with hyperdiploidy? Leukemia. 1988 Apr;2(4):222–5.

[129] Harris MB, Shuster JJ, Carroll A, Look AT, Borowitz MJ, Crist WM, et al. Trisomy of leukemic cell chromosomes 4 and 10 identifies children with B-progenitor cell acute lymphoblastic leukemia with a very low risk of treatment failure: a Pediatric Oncology Group study. Blood. 1992 Jun 15;79(12):3316–24.

[130] Heerema NA, Sather HN, Sensel MG, Zhang T, Hutchinson RJ, Nachman JB, et al. Prognostic impact of trisomies of chromosomes 10, 17, and 5 among children with acute lymphoblastic leukemia and high hyperdiploidy (> 50 chromosomes). J. Clin. Oncol. 2000 May;18(9):1876–87.

[131] Moorman AV, Richards SM, Martineau M, Cheung KL, Robinson HM, Jalali GR, et al. Outcome heterogeneity in childhood high-hyperdiploid acute lymphoblastic leukemia. Blood. 2003 Oct 15;102(8):2756–62.

[132] Sutcliffe MJ, Shuster JJ, Sather HN, Camitta BM, Pullen J, Schultz KR, et al. High concordance from independent studies by the Children's Cancer Group (CCG) and Pediatric Oncology Group (POG) associating favorable prognosis with combined trisomies 4, 10, and 17 in children with NCI Standard-Risk B-precursor Acute Lymphoblastic Leukemia: a Children's Oncology Group (COG) initiative. Leukemia. 2005 May;19(5):734–40.

[133] Treviño LR, Yang W, French D, Hunger SP, Carroll WL, Devidas M, et al. Germline genomic variants associated with childhood acute lymphoblastic leukemia. Nat. Genet. 2009 Sep;41(9):1001–5.

[134] Moorman AV, Harrison CJ, Buck GAN, Richards SM, Secker-Walker LM, Martineau M, et al. Karyotype is an independent prognostic factor in adult acute lymphoblastic leukemia (ALL): analysis of cytogenetic data from patients treated on the Medical Research Council (MRC) UKALLXII/Eastern Cooperative Oncology Group (ECOG) 2993 trial. Blood. 2007 Apr 15;109(8):3189–97.

[135] Raimondi SC, Zhou Y, Shurtleff SA, Rubnitz JE, Pui C-H, Behm FG. Near-triploidy and near-tetraploidy in childhood acute lymphoblastic leukemia: association with B-lineage blast cells carrying the ETV6-RUNX1 fusion, T-lineage immunophenotype, and favorable outcome. Cancer Genet. Cytogenet. 2006 Aug;169(1):50–7.

[136] Raimondi SC, Zhou Y, Mathew S, Shurtleff SA, Sandlund JT, Rivera GK, et al. Reassessment of the prognostic significance of hypodiploidy in pediatric patients with acute lymphoblastic leukemia. Cancer. 2003 Dec 15;98(12):2715–22.

[137] Cavé H, Suciu S, Preudhomme C, Poppe B, Robert A, Uyttebroeck A, et al. Clinical significance of HOX11L2 expression linked to t(5;14)(q35;q32), of HOX11 expression, and of SIL-TAL fusion in childhood T-cell malignancies: results of EORTC studies 58881 and 58951. Blood. 2004 Jan 15;103(2):442–50.

[138] Zhu Y-M, Zhao W-L, Fu J-F, Shi J-Y, Pan Q, Hu J, et al. NOTCH1 mutations in T-cell acute lymphoblastic leukemia: prognostic significance and implication in multifactorial leukemogenesis. Clin. Cancer Res. 2006 May 15;12(10):3043–9.

[139] van Grotel M, Meijerink JPP, van Wering ER, Langerak AW, Beverloo HB, Buijs-Gladdines JGCAM, et al. Prognostic significance of molecular-cytogenetic abnormalities in pediatric T-ALL is not explained by immunophenotypic differences. Leukemia. 2008 Jan;22(1):124–31.

[140] Ferrando AA, Neuberg DS, Staunton J, Loh ML, Huard C, Raimondi SC, et al. Gene expression signatures define novel oncogenic pathways in T cell acute lymphoblastic leukemia. Cancer Cell. 2002 Feb;1(1):75–87.

[141] Ballerini P, Landman-Parker J, Cayuela JM, Asnafi V, Labopin M, Gandemer V, et al. Impact of genotype on survival of children with T-cell acute lymphoblastic leukemia treated according to the French protocol FRALLE-93: the effect of TLX3/HOX11L2 gene expression on outcome. Haematologica. 2008 Nov;93(11):1658–65.

[142] Aifantis I, Raetz E, Buonamici S. Molecular pathogenesis of T-cell leukaemia and lymphoma. Nat. Rev. Immunol. 2008 May;8(5):380–90.

[143] Bergeron J, Clappier E, Radford I, Buzyn A, Millien C, Soler G, et al. Prognostic and oncogenic relevance of TLX1/HOX11 expression level in T-ALLs. Blood. 2007 Oct 1;110(7):2324–30.

[144] Asnafi V, Beldjord K, Libura M, Villarese P, Millien C, Ballerini P, et al. Age-related phenotypic and oncogenic differences in T-cell acute lymphoblastic leukemias may reflect thymic atrophy. Blood. 2004 Dec 15;104(13):4173–80.

[145] 145. De Keersmaecker K, Real PJ, Gatta GD, Palomero T, Sulis ML, Tosello V, et al. The TLX1 oncogene drives aneuploidy in T cell transformation. Nat. Med. 2010 Nov; 16(11):1321–7.

[146] O'Neil J, Shank J, Cusson N, Murre C, Kelliher M. TAL1/SCL induces leukemia by inhibiting the transcriptional activity of E47/HEB. Cancer Cell. 2004 Jun;5(6):587–96.

[147] Mansur MB, Hassan R, Barbosa TC, Splendore A, Jotta PY, Yunes JA, et al. Impact of complex NOTCH1 mutations on survival in paediatric T-cell leukaemia. BMC Cancer. 2012;12:9.

[148] Mansur MB, Emerenciano M, Brewer L, Sant'Ana M, Mendonça N, Thuler LCS, et al. SIL-TAL1 fusion gene negative impact in T-cell acute lymphoblastic leukemia outcome. Leuk. Lymphoma. 2009 Aug;50(8):1318–25.

[149] Real PJ, Tosello V, Palomero T, Castillo M, Hernando E, de Stanchina E, et al. Gamma-secretase inhibitors reverse glucocorticoid resistance in T cell acute lymphoblastic leukemia. Nat. Med. 2009 Jan;15(1):50–8.

[150] Kittler R, Putz G, Pelletier L, Poser I, Heninger A-K, Drechsel D, et al. An endoribonuclease-prepared siRNA screen in human cells identifies genes essential for cell division. Nature. 2004 Dec 23;432(7020):1036–40.

[151] Choi YH, Kim KB, Kim HH, Hong GS, Kwon YK, Chung CW, et al. FLASH coordinates NF-kappa B activity via TRAF2. J. Biol. Chem. 2001 Jul 6;276(27):25073–7.

[152] Jun J-I, Chung C-W, Lee H-J, Pyo J-O, Lee KN, Kim N-S, et al. Role of FLASH in caspase-8-mediated activation of NF-kappaB: dominant-negative function of FLASH mutant in NF-kappaB signaling pathway. Oncogene. 2005 Jan 20;24(4):688–96.

[153] Alm-Kristiansen AH, Saether T, Matre V, Gilfillan S, Dahle O, Gabrielsen OS. FLASH acts as a co-activator of the transcription factor c-Myb and localizes to active RNA polymerase II foci. Oncogene. 2008 Aug 7;27(34):4644–56.

[154] Alm-Kristiansen AH, Lorenzo PI, Molværsmyr A-K, Matre V, Ledsaak M, Sæther T, et al. PIAS1 interacts with FLASH and enhances its co-activation of c-Myb. Mol. Cancer. 2011;10:21.

[155] Barcaroli D, Dinsdale D, Neale MH, Bongiorno-Borbone L, Ranalli M, Munarriz E, et al. FLASH is an essential component of Cajal bodies. Proc. Natl. Acad. Sci. U.S.A. 2006 Oct 3;103(40):14802–7.

[156] Barcaroli D, Bongiorno-Borbone L, Terrinoni A, Hofmann TG, Rossi M, Knight RA, et al. FLASH is required for histone transcription and S-phase progression. Proc. Natl. Acad. Sci. U.S.A. 2006 Oct 3;103(40):14808–12.

[157] Yang X, Xu B, Sabath I, Kunduru L, Burch BD, Marzluff WF, et al. FLASH is required for the endonucleolytic cleavage of histone pre-mRNAs but is dispensable for the 5′ exonucleolytic degradation of the downstream cleavage product. Mol. Cell. Biol. 2011 Apr;31(7):1492–502.

[158] Flotho C, Coustan-Smith E, Pei D, Iwamoto S, Song G, Cheng C, et al. Genes contributing to minimal residual disease in childhood acute lymphoblastic leukemia: prognostic significance of CASP8AP2. Blood. 2006 Aug 1;108(3):1050–7.

[159] Flotho C, Coustan-Smith E, Pei D, Cheng C, Song G, Pui C-H, et al. A set of genes that regulate cell proliferation predicts treatment outcome in childhood acute lymphoblastic leukemia. Blood. 2007 Aug 15;110(4):1271–7.

[160] Jiao Y, Cui L, Gao C, Li W, Zhao X, Liu S, et al. CASP8AP2 is a promising prognostic indicator in pediatric acute lymphoblastic leukemia. Leuk. Res. 2012 Jan;36(1):67–71.

[161] Remke M, Pfister S, Kox C, Toedt G, Becker N, Benner A, et al. High-resolution genomic profiling of childhood T-ALL reveals frequent copy-number alterations affecting the TGF-beta and PI3K-AKT pathways and deletions at 6q15-16.1 as a genomic marker for unfavorable early treatment response. Blood. 2009 Jul 30;114(5):1053–62.

[162] Molnár A, Georgopoulos K. The Ikaros gene encodes a family of functionally diverse zinc finger DNA-binding proteins. Mol. Cell. Biol. 1994 Dec;14(12):8292–303.

[163] Sun L, Liu A, Georgopoulos K. Zinc finger-mediated protein interactions modulate Ikaros activity, a molecular control of lymphocyte development. EMBO J. 1996 Oct 1;15(19):5358–69.

[164] Sun L, Goodman PA, Wood CM, Crotty ML, Sensel M, Sather H, et al. Expression of aberrantly spliced oncogenic ikaros isoforms in childhood acute lymphoblastic leukemia. J. Clin. Oncol. 1999 Dec;17(12):3753–66.

[165] Sun L, Heerema N, Crotty L, Wu X, Navara C, Vassilev A, et al. Expression of dominant-negative and mutant isoforms of the antileukemic transcription factor Ikaros in infant acute lymphoblastic leukemia. Proc. Natl. Acad. Sci. U.S.A. 1999 Jan 19;96(2): 680–5.

[166] Sun L, Crotty ML, Sensel M, Sather H, Navara C, Nachman J, et al. Expression of dominant-negative Ikaros isoforms in T-cell acute lymphoblastic leukemia. Clin. Cancer Res. 1999 Aug;5(8):2112–20.

[167] Mullighan CG, Su X, Zhang J, Radtke I, Phillips LAA, Miller CB, et al. Deletion of IKZF1 and prognosis in acute lymphoblastic leukemia. N. Engl. J. Med. 2009 Jan 29;360(5):470–80.

[168] Mullighan CG, Miller CB, Radtke I, Phillips LA, Dalton J, Ma J, et al. BCR-ABL1 lymphoblastic leukaemia is characterized by the deletion of Ikaros. Nature. 2008 May 1;453(7191):110–4.

[169] Olivero S, Maroc C, Beillard E, Gabert J, Nietfeld W, Chabannon C, et al. Detection of different Ikaros isoforms in human leukaemias using real-time quantitative polymerase chain reaction. Br. J. Haematol. 2000 Sep;110(4):826–30.

[170] Meleshko AN, Movchan LV, Belevtsev MV, Savitskaja TV. Relative expression of different Ikaros isoforms in childhood acute leukemia. Blood Cells Mol. Dis. 2008 Dec; 41(3):278–83.

[171] Ruiz A, Jiang J, Kempski H, Brady HJM. Overexpression of the Ikaros 6 isoform is restricted to t(4;11) acute lymphoblastic leukaemia in children and infants and has a role in B-cell survival. Br. J. Haematol. 2004 Apr;125(1):31–7.

[172] Yang JJ, Bhojwani D, Yang W, Cai X, Stocco G, Crews K, et al. Genome-wide copy number profiling reveals molecular evolution from diagnosis to relapse in childhood acute lymphoblastic leukemia. Blood. 2008 Nov 15;112(10):4178–83.

[173] Kuiper RP, Waanders E, van der Velden VHJ, van Reijmersdal SV, Venkatachalam R, Scheijen B, et al. IKZF1 deletions predict relapse in uniformly treated pediatric precursor B-ALL. Leukemia. 2010 Jul;24(7):1258–64.

[174] Waanders E, van der Velden VHJ, van der Schoot CE, van Leeuwen FN, van Reijmersdal SV, de Haas V, et al. Integrated use of minimal residual disease classification and IKZF1 alteration status accurately predicts 79% of relapses in pediatric acute lymphoblastic leukemia. Leukemia. 2011 Feb;25(2):254–8.

[175] Den Boer ML, van Slegtenhorst M, De Menezes RX, Cheok MH, Buijs-Gladdines JGCAM, Peters STCJM, et al. A subtype of childhood acute lymphoblastic leukaemia with poor treatment outcome: a genome-wide classification study. Lancet Oncol. 2009 Feb;10(2):125–34.

[176] Pellegrini S, Dusanter-Fourt I. The structure, regulation and function of the Janus kinases (JAKs) and the signal transducers and activators of transcription (STATs). Eur. J. Biochem. 1997 Sep 15;248(3):615–33.

[177] Rawlings JS, Rosler KM, Harrison DA. The JAK/STAT signaling pathway. J. Cell. Sci. 2004 Mar 15;117(Pt 8):1281–3.

[178] Mullighan CG, Collins-Underwood JR, Phillips LAA, Loudin MG, Liu W, Zhang J, et al. Rearrangement of CRLF2 in B-progenitor- and Down syndrome-associated acute lymphoblastic leukemia. Nat. Genet. 2009 Nov;41(11):1243–6.

[179] Bercovich D, Ganmore I, Scott LM, Wainreb G, Birger Y, Elimelech A, et al. Mutations of JAK2 in acute lymphoblastic leukaemias associated with Down's syndrome. Lancet. 2008 Oct 25;372(9648):1484–92.

[180] Gaikwad A, Rye CL, Devidas M, Heerema NA, Carroll AJ, Izraeli S, et al. Prevalence and clinical correlates of JAK2 mutations in Down syndrome acute lymphoblastic leukaemia. Br. J. Haematol. 2009 Mar;144(6):930–2.

[181] Kearney L, Gonzalez De Castro D, Yeung J, Procter J, Horsley SW, Eguchi-Ishimae M, et al. Specific JAK2 mutation (JAK2R683) and multiple gene deletions in Down syndrome acute lymphoblastic leukemia. Blood. 2009 Jan 15;113(3):646–8.

[182] Mullighan CG, Zhang J, Harvey RC, Collins-Underwood JR, Schulman BA, Phillips LA, et al. JAK mutations in high-risk childhood acute lymphoblastic leukemia. Proc. Natl. Acad. Sci. U.S.A. 2009 Jun 9;106(23):9414–8.

[183] Russell LJ, Capasso M, Vater I, Akasaka T, Bernard OA, Calasanz MJ, et al. Deregulated expression of cytokine receptor gene, CRLF2, is involved in lymphoid transformation in B-cell precursor acute lymphoblastic leukemia. Blood. 2009 Sep 24;114(13): 2688–98.

[184] Ziegler SF, Liu Y-J. Thymic stromal lymphopoietin in normal and pathogenic T cell development and function. Nat. Immunol. 2006 Jul;7(7):709–14.

[185] Akasaka T, Balasas T, Russell LJ, Sugimoto K, Majid A, Walewska R, et al. Five members of the CEBP transcription factor family are targeted by recurrent IGH translocations in B-cell precursor acute lymphoblastic leukemia (BCP-ALL). Blood. 2007 Apr 15;109(8):3451–61.

[186] Hertzberg L, Vendramini E, Ganmore I, Cazzaniga G, Schmitz M, Chalker J, et al. Down syndrome acute lymphoblastic leukemia, a highly heterogeneous disease in which aberrant expression of CRLF2 is associated with mutated JAK2: a report from the International BFM Study Group. Blood. 2010 Feb 4;115(5):1006–17.

[187] Cario G, Zimmermann M, Romey R, Gesk S, Vater I, Harbott J, et al. Presence of the P2RY8-CRLF2 rearrangement is associated with a poor prognosis in non-high-risk precursor B-cell acute lymphoblastic leukemia in children treated according to the ALL-BFM 2000 protocol. Blood. 2010 Jul 1;115(26):5393–7.

[188] Harvey RC, Mullighan CG, Chen I-M, Wharton W, Mikhail FM, Carroll AJ, et al. Rearrangement of CRLF2 is associated with mutation of JAK kinases, alteration of IKZF1, Hispanic/Latino ethnicity, and a poor outcome in pediatric B-progenitor acute lymphoblastic leukemia. Blood. 2010 Jul 1;115(26):5312–21.

[189] Ensor HM, Schwab C, Russell LJ, Richards SM, Morrison H, Masic D, et al. Demographic, clinical, and outcome features of children with acute lymphoblastic leukemia and CRLF2 deregulation: results from the MRC ALL97 clinical trial. Blood. 2011 Feb 17;117(7):2129–36.

[190] Palmi C, Vendramini E, Silvestri D, Longinotti G, Frison D, Cario G, et al. Poor prognosis for P2RY8-CRLF2 fusion but not for CRLF2 over-expression in children with intermediate risk B-cell precursor acute lymphoblastic leukemia. Leukemia: official journal of the Leukemia Society of America, Leukemia Research Fund, U.K [Internet]. 2012 Apr 9 [cited 2012 Jul 30]; Available from: http://www.ncbi.nlm.nih.gov/pubmed/22484421

[191] Yoda A, Yoda Y, Chiaretti S, Bar-Natan M, Mani K, Rodig SJ, et al. Functional screening identifies CRLF2 in precursor B-cell acute lymphoblastic leukemia. Proc. Natl. Acad. Sci. U.S.A. 2010 Jan 5;107(1):252–7.

[192] Buitenkamp TD, Pieters R, Gallimore NE, van der Veer A, Meijerink JPP, Beverloo HB, et al. Outcome in children with Down's syndrome and acute lymphoblastic leukemia: role of IKZF1 deletions and CRLF2 aberrations. Leukemia. 2012. Available from: http://www.ncbi.nlm.nih.gov/pubmed/22441210 (accessed 22 Mar 2012)

[193] Carpino N, Thierfelder WE, Chang M, Saris C, Turner SJ, Ziegler SF, et al. Absence of an essential role for thymic stromal lymphopoietin receptor in murine B-cell development. Mol. Cell. Biol. 2004 Mar;24(6):2584–92.

Chapter 10

Survival of Patients with Acute Lymphoblastic Leukemia

Jorge Organista-Nava, Yazmín Gómez-Gómez,
Berenice Illades-Aguiar and
Marco Antonio Leyva-Vázquez

Additional information is available at the end of the chapter

http://dx.doi.org/10.5772/54261

1. Introduction

Over the past 50 years, the treatment of patients with acute lymphoblastic leukemia (ALL) has significantly improved. This success is measured by the improved survival of ALL patients from less than 10% in the 1960s to more than 80% in more recent reports. However, many factors influence to a good outcome to treatment and subsequently in the improved survival of patients with ALL.

Age is the factor that has been more associated with survival. Younger patients (especially those younger than age 50) have a better survival than older patients. Not only age but also gender and race also are related with survival of ALL patients. The girls have showed a better survival than boys, this partly due to boys' risks for testicular cancer. African-American and Hispanic individuals have lower survival rates than Caucasian and Asian individual, but this may be due to poorer access to treatment. A very important factor in the clinic that somehow predicts good to bad prognosis of the patient and of course has also been linked to survival is the Initial white blood cell (WBC) count; people diagnosed with a WBC count below 50,000/μL tend to be better than people with higher WBC counts. Even, ALL subtype plays a role very important. For example, patients with T-cell ALL tend to have a better prognosis and survival than those with mature B-cell ALL (Burkitt leukemia). Nowadays, the identification of chromosome translocations help to prognosis of ALL patients; people who have Philadelphia chromosome-positive ALL tend to have a poorer prognosis, although is important to note that new treatments are helping many of these patients achieve remission.

Effectively, all the above factors (age, gender, race, Initial white blood cell (WBC) count, ALL subtype, and chromosome translocations) have an impact on treatment and survival of patients with leukemia. Since several years it is known that single nucleotide polymorphisms (SNPs) are some of the population genetic variations that greatly influence in the response to treatment of patients with ALL. It has been shown to SNPs modify the metabolism of chemical agents used in chemotherapy by affect the normal activity of enzymes involved in drug metabolism. This speaks of a very important role of these SNPs in the adequately outcome and survival of patients with ALL under treatment. This chapter shows how all the above factors play an important role in the survival to ALL and as the survival of patients with ALL varies according to these factors in different populations. The challenge remains to optimize the treatments according to population groups.

2. Age

Survival rates for children with ALL have increased dramatically over the past 4 decades, with 5-year survival rates of >90% in recent trials [1]. Data emerging from the surveillance, epidemiology and end results (SEER) database suggest that patients' age serves as a significant prognostic factor that affects clinical outcomes such as overall survival (OS) [2]. The SEER 9 (Atlanta, Connecticut, Detroit, Hawaii, Iowa, New Mexico, San Francisco-Oakland, Seattle-Puget Sound, Utah) showed that the 5-year survival rates for children younger than age 15 years with ALL improved from 61.0% in 1975-1978 to 88.5% in 1999-2002. Adolescents 15 to 19 years of age also showed improvement in survival over the same period, although their outcome in recent periods (50.1% 5-year survival in 1999-2002) was lower than that among children younger than age 15 years [3]. This lower survival rate partially reflects differences in tumor biology between children and older adolescents and likely also reflects differences in the way medical oncologists and pediatric oncologists have historically treated ALL arising in this age group [4, 5]. Survival for infants remains poor compared with that for children 1 to 14 years of age, although 5-year survival rates have increased from 22% in 1975-1978 to 62% in 1999-2002 [3].

In 2005, estimates derived SEER program of the National Cancer Institute placed the number of survivors of childhood ALL in the United States at 49 271 (0-19 years of age) being one of the cancer types with the largest number of survivors to 5-years. However, survival decreased with increasing age, with a relatively notable decline in survival beginning at ages 20 o more years [6]. As in Japanese population of aged 15-60 years where survival at 5 years is 35.0% [7] and Japanese children younger than 16 years age had 7-year OS rate of 76.0% [8]. In work done at Department of Epidemiology and Cancer Control, St Jude Children's Research Hospital, Memphis, TN of 1991 to 2006 in children with acute lymphoblastic leukemia; 5-year event-free survival (EFS) estimates were 88% for children aged 1–9 years, 73% for adolescents aged 10–15 years, 69% for those older than 15 years, and 44% for babies younger than 12 months [9, 10]. Today, the long-term survival has increased from approximately 10% in the early- to mid-1960s to more than 90% at St Jude Children's Research Hospital, Memphis, TN [1].

In Italian children between 1 and 18 years of age with newly diagnosed of ALL, enrolled in the AIEOP-BFM ALL 2000 study, had a 7-year EFS and survival of 80.4% and 91.8%, respectively. However when the children were stratified by minimal residual disease (MRD) their overall 7-year estimates for EFS and survival were 80.7% and 92.8%, respectively [11]. In United Kingdom, children aged 1–18 years survival estimates at 5 years were 87% [12]. In Pakistani population aged > 15 years their median survival was 12.7 months and disease-free survival was 6.2 months [13].

Currently, due to intensive chemotherapy regimens, the outcome of adult ALL has improved markedly. The complete response rates now are more than 80% [14] and the long-term survival rate is 30%–45% [15]. Based on a study by Stephen Hunger and colleagues, 5-year OS rates now above 90% for the first time (83.7% in the period 1990-1994; 90.4% in the most recent period 2000-2005). This study is based on information on 21,626 ALL patients between 0 and 22 years who were enrolled onto the Children's Oncolocy Group (COG) ALL clinical trials from 1990 to 2005. It is clear that survival improved in all subgroups of ALL (1-9 years), except for infants under the age of 1 year. Besides, 5-year OS also remains significantly lower (81.6%) for children over the age of 10 years [16]. Childhood ALL reflects one of the diagnosis for which the most impressive improvements have been realized [1].

The better results seen among the childhood population as compared to adults with ALL have been attributed to a number of prognostic factors. It is important to consider a number of important differences between younger and older patients with ALL exist. First, the biology of both, underlying disease and the patients' metabolic changes with age are very different between two cohorts [17]. The second major difference is the difference in therapy related toxicity [18]. The third potential cause for a superior outcome in the younger population is relates to the protocols administered. It is important to consider that the treatment protocols from each institution, the dose adjustments and many others factors can increase long-term survival, but the factor toxicity could have a negative effect on long-term.

3. Gender

Survival disparity by the sex of the patient with leukemia has been observed since the nineteen sixties; however, what remains to be fully grasped are the factors responsible for this persisting survival difference between boys and girls. Girls continue to demonstrate survival advantage relative to boys. Studies over the past years have repeatedly shown that after diagnosis of pediatric leukemia, boys present with poorer survival that the girls (Table 2).

In 2012 using a large sample and long-term data could help explain the ongoing variance in leukemia survival comparing boys to girls and found that boys are more likely to die from leukemia (Table 1). The explanation to the observed disparity in survival by sex, since most of the patients who had T-cell type were boys, and survival was poorer among boys in this study [19]. A biological explanation for sex disparity in leukemia survival, it is plausible to suspect XY chromosomal instability as a possible contribution to abnormal cellular proliferation, thus resulting in a biologically aggressive leukemia among male patients. Also, it might be possible that testosterone or estrogen may play a small role in pediatric leukemia, this partly due to boys' risks for develop testicular cancer [19].

Population			Survival estimated	% of Overall Survival	Number of patients	Ref.
		Sex				
U.S.	Male	Children	At 5 years	53.9	8,622	[19]
	Female			58.0	6,593	
European	Male	Children	At 5 years	63.0	401	[20]
	Female			67.0	299	
U.S.	Male	Children	At 5 years	63.5	1,151	[21]
	Female			73.4	904	
		WBC count				
Japanese	$< 10.0x10^9/L$	Children	At 7 years	71.5	300	[22]
	$10.0\text{-}49.9x10^9/L$			62.7	206	
	$50.0\text{-}99.9x10^9/L$			52.9	35	
	$\geq 100.0x10^9/L$			19.3	48	
Japanese	$<3x10^9/L$	Adults	At 5 years	20.0	15	[23]
	$3x10^9\text{-}50x10^9/L$			48.8	45	
	$>50x10^9/L$			19.2	27	
Korean	$<100.0x10^3/\mu L$	Children	At 4 years	87.5	83	[24]
	$\geq 100.0x10^3/\mu L$			57.1	17	
European	$<50x10^9/L$	Children	At 5 years	92.3	1,348	[11]
	$50.0\text{-}99.9x10^9/L$			77.6	1,647	
	$\geq 100.0x10^9/L$			50.1	189	
European	$<50x10^9/L$	Children	At 5 years	94.0	923	[12]
	$>50x10^9/L$			61.0	166	
U.S.	$<50,000/\mu L$	Children	At 4 years	80.3	68	[25]

Table 1. Recent studies on survival of ALL patients by gender and Initial white blood cell (WBC) count

4. Initial White Blood Cell (WBC) count

Along with age, the initial peripheral blood leukocyte count is another of the firsts identified prognostic factors in every study of ALL. The WBC at diagnosis is a crucial variable for describing the nature of the patient's leukemia and especially the tumor burden. The other measures of the tumor burden are the size of a mediastinal mass, hepatosplenomegaly, and enlargement of lymph nodes. Children with WBC of more than $50x10^9/L$ are commonly considered to be at high risk of relapse and receive intensive treatment [1, 2]. In retrospective analysis was found that patients with hyperleukocytosis (WBC count

http://dx.doi.org/10.5772/54261

>50 10^9/L) were significantly related to lower survival. Similar findings are the rule in reports from various study groups (Table 1).

The cytogenetic features are closely linked to the WBC and at least partly explain the prognostic of WBC, although there is evidence that children with similar cytogenetic aberrations may have very different WBCs, and their prognostic value is related partly to the WBC [26-28].

Race/ethnicity		Survival estimated	% of Overall Survival	Number of patients	Ref.
Non-Hispanic white	Children	At 5 years	70	1,529	[29]
Hispanic			56	178	
Asian/Pasific islander			56	2,542	
Non-Hispanic black			46	408	
Whites	Children	At 5 years	78	6703	[30]
Blacks			65	506	
Hispanics			69	1071	
Asians			84	167	
Whites	Children	At 5 years	70	3621	[31]
Blacks			57	356	
Asians			71	410	
Native American			54	61	
Hispanics			63	504	

Table 2. Recent studies on survival of ALL patients by race/ethnicity

5. Race/ethnicity

Variability in survival outcome across racial and ethnic groups (hereafter referred to as race/ethnicity) also has been identified in some, but not all, clinical research. Survival rates in Black, Hispanic and Native American children with ALL have been somewhat lower than the rates in White children with ALL (Table 2). This difference may be therapy-dependent [32]. Asian children with ALL fare slightly better than white children [33]. The reason for better outcome in White and Asian children compared with Black, Native American and Hispanic children is at least partially explained by the different spectrum of ALL subtypes. For example, blacks have a higher incidence of T-cell ALL and lower rates of favorable genetic subtypes of ALL. However, these differences do not completely explain the observed racial differences in outcome [33].

Population		Survival estimated	% of Overall Survival	Number of patients	Ref.
		ETV6-RUNX1 [t(12;21)]			
Brazilian	Children	At 5 years	77.6	58	[34]
Nordic countries	Children	At 5 years	65.0	669	[35]
U.S.	Children	At 5 years	93.7	662	[36]
French	Children	At 5 years	50.0	73	[37]
		BCR-ABL [t(9;22)]			
Spanish	Adults	At 4 years	16.0	30	[38]
Europe and U.S.	Children	At 2 years	35.5 - 46.3	267	[39]
U.S.	Children	At 4 years	35.0	120	[40]
Japanese	Adults	At 2 years	12.5	80	[41]
		MLL-AF4[t(4;11) (q21;q23)]			
Europe	Adults	At 5 years	39.0	236	[42]
Japanese	Infants	At 3 years	43.5	54	[43]
Europe	Adults	At 5 years	13.0	24	[44]
Spanish	Infants, Children, Adults	At 5 years	36.0	51	[45]
		PBX1/E2A[t(1;19)(q23;p13.3)/der(19)t(1;19)(q23;p13.3)]			
Caucasian	Children	At 5 years	90.0	31	[46]
U.S.	Children	At 5 years	84.2	41	[47]
Europe	Children	At 5 years	84.0	50	[12]
Europe	Adults	At 5 years	79.0	47	[48]

Table 3. Studies on survival of ALL patients with genetic rearrangements

6. Survival by ALL Immunophenotype

The World Health Organization (WHO) classifies ALL as either B lymphoblastic leukemia or T lymphoblastic leukemia [49]. Historically, T-cell ALL patients have had a worse prognosis than other ALL, the relapse rate of T-cell ALL is greater than B-cell ALL cases, and T-cell ALL cases have shown less EFS than B-ALL cases [50, 51]. Patients with T-cell ALL treated on Dana-Farber Cancer Institute (DFCI) Boston, MA had an overall survival at 5 years of 78 % compared with 86 % for B progenitor ALL patients [50]. A study based cancer registry areas of the Surveillance, Epidemiology and End Results (SEER) Program (SEER-17) during 2001 to 2007 reported that infants with B-cell ALL and ALL of unknown lineage had intermediate survival to 5-years compared with 5- to 19-year and 20- to 39-year age groups.

Notably, children and young adults 1 to 4 and 5 to 19 years of age with B-cell ALL had more favorable survival (Approximately 99% and 88%) than those with T-cell ALL (Approximately 84% and 78%). In contrast, survival for T-cell ALL was substantially higher than B-cell ALL among adults 20 to 39, 40 to 59, and 60 years or older of age [52].

7. *Chromosomal translocations in* B-cell acute lymphoblastic leukemia (B-cell ALL)

Acute lymphoblastic leukemia is a heterogeneous disease that originates from lymphocyte progenitor cells of B- or T-cell origin. ALL comprises multiple distinct subtypes that are characterized by recurrent copy number alterations and structural chromosomal rearrangements, which have important clinical implications. Such cytogenetically distinct subtypes include B-cell precursor (BCP) leukemia with the chromosomal translocations t(12;21)(p13;q22) [ETV6/RUNX1], t(9;22)(q11;q34) [BCR/ABL1], (4;11)(q21;q23)/MLL-AF4, *t(11;19)/MLL-ENL, t(1;19)(q23;p13)/PBX1/E2A* karyotypes. It is well established that ALL subtypes differ from a clinical perspective, but the underlying molecular consequences of most of the recurrent chromosomal abnormalities are poorly understood [53].

8. ETV6-RUNX1 [t(12;21) cryptic translocation, formerly known as TEL-AML1]

The translocation t(12;21)(p13;q22) is the most frequent chromosomal alteration in childhood B-lineage ALL (B-ALL) [54], which involves the fusion of the ETV6 (alias TEL) gene on chromosome 12 to the RUNX1 gene on chromosome 21. It is identified in 20% to 25% of the cases of B-precursor ALL and is rarely observed in T-lineage ALL [55]. The t(12;21) is most commonly found in children aged 2 to 9 years [56]. Reports generally indicate favorable OS in children with the ETV6-RUNX1 fusion (Table 3); however, the prognostic impact of this genetic feature is modified by factors such as early response to treatment and treatment regimen [57].

9. Philadelphia chromosome (Ph) or t(9;22) translocation

The Ph results from a reciprocal translocation (t) between chromosomes 9 and 22 (t [9,22] [q34;q11]) [58, 59], occurs in approximately 3 to 5% of children, as compared with up to 30 percent of adults with ALL [60, 61].

The Ph produces a fusion gene on chromosome 22, namely, the breakpoint cluster region Abelson leukemia viral proto-oncogene (BCR-ABL). The translocation can result in 3 fusion protein of different sizes: p190, p210, and p230 [62]. The p190 BCR-ABL fusion gene occurs in about 90% of children with Ph-positive ALL [63] and between 50% and 80% of adults with Ph-positive ALL [64, 65].

Ph-positive ALL has an extremely poor prognosis overall (rates of EFS are 30 to 46 percent in children and less than 20 percent in adults) Table 3. However, some investigators suggest that in this type of ALL, the prognosis is influenced by the treatment with glucocorticoids (and intrathecal methotrexate) [66], or by other factors (such as age and leukocyte count at diagnosis) [67, 68]. These variations in the response to therapy suggest that Ph-positive ALL is heterogeneous with regard to sensitivity to treatment [39].

10. MLL translocations

10.1. MLL-AF4; t(4;11) (q21;q23) translocation

The incidence of t(4;11)(q21;q23)/MLL-AF4, occurring in over 50% ALL cases in infants aged less than 6 months, in 10–20% of older infants, in about 2% of children, and in almost 10% of adults [69, 70]. The presence of the translocation t(4;11)(q21;q23) or a fusion gene MLL-AF4 is detected in almost 10% of newly diagnosed B-cell ALL and in about 30–40% of pro-B ALL subtypes [71, 72].

A t(4;11)(q21;q23)/MLL-AF4 positive ALL is generally considered as a high risk leukemia, characterized by a poor clinical outcome respect to other cytogenetic risk groups [73]. Moreover, in several studies it has been demonstrated that cytogenetic-molecular risk and WBC count at diagnosis were the main prognostic factors that influenced OS in ALL patients (Table 3).

10.2. MLL-ENL; t(11;19) translocation

The t(11;19)/ MLL-ENL is present in approximately 1% of cases and occurs in both early B-cell and T-cell ALL [74]. Outcome for infants with t(11;19) is poor, but outcome appears relatively favorable in older children with T-cell ALL and the t(11;19) translocation [74].

10.3. PBX1/E2A; t(1;19)(q23;p13) translocation

The translocation t(1;19)(q23;p13), and its unbalanced variant del(19)t(1;19)(q23;p13), is a primary and well known chromosome abnormality in childhood B-cell precursor ALL, being present in 3–5% of all such cases [75, 76].

The t(1;19) produces a fusion between TCF3 gene on 19p13 and PBX1 on 1q23 [77], with the TCF3-PBX1 fusion transcript being expressed from the chromosome 19 [78]. Initially, t(1;19) was associated with a poor prognosis in ALL [79, 80], however most patients treated by contemporary therapies now achieve improved outcomes (Table 6).

11. *Chromosomal translocations in* T-cell acute lymphoblastic leukemia (T-cell ALL)

T-cell ALL accounts for about 15% and 25% of ALL in pediatric and adult cohorts respectively [69]. Cytogenetic abnormalities are rare in T-cell ALL. Multiple chromosomal translocations have been identified in T-cell ALL, with many genes encoding for transcription factors (e.g., TAL1; [t(1;14)(p32;q11) and t(1;7)(p32;q34)], LMO1; [t(11;14)(p15;q11)], LMO2; [t(11;14)(p13;q11) and t(7;11)(q35;p13)], LYL1; [t(7;19)(q34;p13)], TLX1/HOX11 [t(7;10)(q34;q24) and t(10;14)(q24;q11)], and TLX3/HOX11L2 [t(5;14)(q35;q32)]) fusing to one of the T-cell receptor (TCR) loci and resulting in aberrant expression of these transcription factors in leukemia cells [81]. Historically, T-cell ALL in children has been associated with a worse prognosis than other sub-types of childhood ALL [82, 83].

High expression of TLX1/HOX11 resulting from translocations involving this gene occurs in 5% to 10% of pediatric T-cell ALL cases and is associated with more favorable outcome in both adults and children with T-cell ALL [84-86]. Overexpression of TLX3/HOX11L2 resulting from the t(5;14)(q35;q32) translocation occurs in approximately 20% of pediatric T-cell ALL cases and appears to be associated with increased risk of treatment failure [85].

12. Gene polymorphisms associated to poor survival in ALL patients

It is difficult to define which component of the protocol/regimen is the responsible for the improved outcome of patients with ALL. Antifolates, such as methotrexate (MTX), are competitive inhibitors of folate-dependent enzymes and are widely used in the treatment of many human cancers [87]. In last decades, the MTX has been a key agent for the treatment of ALL and the benefit of high-dose MTX is well established as it significantly increases cure rates and improves patients' prognosis [88]. MTX exerts its cytotoxic effects by competitively inhibiting dihydrofolate reductase (DHFR), the enzyme responsible for converting folates to tetrahydrofolate, the reduced folate carriers which function in the transfer of carbon units. These carbon units are required for de novo purine synthesis and the methylation of uracil to thymine in DNA synthesis [89].

MTX enters the cells and is metabolized into 7-hydroxymethotrexate (7-OHMTX), 2,4-diamino-N^{10}-methylpteroic acid (DAMPA) and more active derivatives as methotrexate polyglutamates (MTXPG) with sequential gamma-linkage of 2 to 6 glutamyl residues by the folylpolyglutamate synthetase (FPGS) [88]. MTXPG retained in cells for a longer time result in prolonged MTX antifolate effect [89]. However, accumulation of MTXPG is a critical factor associated with cytotoxicity and response of ALL patients to the therapy [89]. On the other hand, the polyglutamation process competes with deconjugation that converts MTXPG back into MTX by gamma-glutamyl hydrolase (GGH). Long chain MTXPG have higher affinity than MTX for the enzymes involved in de novo purine synthesis such as 5-aminoimidazole-4-carboxamide ribonucleotide transformylase (ATIC) and thymidilate synthase (TS), which results in a reinforcement of MTX inhibition (Figure 1) [88]. Thus, intracellular formation of MTXPG enhances the cytotoxic and antileukemic effect of MTX.

The disease-free survival of childhood ALL has improved steadily the last decades, reaching 80% in the developed countries [17]. Despite the advances, almost 20% of the children either relapse or do not respond to treatment. This seems to be related to various parameters, including the presence of polymorphisms of drug transporters, receptors, targets, and drug-metabolizing enzymes, hence influencing the efficacy, the toxicity of therapy [91].

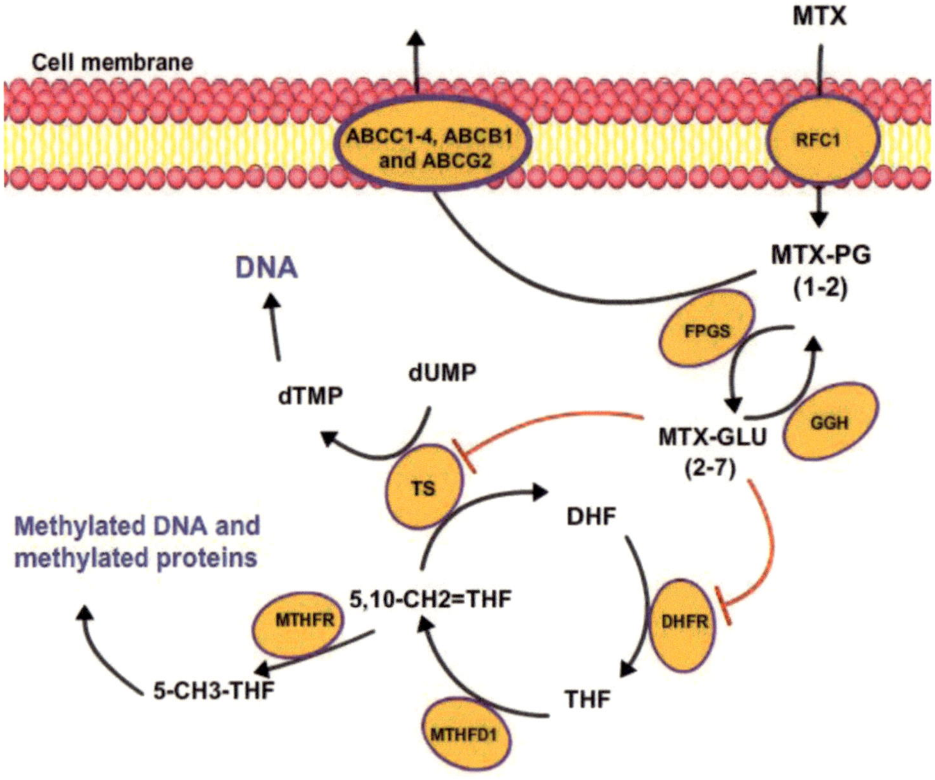

Figure 1. Methotrexate enters cells through the reduced **folate carrier** (RFC1) or other transport systems. Its main intracellular target is **dihydrofolate reductase** (DHFR), inhibition of which results in accumulation of dihydrofolate (DHF) and depletion of cellular folates. Cytosolic **folylpolyglutamyl synthase** (FPGS) adds glutamate residues to methotrexate to produce methotrexate polyglutamates (MTXPGs), they are retained by the cell, and the resulting increase the efficacy of methotrexate. The addition of glutamate residues to methotrexate also increases its affinity for other target enzymes (**thymidylate synthetase** (TS) and **dihydrofolate reductase** (DHFR). Other enzymes that are indirectly affected by methotrexate are **5,10-methylenetetrahydrofolate reductase** (MTHFR) and **methylenetetrahydrofolate dehydrogenase** (MTHFD1). dTMP, deoxythymidine monophospate; dUMP, deoxyuridine monophospate; THF, tetrahydrofolate. Figure modified with permission from Ref. [90] © PharmGKB and Stanford University (2011).

Recently, attention has been drawn on genes involved in diverse metabolic pathways, which are known to be polymorphic at various sites and can affect both the susceptibility for leukemia, the treatment outcome and survival in patients with ALL [91].

13. The reduced folate carrier (RFC1/SLC19A1)

Several polymorphisms in enzymes of the folate cycle as well as in the MTX transporters have been described. The reduced folate carrier gene (RFC1) is a major MTX transporter whose impaired function was recognized as a frequent mechanism of antifolate resistance [92]. The most common SNP in RFC1, 80A>G, which results in the amino acid substitution of Arg with His at position 27 of the RFC1 protein, may alter the affinity of the transporter [93]. Several investigators had studied the association of the SNP of RFC G80A and the outcome in ALL. Reports generally indicate association between the G/G and/or A/G genotypes of the G80A polymorphism with a poorer survival in patient's children and adults con ALL. Survival rates in Italian and Mexican population with ALL have been somewhat lower than the rates in European and French-Canadian population (Table 4).

14. Folypolyglutamate Hydrolase (GGH)

GGH is a lysosomal peptidase that catalyses the removal of gamma-linked polyglutamates and convert long-chain polyglutamates (n=4–7) into short-chain polyglutamates (n=2–3) and ultimately MTX, allowing folate to be exported from the cell [94].

Several SNPs have been identified in the GGH gene at bases −401C>T, −354G>T, −124T>G, +16T>C, +452C>T, and +1102A>G; these sites comprise both the promoter and the coding region [95, 96]. Nevertheless, few SNPs have been associated with catalytic activity of the GGH in B- and T-lineage ALL cells, and greater accumulation of long-chain MTX in these cells [97].

The polymorphism +452C>T in the transcribed region of GGH gene alters Thr-127 to Ile-1271, and has been associated with reduced catalytic activity in hyperdiploid B- and T-lineage acute lymphocytic leukemia (ALL) cells, and greater accumulation of long-chain MTXPG in these cells [97]. In contrast, all of the promoter polymorphisms enhanced GGH expression and an increased GGH activity may lead to decreased accumulation of MTXPG and to MTX resistance. At least one of these, −401C>T, has been shown to be correlated with decreased accumulation of long-chain MTX-Glu3–5 in rheumatoid arthritis patients treated with MTX [98].

Only polymorphism -354G>T has been associated with survival of children with ALL. -354GT or -354TT genotypes carrier have better probability of 5-year post-treatment OS compared to -354GG genotypes (p = 0.04) (Table 4) [99]. This shows the enzyme GGH clearly plays an important role in the metabolism of folates and anti-folates. However, unambiguous demonstration of a direct role of GGH in anti-folate drug resistance has been difficult. Part of the difficulty is that GGH is only one of several factors that can affect anti-folate levels, and its role presumably is directly linked to those of the other enzymes. [100]. However, these studies have demonstrated that polymorphisms in GGH increase promoter activity and an increased GGH activity may lead to decreased accumulation of MTXPG and to MTX resistance [101]

Genotypes	Population	Survival estimated	% of Overall Survival	Number of patients	Ref.
80A>G polymorphism in RFC1 gene					
G/G	Italian (adults)	At 5 years	59.0	13	[102]
A/G + A/A			28.0	34	
G/G	Mexican (children)	At 5 years	76.0	20	[103]
A/G + A/A			42.0	50	
G/G	European (children)	At 5 years	97.0	160	[104]
A/G + A/A			75.0	305	
G/G	French-Canadian origin (children)	At 5 years	89.0	61	[93]
A/G + A/A			76.0	143	
-354G>T polymorphism in GGH gene					
GG	European (children)	At 5 years	90.0	123	[99]
GT+TT			>90.0	116	
-317A>G polymorphism in DHFR gene					
A/A	Mexican (children)	At 5 years	78.0	14	[105]
A/G + G/G			41.0	56	
A/A	Canadian (children)	At 5 years	92.0	24	[106]
A/G + G/G			76.0	31	
829C>T polymorphism in DHFR gene					
C/C	Mexican (children)	At 5 years	80.0	10	[105]
C/T + T/T			38.0	60	
Polymorphism in TS gene					
3R/3R-negative	Canadian (children)	At 5 years	82.0	193	[107]
3R/3R-positive			71.0	66	
2R/2R or 2R/3R	French-Canadian (children)	At 5 years	87.0	155	[108]
3R/3R			68.0	50	
677C>T polymorphism in MTHFR gene					
C	Italian (Adults)	At 2 years	55.0	118	[109]
TT			14.0		
C	Spanish (children)	At 4 years	98.0	106	[110]
TT			52.0	35	
C	Egyptian (children)	At 2 years	90.9	22	[111]
TT			50.0	4	
T677A1298 haplotype of the MTHFR gene					
T677A1298 (-)	French–Canadian origin (Children)	At 5 years	89.0	84	[112]
T677A1298 (+)			74.0	117	

Table 4. Genetic polymorphism and its relationship to survival in ALL

15. Dihydrofolate Reductase (DHFR)

DHFR is responsible to catalyze the reduction of dihydrofolate (DHF) to tetrahydrofolate (THF) [113]. The major mechanism of MTX action involves competitive inhibition of DHFR, leading to the impaired regeneration of THF from DHF; essential for the biosynthesis of purines and thymidylate, thus it also blocks the novo synthesis of DNA [114, 115].

Changes in the levels of DHFR expression and consequently in the sensitivity to MTX can also be due to single SNPs, particularly those located in the regulatory elements [105]. The C829T SNP is located at the 223 nucleotide downstream from the stop codon between the first and second polyadenylation sites in the 3'UTR of the DHFR gene, which leads to the stability of mRNA [116]. A previous study reported that the -A317G SNP in the DHFR promoter region results in higher transcriptional activity [106]. Recently demonstrated an association between G/G and T/T genotypes of the -A317G and C829T polymorphisms and reduced survival in pediatric patients with ALL (Table 4).

16. Thymidylate Synthase (TS)

The TS is a key enzyme in the nucleotide biosynthesis and important target of several chemotherapeutics. TS provides the only source for de novo thymidylate production by catalyzing the methylation of deoxyuridine monophosphate (dUMP) to deoxythymidine monophosphate (dTMP) [107]. TS is efficiently inhibited by the uracil analog, 5-fluorouracil (5-FU) and MTX, used for many years as a treatment for a variety of cancers.

The most common polymorphism in TS is a unique double (2R) or triple (3R) 28-bp tandem repeat sequence in the 5' untranslated region (5'-UTR) of the TS gene also called TS enhancer region (TSER), immediately upstream from the initiation site, which influences protein expression in cancer cells [117]. The presence of a triple versus double 28-bp repeat in the enhancer region has been associated with an increased TS expression both in *in vivo* and *in vitro* studies [118, 119].

Previous studies have shown that pediatric patients who were homozygous for the triple repeat (3R/3R) had a poorer prognostic (odds ratio 4.1, 95% CI 1.9–9.0, p=0.001) [108] and shorter survival than those patients with other genotypes (Table 4).

17. Methylenetetrahydrofolate Reductase (MTHFR)

The MTHFR is a key folate enzyme that catalyzes the conversion of 5,10-methylenetetrahydrofolate to 5-methyltetrahydrofolate in the folic acid cycle, and is interrupted by methotrexate (MTX), a critical chemotherapy agent in ALL therapy [120].

Despite the fact that several MTHFR polymorphisms have been described thus far, only two polymorphisms, C677T and A1298C, have been intensively investigated. The C-to-T transition at the nucleotide position 677 in exon 4 of MTHFR generates an alanine-to-valine substitution at amino acid 222 [121]. As a result, carriers of the MTHFR 677TT genotype possess a thermolabile enzyme of reduced activity [122]. The second most studied polymorphism in MTHFR is an A-to-C transversion substitution at nucleotide 1,298 (exon 7) that results in an amino acid substitution of glutamate for alanine at codon 429 [123]. Once this amino acid substitution takes place at the S-adenosylmethionine regulatory domain of the MTHFR, the A1298C polymorphism also generates an enzyme with a decreased activity [123]. Other investigators have reported that A1298C and C677T polymorphisms in MTHFR gene are associated with disease outcomes and survival both in children and adults (table 4).

The overall survival rate of MTHFR 677TT and 1298CC carriers was lower than that of patients carrying MTHFR C or A alleles respectively. A limited amount of evidence has been reported on the influence of MTHFR polymorphisms on survival.

18. Methylenetetrahydrofolate Dehydrogenase (MTHFD1)

MTHFD1 is an enzyme involved in folate metabolism, which plays an important role in the generation of the 5,10-methylene-THF and 10-formyl-THF. The last two are the donor cofactors for de novo purine and pyrimidine biosynthesis and, thus, for the biosynthesis of DNA [124]. The G to A substitution at position 1958 of the MTHFD1 gene, causing an alanine to glycine substitution at codon 653 located within the 10-formyl-THF synthetase enzyme domain, which reduces the enzyme's activity [124].

A analysis of 201 children treated with methotrexate showed that patients with the MTHFD1 A1958 variant had a remarkably lower probability of 5-year post-treatment survival, compared to subjects with no event-predisposing genotypes (45.0% vs 95.0%, p=0.0002) [112].

Expression	Population	Survival estimated	% of Overall Survival	Number of patients	Ref.
Negative	Korean (Children and Adults	At 2 years	>85.0	24	[125]
Positive			<55.0	8	
Low	Brazilian (Childen)	At 5 years	81.0	150	[126]
High			54.0		
Low	European (Children)	At 5 years	87.2	56	[127]
High			60.0		
Low	European (Adults)	At 5 years	80.0	49	[127]
High			52.0		

Table 5. Expression of MRP1 and its relationship to survival in ALL

http://dx.doi.org/10.5772/54261

19. Multidrug Resistance-Associated Protein 1 (MRP1/ABCC1)

Multidrug resistance (MDR) is one of the major obstacles in cancer chemotherapy. Over-expression of ATP-binding cassette (ABC) transporters, such as P-glycoprotein (Pgp/MDR1/ABCB1) and multidrug resistance-associated protein 1 (MRP1/ABCC1), have been shown to cause MDR in model cell lines and in clinical settings [128-130]. Currently, eight MRP genes have been identified, of which the MRP transporters (MRP1-6) are known to be involved in extruding substrates that are generally used in the treatment of ALL, including doxorubicin, vincristine, etoposide, 6-mercaptopurine, and methotrexate [131-134].

Recent studies have shown that in ALL patients, high expression of MRP1, is a highly significant indicator of poor response to chemotherapy and poor overall survival in both in children and adults (Table 5).

20. Summary and future directions

Several clinical and biological features have been associated with the improved survival of patients with ALL, including age, sex, WBC, race/ethnicity, immunophenotype, recurrent chromosomal abnormalities, and genetics polymorphisms. The application of risk-stratified therapy utilizing these prognostic factors has resulted in long-term event-free survival in up to 80-85% of patients with ALL. Further improvement in outcome will require, in part, the discovery of novel prognostic factors, (such as, genetic variation in the folate pathway, transport of drugs, as well as miRNAs expression) to identify the 15-20% of patients who are not cured with current therapies. Recent advances in our understanding of underlying leukemia biology, including the identification of prognostically distinctive subsets of patients, and of host pharmacogenomics may allow for more precise risk stratification and more targeted, individualized treatment planning that will lead to higher survival of the patients with ALL.

Author details

Jorge Organista-Nava[1], Yazmín Gómez-Gómez[1], Berenice Illades-Aguiar[2] and Marco Antonio Leyva-Vázquez[2*]

*Address all correspondence to: leyvamarco13@gmail.com

1 Institute of Cellular Physiology, National Autonomous University of Mexico (UNAM), D.F., Mexico

2 Molecular Biomedicine Laboratory, School of Biological Sciences, Guerrero State University, Chilpancingo, Guerrero, Mexico

References

[1] Robison LL. Late Effects of Acute Lymphoblastic Leukemia Therapy in Patients Diagnosed at 0-20 Years of Age. ASH Education Program Book 2011, 2011;2011(1): 238-42.

[2] Pulte D, Gondos A, Brenner H. Improvement in survival in younger patients with acute lymphoblastic leukemia from the 1980s to the early 21st century. Blood 2009, 2009;113(7):1408-11.

[3] Smith MA, Seibel NL, Altekruse SF, Ries LAG, Melbert DL, O'Leary M, et al. Outcomes for Children and Adolescents With Cancer: Challenges for the Twenty-First Century. Journal of Clinical Oncology 2010, 2010;28(15):2625-34.

[4] Nachman J. Clinical characteristics, biologic features and outcome for young adult patients with acute lymphoblastic leukaemia. British Journal of Haematology 2005;130(2):166-73.

[5] Stock W, La M, Sanford B, Bloomfield CD, Vardiman JW, Gaynon P, et al. What determines the outcomes for adolescents and young adults with acute lymphoblastic leukemia treated on cooperative group protocols? A comparison of Children's Cancer Group and Cancer and Leukemia Group B studies. Blood 2008, 2008;112(5): 1646-54.

[6] Mariotto AB, Rowland JH, Yabroff KR, Scoppa S, Hachey M, Ries L, et al. Long-Term Survivors of Childhood Cancers in the United States. Cancer Epidemiology Biomarkers & Prevention 2009, 2009;18(4):1033-40.

[7] Yanada M, Jinnai I, Takeuchi J, Ueda T, Miyawaki S, Tsuzuki M, et al. Clinical features and outcome of T-lineage acute lymphoblastic leukemia in adults: A low initial white blood cell count, as well as a high count predict decreased survival rates. Leukemia Research 2007;31(7):907-14.

[8] Keizo Horibe a, Junichi Hara, Keiko Yagi, Akio Tawa, Yoshihiro Komada, Megumi Oda, et al. Prognostic Factors in Childhood Acute Lymphoblastic Leukemia in Japan. International Journal of Hematology 2000;72:61-8.

[9] Hilden JM, Dinndorf PA, Meerbaum SO, Sather H, Villaluna D, Heerema NA, et al. Analysis of prognostic factors of acute lymphoblastic leukemia in infants: report on CCG 1953 from the Children's Oncology Group. Blood 2006, 2006;108(2):441-51.

[10] Pieters R, Schrappe M, De Lorenzo P, Hann I, De Rossi G, Felice M, et al. A treatment protocol for infants younger than 1 year with acute lymphoblastic leukaemia (Interfant-99): an observational study and a multicentre randomised trial. The Lancet 2007;370(9583):240-50.

[11] Conter V, Bartram CR, Valsecchi MG, Schrauder A, Panzer-Grümayer R, Möricke A, et al. Molecular response to treatment redefines all prognostic factors in children and

adolescents with B-cell precursor acute lymphoblastic leukemia: results in 3184 patients of the AIEOP-BFM ALL 2000 study. Blood 2010;115(16):3206-14.

[12] Moorman AV, Ensor HM, Richards SM, Chilton L, Schwab C, Kinsey SE, et al. Prognostic effect of chromosomal abnormalities in childhood B-cell precursor acute lymphoblastic leukaemia: results from the UK Medical Research Council ALL97/99 randomised trial. The Lancet Oncology 2010;11(5):429-38.

[13] Shaikh M U, Ali N ASN, M K. Outcome of adult patients with acute lymphoblastic leukaemia receiving the MRC UKALL XII protocol: a tertiary care centre experience. Singapore Medical Journal 2011;52(5):370-74.

[14] Durrant IJ, Richards SM, Prentice HG, Goldstone AH. The medical research council trials in adult acute lyphoblastic leukemia. Hematology/Oncology Clinics of North America 2000;14(6):1327-52.

[15] Larson R. Recent clinical trials in acute lyphoblastic leukemia by the cancer and leukemia group B Hematology/Oncology Clinics of North America 2000;14(6):1367-79.

[16] Hunger SP, Lu X, Devidas M, Camitta BM, Gaynon PS, Winick NJ, et al. Improved survival for children and adolescents with acute lymphoblastic leukemia between 1990 and 2005: a report from the hildren's oncology group. J Clin Oncol 2012;10;30(14):1663-9.

[17] Pui C-H, Evans WE. Treatment of Acute Lymphoblastic Leukemia. New England Journal of Medicine 2006;354(2):166-78.

[18] Hunault-Berger M, Chevallier P, Delain M, Bulabois C-E, Bologna S, Bernard M, et al. Changes in antithrombin and fibrinogen levels during induction chemotherapy with L-asparaginase in adult patients with acute lymphoblastic leukemia or lymphoblastic lymphoma. Use of supportive coagulation therapy and clinical outcome: the CAPE-LAL study. Haematologica 2008, 2008;93(10):1488-94.

[19] Holmes L, Hossain J, desVignes-Kendrick M, Opara F. Sex variability in pediatric leukemia survival: Large cohort evidence. ISRN Oncology 2012:1-9.

[20] Moorman AV, Richards SM, Martineau M, Cheung KL, Robinson HM, Jalali GR, et al. Outcome heterogeneity in childhood high-hyperdiploid acute lymphoblastic leukemia. Blood 2003;102(8):2756-62.

[21] Pui CH, Boyett JM, Relling MV, Harrison PL, Rivera GK, Behm FG, et al. Sex differences in prognosis for children with acute lymphoblastic leukemia. Journal of Clinical Oncology 1999;17(3):818-24.

[22] Horibe K, Hara J, Yagi K, Tawa A, Komada Y, Oda M, et al. Prognostic factors in childhood acute lymphoblastic leukemia in Japan. International Journal of Hematology 2000;72(1):61-8.

[23] [23] Yanada M, Jinnai I, Takeuchi J, Ueda T, Miyawaki S, Tsuzuki M, et al. Clinical features and outcome of T-lineage acute lymphoblastic leukemia in adults: A low ini-

tial white blood cell count, as well as a high count predict decreased survival rates. Leukemia Research 2007;31(7):907-14.

[24] [24] Park J, Park SS, Lim YT. A clinical characteristics and prognosis in children of acute lymphoblastic leukemia with hyperleukocytosis. Clinical Pediatric Hematology-Oncology 2006;13(1):1-8.

[25] Friedmann AM, Weinstein HJ. The role of prognostic features in the treatment of childhood acute lymphoblastic leukemia. The Oncologist 2000;5(4):321-8.

[26] Wood AJJ, Pui CH, Evans WE. Acute lymphoblastic leukemia. New England Journal of Medicine 1998;339(9):605-15.

[27] Ribeiro RC, Broniscer A, Rivera GK, Hancock ML, Raimondi SC, Sandlund JT, et al. Philadelphia chromosome-positive acute lymphoblastic leukemia in children: durable responses to chemotherapy associated with low initial white blood cell counts. Leukemia: official journal of the Leukemia Society of America, Leukemia Research Fund, UK 1997;11(9):1493.

[28] Schrappe M, Arico M, Harbott J, Biondi A, Zimmermann M, Conter V, et al. Philadelphia chromosome-positive (Ph+) childhood acute lymphoblastic leukemia: good initial steroid response allows early prediction of a favorable treatment outcome. Blood 1998;92(8):2730-41.

[29] Kent EE, Sender LS, Largent JA, Anton-Culver H. Leukemia survival in children, adolescents, and young adults: influence of socioeconomic status and other demographic factors. Cancer Causes & Control: An International Journal of Studies of Cancer in Human Populations 2009;20(8):1409-20.

[30] Bhatia S, Sather HN, Heerema NA, Trigg ME, Gaynon PS, Robison LL. Racial and ethnic differences in survival of children with acute lymphoblastic leukemia. Blood 2002;100(6):1957-64.

[31] Kadan-Lottick Ns NKKBSGJG. SUrvival variability by race and ethnicity in childhood acute lymphoblastic leukemia. JAMA 2003;290(15):2008-14.

[32] Pui CH, Sandlund JT, Pei D, Rivera GK, Howard SC, Ribeiro RC, et al. Results of therapy for acute lymphoblastic leukemia in black and white children. JAMA 2003;290(15):2001-7.

[33] Kadan-Lottick NS, Ness KK, Bhatia S, Gurney JG. Survival variability by race and ethnicity in childhood acute lymphoblastic leukemia. JAMA 2003;290(15):2008-14.

[34] Zen PRG, Capra MEZ, Silla LcMR, Loss JF, Fernandes MrS, Jacques SMC, et al. ETV6/RUNX1 fusion lacking prognostic effect in pediatric patients with acute lymphoblastic leukemia. Cancer Genetics and Cytogenetics 2009;188:112-7.

[35] Forestier E, Heyman M, Andersen MK, Autio K, Blennow E, Borgström G, et al. Outcome of ETV6/RUNX1-positive childhood acute lymphoblastic leukaemia in the NO-

PHO-ALL-1992 protocol: frequent late relapses but good overall survival. British Journal of Haematology 2008;140(6):665-72.

[36] Bhojwani D, Pei D, Sandlund JT, Jeha S, Ribeiro RC, Rubnitz JE, et al. ETV6-RUNX1-positive childhood acute lymphoblastic leukemia: improved outcome with contemporary therapy. Leukemia 2012;26(2):265-70.

[37] Gandemer V, Chevret S, Petit A, Vermylen C, Leblanc T, Michel G, et al. Excellent prognosis of late relapses of ETV6/RUNX1-positive childhood acute lymphoblastic leukemia: lessons from the FRALLE 93 protocol. Haematologica 2012;DOI: 10.3324/haematol.2011.059584.

[38] Ribera JM, Oriol A, González M, Vidriales B, Brunet S, Esteve J, et al. Concurrent intensive chemotherapy and imatinib before and after stem cell transplantation in newly diagnosed Philadelphia chromosome-positive acute lymphoblastic leukemia. Final results of the CSTIBES02 trial. Haematologica 2010;95(1):87-95.

[39] Aricó M, Valsecchi MG, Camitta B, Schrappe M, Chessells J, Baruchel A, et al. Outcome of treatment in children with Philadelphia chromosome-positive acute lymphoblastic leukemia. New England Journal of Medicine 2000;342(14):998-1006.

[40] Schultz KR, Bowman WP, Aledo A, Slayton WB, Sather H, Devidas M, et al. Improved early event-free survival with imatinib in Philadelphia chromosome-positive acute lymphoblastic leukemia: A Children's Oncology Group study. Journal of Clinical Oncology 2009;27(31):5175-81.

[41] Yanada M, Takeuchi J, Sugiura I, Akiyama H, Usui N, Yagasaki F, et al. Karyotype at diagnosis is the major prognostic factor predicting relapse-free survival for patients with Philadelphia chromosome-positive acute lymphoblastic leukemia treated with imatinib-combined chemotherapy. Haematologica 2008;93(2):287-90.

[42] Bassan R, Spinelli O, Oldani E, Intermesoli T, Tosi M, Peruta B, et al. Improved risk classification for risk-specific therapy based on the molecular study of minimal residual disease (MRD) in adult acute lymphoblastic leukemia (ALL). Blood 2009;113(18):4153-62.

[43] Kosaka Y, Koh K, Kinukawa N, Wakazono Y, Isoyama K, Oda T, et al. Infant acute lymphoblastic leukemia with MLL gene rearrangements: outcome following intensive chemotherapy and hematopoietic stem cell transplantation. Blood 2004;104(12):3527-34.

[44] Moorman AV, Harrison CJ, Buck GAN, Richards SM, Secker-Walker LM, Martineau M, et al. Karyotype is an independent prognostic factor in adult acute lymphoblastic leukemia (ALL): analysis of cytogenetic data from patients treated on the Medical Research Council (MRC) UKALLXII/Eastern Cooperative Oncology Group (ECOG) 2993 trial. Blood 2007;109(8):3189-97.

[45] del Carmen Chillon M, Gomez-Casares MT, Lopez-Jorge CE, Rodriguez-Medina C, Molines A, Sarasquete ME, et al. Prognostic significance of FLT3 mutational status

and expression levels in MLL-AF4+ and MLL-germline Acute Lymphoblastic leukemia. Leukemia 2012.

[46] Kager L, Lion T, Attarbaschi A, Koenig M, Strehl S, Haas OA, et al. Incidence and outcome of TCF3-PBX1-positive acute lymphoblastic leukemia in Austrian children. Haematologica 2007;92(11):1561-4.

[47] Jeha S, Pei D, Raimondi SC, Onciu M, Campana D, Cheng C, et al. Increased risk for CNS relapse in pre-B cell leukemia with the t(1;19)/TCF3-PBX1. Leukemia 2009;23(8): 1406-9.

[48] Moorman AV, Chilton L, Wilkinson J, Ensor HM, Bown N, Proctor SJ. A population-based cytogenetic study of adults with acute lymphoblastic leukemia. Blood 2010;115(2):206-14.

[49] Swerdlow SH, Cancer. IAfRo, Organization. WH. WHO classification of tumours of haematopoietic and lymphoid tissues. Book 2008;4th ed.: 380-428.

[50] Goldberg JM, Silverman LB, Levy DE, Dalton VK, Gelber RD, Lehmann L, et al. Childhood T-Cell Acute Lymphoblastic Leukemia: The Dana-Farber Cancer Institute Acute Lymphoblastic Leukemia Consortium Experience. Journal of Clinical Oncology 2003, 2003;21(19):3616-22.

[51] Zhang YL, Zhao WL, Nie SS, Guo DD, Ji ZH, Chai YH. Analysis of Clinical Features and Prognostic Significance of Childhood T-lineage Acute Lymphoblastic Leukemia. Journal of experimental hematology/Chinese Association of Pathophysiology 2011;19(6):1496-500.

[52] Dores GM, Devesa SS, Curtis RE, Linet MS, Morton LM. Acute leukemia incidence and patient survival among children and adults in the United States, 2001-2007. Blood 2011, 2012;119(1):34-43.

[53] Nordlund J, Kiialainen A, Karlberg O, Berglund EC, Goransson-Kultima H, Sonderkar M, et al. Digital gene expression profiling of primary acute lymphoblastic leukemia cells. Leukemia 2012;26(6):1218-27.

[54] Forestier E, Andersen MK, Autio K, Blennow E, Borgström G, Golovleva I, et al. Cytogenetic patterns in ETV6/RUNX1-positive pediatric B-cell precursor acute lymphoblastic leukemia: A Nordic series of 245 cases and review of the literature. Genes, Chromosomes and Cancer 2007;46(5):440-50.

[55] Nachman JB, Heerema NA, Sather H, Camitta B, Forestier E, Harrison CJ, et al. Outcome of treatment in children with hypodiploid acute lymphoblastic leukemia. Blood 2007;110(4):1112-5.

[56] Rubnitz JE, Wichlan D, Devidas M, Shuster J, Linda SB, Kurtzberg J, et al. Prospective Analysis of TEL Gene Rearrangements in Childhood Acute Lymphoblastic Leukemia: A Children's Oncology Group Study. Journal of Clinical Oncology 2008;26(13):2186-91.

[57] Borowitz MJ, Devidas M, Hunger SP, Bowman WP, Carroll AJ, Carroll WL, et al. Clinical significance of minimal residual disease in childhood acute lymphoblastic leukemia and its relationship to other prognostic factors: a Children's Oncology Group study. Blood 2008;111(12):5477-85.

[58] Nowell PC, Hungerford DA. A minute chromosome in human chronic granulocytic leukemia. Science 1960;132:1497-501.

[59] Rowley JD. A new consistent chromosomal adnormality in chronic myelogeneus leukaemia identified by quinacrine fluorescence and Giemsa staining Nature 1973;243(51):290-93.

[60] Gleißner B, Gökbuget N, Bartram CR, Janssen B, Rieder H, Janssen JWG, et al. Leading prognostic relevance of the BCR-ABL translocation in adult acute B-lineage lymphoblastic leukemia: a prospective study of the German Multicenter Trial Group and confirmed polymerase chain reaction analysis. Blood, 2002;99(5):1536-43.

[61] Schlieben S, Borkhardt A, Reinisch I, Ritterbach J, Janssen JW, Ratei R, et al. Incidence and clinical outcome of children with BCR/ABL-positive acute lymphoblastic leukemia (ALL). A prospective RT-PCR study based on 673 patients enrolled in the German pediatric multicenter therapy trials ALL-BFM-90 and CoALL-05-92. Leukemia 1996;10(6):957-63.

[62] Melo JV. The diversity of BCR-ABL fusion proteins and their relationship to leukemia phenotype. Blood 1996;88(7):2375-84.

[63] Russo C, Carroll A, Kohler S, Borowitz M, Amylon M, Homans A, et al. Philadelphia chromosome and monosomy 7 in childhood acute lymphoblastic leukemia: a Pediatric Oncology Group study. Blood 1991;77(5):1050-6.

[64] Kantarjian HM, Talpaz M, Dhingra K, Estey E, Keating MJ, Ku S, et al. Significance of the P210 versus P190 molecular abnormalities in adults with Philadelphia chromosome-positive acute leukemia. Blood 1991;78(9):2411-8.

[65] Melo JV, Gordon DE, Tuszynski A, Dhut S, Young BD, Goldman JM. Expression of the ABL-BCR fusion gene in Philadelphia-positive acute lymphoblastic leukemia. Blood 1993;81(10):2488-91.

[66] Schrappe M, Aricó M, Harbott J, Biondi A, Zimmermann M, Conter V, et al. Philadelphia chromosome-positive (Ph+) childhood acute lymphoblastic leukemia: good initial steroid response allows early prediction of a favorable treatment outcome. Blood 1998;92(8):2730.

[67] Ribeiro RC, Broniscer A, Rivera GK, Hancock ML, Raimondi SC, Sandlund JT, et al. Philadelphia chromosome-positive acute lymphoblastic leukemia in children: durable responses to chemotherapy associated with low initial white blood cell counts. Leukemia 1997;11(9):1493-6.

[68] Thomas X, Thiebaut A, Olteanu N, Danaila C, Charrin C, Archimbaud E, et al. Philadelphia chromosome positive adult acute lymphoblastic leukemia: characteristics,

prognostic factors and treatment outcome. Hematology and Cell Therapy 1998;40(3): 119-28.

[69] Pui CH, Relling MV, Downing JR. Acute lymphoblastic leukemia. New England Journal of Medicine 2004;350(15):1535-48.

[70] Pui CH, Frankel LS, Carroll AJ, Raimondi SC, Shuster JJ, Head DR, et al. Clinical characteristics and treatment outcome of childhood acute lymphoblastic leukemia with the t (4; 11)(q21; q23): a collaborative study of 40 cases. Blood 1991;77(3):440-7.

[71] Cimino G, Elia L, Mancini M, Annino L, Anaclerico B, Fazi P, et al. Clinico-biologic features and treatment outcome in the GIMEMA 0496 study: absence of the ALL1/AF4 and of the BCR/ABL fusion genes correlates with a significantly better clinical outcome. Blood 2003;102(6):2014-20.

[72] Mancini M, Scappaticci D, Cimino G, Nanni M, Derme V, Elia L, et al. A comprehensive genetic classification of adult acute lymphoblastic leukemia (ALL): analysis of the GIMEMA 0496 protocol. Blood 2005;105(9):3434-41.

[73] Marchesi F, Girardi K, Avvisati G. Pathogenetic, Clinical, and Prognostic Features of Adult t (4; 11)(q21; q23)/MLL-AF4 Positive B-Cell Acute Lymphoblastic Leukemia. Advances in Hematology 2011:1-8.

[74] [74] Rubnitz JE, Camitta BM, Mahmoud H, Raimondi SC, Carroll AJ, Borowitz MJ, et al. Childhood Acute Lymphoblastic Leukemia With the MLL-ENL Fusion and t(11;19)(q23;p13.3) Translocation. Journal of Clinical Oncology 1999;17(1):191-6.

[75] Moorman AV, Ensor HM, Richards SM, Chilton L, Schwab C, Kinsey SE, et al. Prognostic effect of chromosomal abnormalities in childhood B-cell precursor acute lymphoblastic leukaemia: results from the UK Medical Research Council ALL97/99 randomised trial. The Lancet Oncology;11(5):429-38.

[76] Schmiegelow K, Forestier E, Hellebostad M, Heyman M, Kristinsson J, Soderhall S, et al. Long-term results of NOPHO ALL-92 and ALL-2000 studies of childhood acute lymphoblastic leukemia. Leukemia 2010;24(2):345-54.

[77] Mellentin JD, Murre C, Donlon TA, McCaw PS, Smith SD, Carroll AJ, et al. The gene for enhancer binding proteins E12/E47 lies at the t (1; 19) breakpoint in acute leukemias. Science 1989;246(4928):379-82.

[78] Andersen MK, Autio K, Barbany G, Borgström G, Cavelier L, Golovleva I, et al. Paediatric B-cell precursor acute lymphoblastic leukaemia with t(1;19)(q23;p13): clinical and cytogenetic characteristics of 47 cases from the Nordic countries treated according to NOPHO protocols. British Journal of Haematology 2011;155:235–43

[79] Secker-Walker LM, Berger R, Fenaux P, Lai JL, Nelken B, Garson M, et al. Prognostic significance of the balanced t (1; 19) and unbalanced der (19) t (1; 19) translocations in acute lymphoblastic leukemia. Leukemia 1992;6(5):363-9.

[80] Uckun FM, Sensel MG, Sather HN, Gaynon PS, Arthur DC, Lange BJ, et al. Clinical significance of translocation t(1;19) in childhood acute lymphoblastic leukemia in the

context of contemporary therapies: a report from the Children's Cancer Group. Journal of Clinical Oncology 1998;16(2):527-35.

[81] Chiaretti S, Foá R. T-cell acute lymphoblastic leukemia. Haematologica 2009;94(2): 160-2.

[82] Sen L, Borella L. Clinical Importance of Lymphoblasts with T Markers in Childhood Acute Leukemia. New England Journal of Medicine 1975;292(16):828-32.

[83] Sallan SE. T-cell acute lymphoblastic leukemia in children. Haematology and Blood Transfusion 1981;26:121-3.

[84] Bergeron J, Clappier E, Radford I, Buzyn A, Millien C, Soler G, et al. Prognostic and oncogenic relevance of TLX1/HOX11 expression level in T-ALLs. Blood 2007;110(7): 2324-30.

[85] Cavé H, Suciu S, Preudhomme C, Poppe B, Robert A, Uyttebroeck A, et al. Clinical significance of HOX11L2 expression linked to t (5; 14)(q35; q32), of HOX11 expression, and of SIL-TAL fusion in childhood T-cell malignancies: results of EORTC studies 58881 and 58951. Blood 2004;103(2):442-50.

[86] Ferrando AA, Neuberg DS, Dodge RK, Paietta E, Larson RA, Wiernik PH, et al. Prognostic importance of TLX1 (HOX11) oncogene expression in adults with T-cell acute lymphoblastic leukaemia. The Lancet 2004;363(9408):535-6.

[87] Zhao R, Goldman ID. Resistance to antifolates. Oncogene 2003;22(47):7431-57.

[88] Tiphaine Adam de Beaumais, Jacqz-Aigrain E. Intracellular disposition of methotrexate in acute lymphoblastic leukemia in children. Current Drug Metabolism 2012;13(6):822-34.

[89] Lennard L. Therapeutic drug monitoring of cytotoxic drugs. Br J Clin Pharmacol 2001;52:75–87.

[90] Mikkelsen Torben S TCF, Yang Jun J, Ulrich Cornelia M, French Deborah, Zaza Gianluigi, Dunnenberger Henry M, Marsh Sharon, McLeod Howard L, Giacomini Kathy, Becker Mara L, Gaedigk Roger, Leeder James Steven, Kager Leo, Relling Mary V, Evans William, Klein Teri E, Altman Russ B. "PharmGKB summary: methotrexate pathway" Pharmacogenetics and genomics (2011).

[91] Karathanasis NV, Choumerianou DM, Kalmanti M. Gene polymorphisms in childhood ALL. Pediatric Blood & Cancer 2009;52(3):318-23.

[92] Sierra E, Goldman ID. Recent advances in the understanding of the mechanism of membrane transport of folates and antifolates. Seminars Oncology 1999;26:11-23.

[93] Laverdiére C, Chiasson S, Costea I, Moghrabi A, Krajinovic M. Polymorphism G80A in the reduced folate carrier gene and its relationship to methotrexate plasma levels and outcome of childhood acute lymphoblastic leukemia. Blood 2002;100(10):3832-4.

[94] Ansari M, Krajinovic M. Pharmacogenomics of acute leukemia. Pharmacogenomics 2007;8(7):817-34.

[95] Chave KJ, Ryan TJ, Chmura SE, Galivan J. Identification of single nucleotide polymorphisms in the human gamma-glutamyl hydrolase gene and characterization of promoter polymorphisms. Gene 2003;319(0):167-75.

[96] Organista-Nava J, Gómez-Gómez Y, Saavedra-Herrera MV, Rivera-Ramírez AB, Terán-Porcayo MA, Alarcón-Romero LdC, et al. Polymorphisms of the gamma-glutamyl hydrolase gene and risk of relapse to acute lymphoblastic leukemia in Mexico. Leukemia Research 2009;34(6):728-32.

[97] Cheng Q, Wu B, Kager L, Panetta J, Zheng J, Pui C, et al. A substrate specific functional polymorphism of human gamma-glutamyl hydrolase alters catalytic activity and methotrexate polyglutamate accumulation in acute lymphoblastic leukaemia cells. Pharmacogenetics 2004;14(8):557-67.

[98] Dervieux T, Kremer J, Lein D, Capps R, Barham R, Meyer G, et al. Contribution of common polymorphisms in reduced folate carrier and gamma-glutamylhydrolase to methotrexate polyglutamate levels in patients with rheumatoid arthritis. Pharmacogenetics 2004;14(11):733-9.

[99] Garcia-Bournissen F, Moghrabi A, Krajinovic M. Therapeutic responses in childhood acute lymphoblastic leukemia (ALL) and haplotypes of gamma glutamyl hydrolase (GGH) gene. Leukemia Research 2007;31(7):1023-5.

[100] Schneider E, Ryan TJ. Gamma-glutamyl hydrolase and drug resistance. Clinica Chimica Acta 2006;374:25-32.

[101] Chave KJ, Ryan TJ, Chmura SE, Galivan J. Identification of single nucleotide polymorphisms in the human g-glutamyl hydrolase gene and characterization of promoter polymorphisms. Gene 2003;319(0):167-75.

[102] Chiusolo P, Giammarco S, Bellesi S, Metafuni E, Piccirillo N, De Ritis D, et al. The role of MTHFR and RFC1 polymorphisms on toxicity and outcome of adult patients with hematological malignancies treated with high-dose methotrexate followed by leucovorin rescue. Cancer Chemotherapy and Pharmacology 2012;69(3):691-6.

[103] Leyva-Vázquez M, Organista-Nava J, Gómez-Gómez Y, Contreras-Quiroz A, Flores-Alfaro E, Illades-Aguiar B. Polymorphism G80A in the reduced folate carrier gene and its relationship to survival and risk of relapse in acute lymphoblastic leukemia. Journal of Investigative Medicine;2012, 60:1064-7.

[104] Gregers J, Christensen IJ, Dalhoff K, Lausen B, Schroeder H, Rosthoej S, et al. The association of reduced folate carrier 80G> A polymorphism to outcome in childhood acute lymphoblastic leukemia interacts with chromosome 21 copy number. Blood 2010;115(23):4671-7.

[105] Gómez-Gómez Y, Organista-Nava J, Saavedra-Herrera MV, Rivera-Ramírez AB, Terán-Porcayo MA, Alarcón-Romero LdC, et al. Survival and risk of relapse of acute

lymphoblastic leukemia in a Mexican population is affected by dihydrofolate reductase gene polymorphisms. Experimental and Therapeutic Medicine 2012;3(4):665-72.

[106] Dulucq S, St-Onge G, Gagné V, Ansari M, Sinnett D, Labuda D, et al. DNA variants in the dihydrofolate reductase gene and outcome in childhood ALL. Blood 2008;111(7):3692-700.

[107] Krajinovic M, Costea I, Primeau M, Dulucq S, Moghrabi A. Combining several polymorphisms of thymidylate synthase gene for pharmacogenetic analysis. Pharmacogenomics Journal 2005;5(6):374-80.

[108] Krajinovic M, Costea I, Chiasson S. Polymorphism of the thymidylate synthase gene and outcome of acute lymphoblastic leukaemia. The Lancet 2002;359(9311):1033-4.

[109] Ongaro A, De Mattei M, Della Porta MG, Rigolin GM, Ambrosio C, Di Raimondo F, et al. Gene polymorphisms in folate metabolizing enzymes in adult acute lymphoblastic leukemia: effects on methotrexate-related toxicity and survival. Haematologica 2009;94(10):1391-8.

[110] Salazar J, Altés A, Del Río E, Estella J, Rives S, Tasso M, et al. Methotrexate consolidation treatment according to pharmacogenetics of MTHFR ameliorates event-free survival in childhood acute lymphoblastic leukaemia. The Pharmacogenomics Journal 2011;doi:10.1038/tpj.2011.25.

[111] El-Khodary N, El-Haggar S, Eid M, Ebeid E. Study of the pharmacokinetic and pharmacogenetic contribution to the toxicity of high-dose methotrexate in children with acute lymphoblastic leukemia. Medical Oncology 2011:1-10.

[112] Krajinovic M, Lemieux-Blanchard E, Chiasson S, Primeau M, Costea I, Moghrabi A. Role of polymorphisms in MTHFR and MTHFD1 genes in the outcome of childhood acute lymphoblastic leukemia. The Pharmacogenomics Journal 2004;4(1):66-72.

[113] Wang L, Goodey NM, Benkovic SJ, Kohen A. Coordinated effects of distal mutations on environmentally coupled tunneling in dihydrofolate reductase. Proceedings of the National Academy of Sciences 2006;103(43):15753-8.

[114] Volpato JP, Fossati E, Pelletier JN. Increasing Methotrexate Resistance by Combination of Active-site Mutations in Human Dihydrofolate Reductase. Journal of Molecular Biology 2007;373(3):599-611.

[115] Allemann RK, Evans RM, Tey L-h, Maglia G, Pang J, Rodriguez R, et al. Protein motions during catalysis by dihydrofolate reductases. Philosophical Transactions of the Royal Society B: Biological Sciences 2006;361(1472):1317-21.

[116] Goto Y, Yue L, Yokoi A, Nishimura R, Uehara T, Koizumi S, et al. A novel single-nucleotide polymorphism in the 3'-untranslated region of the human dihydrofolate reductase gene with enhanced expression. Clinical Cancer Research 2001;7(7):1952-6.

[117] Nazki FH, Masood A, Banday MA, Bhat A, Ganai BA. Thymidylate synthase enhancer region polymorphism not related to susceptibility to acute lymphoblastic leukemia in the Kashmir population. Genetics and Molecular Research 2012;11(2):906-17.

[118] Horie N, Aiba H, Oguro K, Hojo H, Takeishi K. Functional analysis and DNA polymorphism of the tandemly repeated sequences in the 5'-terminal regulatory region of the human gene for thymidylate synthase. Cell Structure and Function 1995;20(3): 191-7.

[119] Rahimi Z, Ahmadian Z, Akramipour R, Vaisi-Raygani A, Rahimi Z, Parsian A. Thymidylate synthase and methionine synthase polymorphisms are not associated with susceptibility to childhood acute lymphoblastic leukemia in Kurdish population from Western Iran. Molecular Biology Reports 2001;39(3):2195-200.

[120] Aplenc R, Thompson J, Han P, La M, Zhao H, Lange B, et al. Methylenetetrahydrofolate Reductase Polymorphisms and Therapy Response in Pediatric Acute Lymphoblastic Leukemia. Cancer Research 2005, 65(6):2482-7.

[121] Guenther BD, Sheppard CA, Tran P, Rozen R, Matthews RG, Ludwig ML. The structure and properties of methylenetetrahydrofolate reductase from Escherichia coli suggest how folate ameliorates human hyperhomocysteinemia. Nature Structural & Molecular Biology 1999;6(4):359-65.

[122] Frosst P, Blom HJ, Milos R, Goyette P, Sheppard CA, Matthews RG, et al. A candidate genetic risk factor for vascular disease: a common mutation in methylenetetrahydrofolate reductase. Nature Genetics 1995;10(1):111-3.

[123] van der Put NMJ, GabreÃ«ls F, Stevens E, Smeitink JAM, Trijbels FJM, Eskes TKAB, et al. A second common mutation in the methylenetetrahydrofolate reductase gene: an additional risk factor for neural-tube defects? The American Journal of Human Genetics 1998;62(5):1044-51.

[124] Hol FA, van der Put NMJ, Geurds MPA, Heil SG, Trijbels FJM, Hamel BCJ, et al. Molecular genetic analysis of the gene encoding the trifunctional enzyme MTHFD(methylenetetrahydrofolate-dehydrogenase, methenyltetrahydrofolate-cyclohydrolase, formyltetrahydrofolate synthetase) in patients with neural tube defects. Clinical Genetics 1998;53(2):119-25.

[125] Huh HJ, Park CJ, Jang S, Seo EJ, Chi HS, Lee JH, et al. Prognostic significance of multidrug resistance gene 1 (MDR1), multidrug resistance-related protein (MRP) and lung resistance protein (LRP) mRNA expression in acute leukemia. Journal of Korean Medical Science 2006;21(2):253-8.

[126] Cortez MAA, Scrideli CA, Yunes JA, Valera ET, Toledo SRC, Pavoni-Ferreira PCB, et al. mRNA expression profile of multidrug resistance genes in childhood acute lymphoblastic leukemia. Low expression levels associated with a higher risk of toxic death. Pediatric Blood & Cancer 2009;53(6):996-1004.

[127] Plasschaert SLA, de Bont ESJM, Boezen M, vander Kolk DM, Daenen SMJG, Faber KN, et al. Expression of Multidrug Resistance-Associated Proteins Predicts Prognosis in Childhood and Adult Acute Lymphoblastic Leukemia. Clinical Cancer Research 2005;11(24):8661-8.

[128] Stride BD, Grant CE, Loe DW, Hipfner DR, Cole SPC, Deeley RG. Pharmacological Characterization of the Murine and Human Orthologs of Multidrug-Resistance Protein in Transfected Human Embryonic Kidney Cells. Molecular Pharmacology 1997;52(3):344-53.

[129] Breuninger LM, Paul S, Gaughan K, Miki T, Chan A, Aaronson SA, et al. Expression of Multidrug Resistance-associated Protein in NIH/3T3 Cells Confers Multidrug Resistance Associated with Increased Drug Efflux and Altered Intracellular Drug Distribution. Cancer Research 1995;55(22):5342-7.

[130] Conseil G, Deeley RG, Cole SPC. Polymorphisms of MRP1 (ABCC1) and related ATP-dependent drug transporters. Pharmacogenetics and Genomics 2005;15(8): 523-33.

[131] Belinsky MG, Chen ZS, Shchaveleva I, Zeng H, Kruh GD. Characterization of the drug resistance and transport properties of multidrug resistance protein 6 (MRP6, ABCC6). Cancer Research 2002;62(21):6172.

[132] Borst P, Evers R, Kool M, Wijnholds J. A family of drug transporters: the multidrug resistance-associated proteins. Journal of the National Cancer Institute 2000;92:1295-302.

[133] Jedlitschky G, Burchell B, Keppler D. The multidrug resistance protein 5 functions as an ATP-dependent export pump for cyclic nucleotides. The Journal of Biological Chemistry 2000;275(39):30069-74.

[134] Kool M, Van Der Linden M, De Haas M, Scheffer GL, De Vree JML, Smith AJ, et al. MRP3, an organic anion transporter able to transport anti-cancer drugs. Proceedings of the National Academy of Sciences 1999;96(12):6914-9.

Chapter 11

Bone Marrow Transplantation (BMT) in Philadelphia-Positive Acute Lymphoblastic Leukemia (Ph+ ALL)

Jorge Milone and Enrico Alicia

Additional information is available at the end of the chapter

http://dx.doi.org/10.5772/55523

1. Introduction

Ph+ ALL represents approximately about 25 to 40% of adults patients with ALL. In children, Ph+ ALL is much less common. Different breakpoint in the bcr gene, major and minor, produce fusion genes resulting in either a 210 or a 190 KDa protein respectively. It appears that major breakpoint fusion (p210) originates in hematopoietic stem cells whereas minor breakpoint fusion (p190) has a B cell progenitor origin, suggesting that p190 ALL and p210 Ph+ ALL may be distinct biological and clinical entities. [1] BMT is the first option for consolidation the complete remission in this patients. The proportion of patients able to undergo BMT in CR1 (Complete Remission) has increased with imatinib-based induction and early post-remission therapy, and there is currently no evidence that imatinib has an adverse effect on transplant-related morbidity or mortality (TMR). In addition, donor availability has benefitted from results showing equivalence of sibling and matched unrelated donors in terms of remission duration, non-relapse mortality and overall survival (OS).[1, 2] Several studies have shown improved post-transplant outcome of patients previously receiving imatinib-based treatment when compared with historic control groups, which have been dealt with in the previous chapter. As a consequence, most ALL study groups currently consider imatinib-based treatment, followed by matched related or unrelated allogeneic SCT (allo-SCT) in CR1, to be the gold standard of first-line therapy for Ph+ ALL. [3], Imatinib-based treatment not followed by SCT has been suggested to achieve OS and Disease Free Survival (DFS) similar to that obtained after SCT in one study, [4] and the results of MDACC study showed only a trend towards better OS in transplanted patients. [5] It still needs to be determined whether therapy based on second generation TKI may be equivalent or superior to BMT in a subset of patients, particularly those at high risk of TRM

The challenges in the treatment of Ph+ ALL are the selection of appropriate pre-transplantation therapy, the minimization of transplantation toxicity, the correct use of TKIs after transplantation and the appropriate use of and response to BCR/ABL monitoring.

2. Allogeneic stem cell transplantation with myeloablative conditioning

Attempts to improve outcome of Ph+ ALL included intensified conditioning regimens in order to reduce the relapse rate. An intensified preparatory regimen consisting of SCT after fractionated total body irradiation and Cyclophosphamide with or without etoposide has been explored by different investigation groups. Kröger et al investigated an intensified conditioning regimen including fractionated total body irradiation (TBI) (12 Gy), etoposide (30-45 mg/kg) and cyclophosphamide (120 mg/kg), followed by autologous (n = 5), allo-related (n = 13) or allo-unrelated (n = 6) bone marrow (n = 22) or peripheral stem cell (n = 2) transplantation in patients with Ph+ALL. One patient received busulfan (16 mg/kg) instead of TBI. Nineteen patients were transplanted in 1CR, two in 2CR, one in 1PR and two in relapse. After a median follow-up of 45 months, nine patients (37.5%) remain alive in CR. Nine patients (37.5%) relapsed and eight (33.3%) of these subsequently died. After autologous transplantation, four of five patients (80%) relapsed and died. In terms of late relapse the authors had seen it after allogeneic, as well as autologous transplantation, at 33 and 59 months, respectively. The Kaplan-Meier estimate of leukemia-free survival for all patients was 38% at 3 years and 35% at 5 years. For allogeneic transplants in first CR (n = 15) the estimate of DFS was 46% at 3 years and 34% at 5 years. Patients aged below 30 years had a better estimated OS at 3 years (61% vs 11%, P < 0.001). The bcr-abl fusion transcript (p210 vs p190 vs p210/190) did not affect DFS OR OS. For the authors an intensified conditioning regimen seems to improve the results of bone marrow transplantation in patients with Ph+ acute lymphoblastic leukemia. [6]

In another study Laport et al. evaluated sixty-seven patients with HLA-matched sibling donor who received fractionated total body irradiation (FTBI) and high-dose VP16, whereas 11 patients received TBI/VP16/cyclophosphamide, and 1 patient received TBI/VP16/busulfan. The median age was 36 years. At the time of BMT, 62% of the patients were in first complete remission and 38% of the patients were beyond CR1 (> CR1). The median follow-up was 75 months The 10-year OS for the CR1 and beyond CR1 patients was 54% and 29%, and event-free survival was 48% and 26%. The authors did not find significant difference in relapse incidence (28% vs 41%, but non relapse mortality was significantly higher in the beyond CR1 patients, (31% vs 54%). In this study the univariate analysis, factors affecting event-free and overall survival were white blood cell count at diagnosis (< 30 _ 109/L vs > 30 _ 109/L) and disease status (CR1 vs > CR1). The median time to relapse for CR1 and for beyond CR1 patients was 12 months and 9 months, respectively. These results showed that FTBI/VP16 with or without cyclophosphamide confers long-term survival in Ph+ ALL patients and that disease status at the time of BMT is an important predictor of outcome. [7]

In these and other studies the factors that identify modifications in the transplant outcome have been analyzed. Complications such as TRM was mainly due to infections or GVHD (graft-versus-host-disease), and was higher in patients with more advanced disease. Factors affecting event-free and overall survival likewise included disease status (CR1 vs > CR1) and higher age, with a cutoff at approximately 30 years, at the time of transplantation. [8] The intensified preparatory regimens confer long-term survival in a subset of patients with Ph+ ALL, relapse and TRM remain important causes of treatment failure, making success unlikely in patients with more advanced disease. Interestingly, comparable survival data were reported for patients with high-risk ALL with the Philadelphia chromosome and those with normal cytogenetic; actuarial disease-free survival (DFS) at 5 years was 43% for patients in first remission. Chronic GVHD appears to reduce the risk of relapse without increasing the risk of TRM, whereas severe acute GVHD increases the risk of TRM without diminishing the risk of relapse. Thus, patients who developed extensive chronic GVHD had better survivals, and those who developed grade III-IV acute GVHD had worse survivals than did the others. [8,9]

3. Reduced-intensity conditioning allogeneic stem cell transplantation

In order to decrease the high TRM associated with myeloablative allogeneic stem cell transplantation but still generate a graft-versus- leukemia effect (GVLE), reduced-intensity conditioning (RIC) regimens were developed for patients unlikely to tolerate the toxicities of intensive preparative regimens. Overall, several retrospective analyses and a single prospective study suggest that BMT with RIC is feasible in adult patients with high-risk ALL but associated with a high probability of treatment failure in patients transplanted beyond CR1. [10,11,12,13] Myeloablative BMT carries considerable risk of TRM and is not applicable to older individuals. Opinions vary on the upper age limit for the procedure; in UKALL12/E2993, a very high TRM of nearly 40% was observed in patients older than 35 years of age receiving myeloablative BMT, resulting in a protocol limit of 40 years of age in the current UK NCRI study, UKALL14. In some studies, patients are offered myeloablative BMT up to the age of 55 years. [14] There are several studies that show the results of the regimens of reduced intensity but with different results, selection and design which must be interpreted with caution.

A comparative study of European Group for Blood and Marrow Transplantation (EBMT) registry report one retrospective study where the outcome of 576 adult acute lymphoblastic leukemia patients aged > 45 years, and who received a reduced-intensity conditioning (RIC; n=127) or myeloablative conditioning (MAC; n=449) allogeneic stem cell transplantation from a human leukocyte antigen-identical sibling while in complete remission is assessed. With a median follow-up of 16 months, at 2 years, the cumulative incidences of non-relapse mortality and relapse incidence were 29% (MAC) versus 21% (RIC), and 31% (MAC) versus 47% (RIC), respectively. In a multivariate analysis, nonrelapse mortality was decreased in RIC recipients, whereas it was associated with higher relapse rate. At 2 years, LFS was 38% (MAC) versus 32% (RIC). In multivariate analysis, the type of conditioning regimen (RIC vs. MAC) was not significantly associated with leukemia-free survival. For this authors the RIC allo-SCT from a human leukocyte antigen identical donor is a potential therapeutic option for acute lymphoblastic leukemia patients aged > 45 years in complete remission and not eligible for MAC allo. [15]

The RIC approaches should be vigorously pursued as part of prospective studies in order to define their role in ALL. In Ph^+ ALL in particular, inquiry into the role of TKIs after alloHSCT is vital. The forthcoming study from the UK NCRI, UKALL14, assigned all patients with ALL of 40 years of age or more to a nonmyeloablative approach with fludarabine, melphalan, and alemtuzumab in an attempt to obtain good disease control with less GVHD. [14] The incidence of TRM and disease progression in these studies was still substantial, however particularly in patients transplanted beyond first CR. The incidence of acute (grades II-IV) and chronic GVHD (43.2% and 65.6%, respectively) was high, but the significantly lower frequency of disease progression in patients with cGVHD highlights the antileukemic activity of cGVHD [15]

4. Autologous stem cell transplantation

The role of autologous stem cell transplantation (ASCT) was studied most extensively in the pre-imatinib era and has attracted little interest since then. While there are no prospective, randomized trials comparing autologous and allogeneic SCT, treatment outcome with conventional ASCT procedures has consistently been inferior to BMT in several retrospective analyses due to a high relapse rate. More recently, some investigators have reevaluated the therapeutic potential of ASCT when given in conjunction with TKI. Shin et al. describe an approach in which Ph+ ALL patients receive imatinib as interim therapy between chemotherapeutic cycles and prior to autologous SCT, followed by maintenance therapy. Small patient numbers and as yet limited duration of follow-up preclude a definite assessment of this strategy, which can be expanded to include the more potent second-generation TKI. [15, 16]

5. Imatinib after SCT

A very important and as yet unanswered question concerns whether TKIs should be administered after BMT and under what circumstances. The high risk of relapse in patients who are MRD positive after SCT makes administration of an ABL-directed TKI conceptually attractive as a measure to prevent relapse and reestablish molecular negativity. [17] Administration of imatinib early after HCT was tested by Carpenter et al in 22 patients, 15 with Ph+ ALL and 7 with high-risk chronic myelogenous leukemia, (CML) who were enrolled in a prospective study and given imatinib from the time of engraftment until 365 days after HCT. Before day 90, adults (n =19) tolerated a median average daily imatinib dose of 400 mg/d, and children (n = 3) tolerated 265 mg/m2/d. The most common adverse events described by the authors were related to imatinib administration with grade 1-3 nausea, emesis, and serum transaminase elevations. [18]

The positive minimal residual disease (MRD) after stem cell transplantation: is associated with a relapse probability exceeding 90%. Starting imatinib in the setting of MRD may decrease this

http://dx.doi.org/10.5772/55523

high relapse rate. This hypothesis was evaluated in another prospective study by Wassmann and al. in 27 Ph+ALL patients that received imatinib upon detection of MRD after SCT. Bcr-abl transcripts became undetectable in 52% of the patients, after a median of 1.5 months, (they called $^{early}CR_{mol}$). All patients who achieved an $^{early}CR_{mol}$ remained in remission for the duration of imatinib treatment; 3 patients relapsed after imatinib was discontinued. The failure to achieve polymerase chain reaction (PCR) negativity shortly after starting imatinib predicted relapse which occurred in 12 of 13 patients after a median of 3 month. The DFS in $^{early\text{-}}CR_{mol}$ patients was 91% and 54% after 12 and 24 months, respectively, compared with 8% after 12 months in patients remaining MRD+. Thus in the post-transplant setting, the molecular response to imatinib discriminates between patients with long-term DFS and patients likely to experience relapse and who therefore should receive additional or alternative antileukemic therapy. [19]

Burke et al between 1999 and 2006, in a single-center analysis of 32 patients with Ph+ ALL, including pediatric patients, who underwent allo-HCT and received imatinib in either the pre- or post-transplant period. The median age at HCT was 21.9 years, of 32 patients, 15 received Imatinib therapy pre- or post-HCT (imatinib group) and 17 patients received either no imatinib (n=11) or only after relapsed (n=6) (non imatinib group) There was a trend towards improved OS, relapse-free survival and relapse at 2 years was, 61%, 67% and 13% for the imatinib group (n = 15) as compared with the 41%, 35% and 35% for the non-imatinib group (n = 17), respectively. Cardiac toxicity and TRM at 2 years were similar between the groups. [20] Overall, further data is needed to define the optimal use and impact of imatinib in the peri-transplant management of patients with Ph+ ALL.

6. Monitoring of *BCR-ABL* in Ph⁺ ALL

Real-time PCR *BCR-ABL* quantification is often used to monitor minimal residual disease in patients with Ph⁺ ALL, but optimal practice and interpretation of results is unclear. In addition, while there is considerable standardization of methodology for p210 quantification, there is less standardization than for p190 quantification.[17] There are conflicting reports on the association between an initial decrease in *BCR-ABL* transcript level and long-term outcome. Preudhomme C et al. In the "pre-imatinib" era, have observed a good correlation between *BCR-ABL* transcript levels and the outcome which had been reported in 17 patients with Ph +ALL. [21]

Ottmann et al. analyzed in elderly patients with de novo Ph+ALL who were randomly assigned to induction therapy with either imatinib Ind(IM)) or multiagent, age-adapted chemotherapy Ind(chemo). Imatinib was subsequently co-administered with consolidation chemotherapy. The *BCR-ABL* transcript levels have also been correlated with response. [22] Unlike in chronic myeloid leukemia, there is no consensus on what represents an optimal response.

Lee et al were able to demonstrate that a 3-log reduction in *BCR-ABL* transcripts after 1 month of imatinib treatment strongly predicted a reduced relapse risk. The outcomes were evaluated for Ph+ ALL in 23 adults patients in remission treated with allogeneic bone marrow transplantation (BMT) [23]

In contrast to the data published by these authors, Yanada et al observed no association between rapid achievement of *BCR-ABL* negativity and long-term outcome after an initial imatinib/chemotherapy induction regimen in 100 patients with Ph+ ALL treated and MRD monitoring [24]

Pfeifer et al examined the prevalence of KD mutations in newly diagnosed and Imatinib-naïve Ph+ ALL patients and assessed their clinical relevance in the setting of uniform frontline therapy with imatinib in combination with chemotherapy. The German Multicenter Study Group for Adult Acute Lymphoblastic Leukemia (GMALL) trial ADE10 for newly diagnosed elderly Ph+ ALL were retrospectively examined for the presence of BCR/ABL KD mutation by denaturing high-performance liquid chromatography (DHPLC),cDNA sequencing and allele-specific polymerase chain reaction (PCR). A KD mutation was detected in a minor subpopulation of leukemic cells in 40% of newly diagnosed and imatinib naïve patients. At relapse the domin cell clone harbored an identical mutation in 90% of the cases, the overall prevalence of mutations at relapse was 80 %. P loop mutations predominated and were not associated with an inferior hematologic or molecular remission rate or shorter rmission duration compared with unmutated BCR/ABL. BCR/ABL mutations conferring high level imatinib resistance are present in a substantial proportion of patients with de novo Ph+ ALL and eventually give rise to relapse.[25]

Soverini et al. analyzed samples collected at diagnosis from 15 patients with Philadelphia-positive acute lymphoblastic leukemia who subsequently received tyrosine kinase inhibitor therapy (dasatinib) by cloning the BCR-ABL kinase domain in a bacterial vector and sequencing 200 independent clones per sample. Mutations at relatively low levels (2-4 clones out of 200) could be detected in all patients--eight who relapsed and seven who achieved persistent remission. Each patient had evidence of two to eight different mutations, the majority of which have never been reported in association with resistance to tyrosine kinase inhibitors. They suggest that the BCR-ABL kinase domain is prone to randomly accumulate point mutations, although the presence of these mutations in a relatively small leukemic subclone does not always preclude a primary response to tyrosine Kinase inhibitor. [26]

So much imatinib or dasatinib regimens can be achieving complete clinical response in 95 -100% of patients.

Eligible patients will be treated with alloHSCT wherever possible, and for these patients, *BCR-ABL* monitoring early in the course of the disease is unlikely to change practice at present. For patients not receiving alloHSCT, serial monitoring during initial therapy is of more relevance because it might prompt a switch of therapy before hematological relapse. [17]

At present, the evidence suggests that *BCR-ABL* by RTQ-PCR should be monitored and must be combined with screening for BCR/ABL domain mutations (in case of suspected resistance) after alloHSCT and that reemergence of *BCR-ABL* is a rational basis for intervention. [27]

7. Resistence

Approximately 80 %to 90% of patients with Ph+ ALL who relapse while on imatinib are found to have BCR/ABL mutation with predominance of P-loop and T315I mutations. With dasatinib relapse is most frequently associated with T315I mutation, whereas P-loop mutations are less common. [28] With variable frequency, the mutations can be present at the time of diagnose. Pfeifer et al detected low levels of mutations in pretreated patients with imatinib with Ph+ ALL who, at the time of relapse, presented the same mutated dominant clone in most of the cases. Soverini et al also reported a high frequency of BCR/ABL mutations which were lately found at the time of relapse. [25,26] Mutations can also be acquired or emerge under the selection pressure of TKI treatment.

Other additional mechanisms of resistance to therapy with TKI have also been suggested, such as cytogenetic abnormalities in addition to Ph chromosome which are present in approximately one third of cases of adult leukemia and have been associated with inferior outcome. Members of the SRC family of kinase have been implicated in leukemogenesis and in the development of imatinib resistance in BCR/ABL positive ALL, suggesting that simultaneous inhibition of Src and Bcr/Abl kinases may benefit individuals with Ph+ acute leukemia. [29, 30]

8. Relapses in Ph+ acute lymphoblastic leukemia

Relapsed ALL is a clinical problem, and outcomes are extremely poor. Fielding et al in the UKALL12/ECOG study, examined 609 adults with recurring ALL, where the OS of newly diagnosed patients was 38% at 5 years, OS at 5 years after relapse was 7%. [31] The CR2 is possible in only ~ 50% of chemotherapy-treated patients. Many young patients with Ph^+ ALL will have already received alloHSCT, making salvage harder and with more toxicity, particularly if chemotherapy reinduction is under consideration. Nevertheless a phase 2 study of dasatinib 140 mg/d in patients who relapsed after imatinib-containing regimens demonstrated that approximately half of the patients could achieve a CR2 with modest toxicity. However, median remission duration was only 3.3 months. Under these circumstances, a second allo-HSCT might be considered.[32] Ishida et published case report which shows a positive outcome for a patient who received dasatinib followed by a RIC alloHSCT after imatinib and myeloablative allo-HSCT which failed to control the disease. All reports of allo-HSCT show less than an ideal outcome in patients beyond CR1. However, many of these were reported before the advent of TKIs, which might, in selected circumstances, allow for second definitive transplantation procedures [33] Among the strategies to treat Ph + ALL relapse after Allo-SCT we will mention donor lymphocyte infusion. This treatment seems to be effective in CML, but it is less useful in ALL maybe due to the immune escape mechanisms of the blastic cells. Likewise, the addition of chemotherapy to ILD is not associated with a better prognosis.

Immunotherapy with donor lymphocyte infusion (DLI) and imatinib appears to be well tolerated but it is rarely and in general only transiently effective. A rationale for the combined use of DLI and second-generation TKIs such as nilotinib is suggested by case reports, but prospectively collected data are as yet not available. [34]

Author details

Jorge Milone and Enrico Alicia

*Address all correspondence to: enrico@netverk.com.ar

Hematology Area, Hospital Italiano de la Plata, La PLata, Argentina

References

[1] Fielding AK; Goldstone AHAllogeneic haematopoietic stem cell transplant in Philadelphia-positive acute lymphoblastic leukemia. Bone marrow transplantation ((2008).

[2] Castor, A, Nilsson, L, et al. distint patterns of hematopoitic stem cell involvement in acute lymphoblastic leukemia. Nature Medicine, 11.630-637 ((2005).

[3] Lee, S, & Yoo-jin, K. Cgang Ki M ey al. The effect of first-line imatinib interin therapy on the outcome of allogeneic stem cell transplantation in adult with newly diagnosed Philadelphia chromosome positive acute lymphoblastic leukemia Blood , 105

[4] Yanada, M, Takeuchi, J, Sugiura, I, et al. High complete remission rate and promising outcome by combination of imatinib and chemotherapy for newly diagnosed BCR-ABL-positive acute lymphoblastic leukemia: a phase II study by the Japan Adult Leukemia Study Group. J Clin Oncol. (2006). Jan 20;, 24(3), 460-6.

[5] De Labarthe, A, Rousselot, P, & Huguet-rigal, F. Imatinib combined with induction or consolidation chemotherapy in patients with de novo Philadelphia chromosome-positive acute lymphoblastic leukemia: results of the GRAAPH-2003 study. Blood. (2007). Feb 15;, 109(4), 1408-13.

[6] Kröger, N, & Krüger, W. Wacker-Backhaus G Intensified conditioning regimen in bone marrow transplantation for Philadelphia chromosome-positive acute lymphoblastic leukemia. Bone Marrow Transplant. (1998). Dec;, 22(11), 1029-33.

[7] Ginna, G. Laport, Joseph C. Alvarnas, Joycelynne M. Long-term remission of Philadelphia chromosome-positive acute lymphoblastic leukemia after allogeneic hematopoietic cell transplantation from matched sibling donors: a year experience with the fractionated total body irradiation-etoposide regimen Blood (2008). , 20.

[8] Yanada, M, Naaoe, T, Iiada, H, et al. Myeloablative allogeneic hematopoietic stem cell transplantation for Philadelphia chromosome-positive acute lymphoblastic leu-

http://dx.doi.org/10.5772/55523

kemia in adults: significant roles of total body irradiation and chronic graft-versus-host disease Bone Marrow Transplantation ((2005).

[9] Doney, K, Hagglun, H, Leisenring, W, et al. Predictive Factors for Outcome of Allogeneic Hematopoietic Cell Transplantation for Adult Acute Lymphoblastic Leukemia. Biology of Blood and Marrow Transplantation 9:472-481 ((2003).

[10] Martino, R, Giralt, S, Caballero, M. D, et al. Allogeneic hematopoietic stem cell transplantation with reduced-intensity conditioning in acute lymphoblastic leukemia: a feasibility study. Haematologica. (2003). , 88, 555-560.

[11] Arnol, R, Massenkeil, G, Bornhauser, M, et al. Nonmyeloablative stem cell transplantation in adults with high risk ALL may be effective in early but not in advanced disease. Leukemia ((2002).

[12] Mohty, M, Labopin, m, Reza, T, et al. Reduced intensity conditioning allegeneic stem cell transplantation for adult patients with acute lymphoblastic leukemia: a retrospective study From the Europeasn Group for Blood and Marrow Transplantation hematologyca , 2008-93.

[13] Hamaki, T, & Kami, M. kanda Y reduced intensity stem cell transplantation for adult acute lymphoblastic leukemia a retrospective study of 33 patients. Bone marrow transplantation (2005). , 2005, 35-549.

[14] Fielding, A, & Rowe, M. Richards G prospective outcome data 267 unselected adult patients with Philadelphia chromosome-positive acute lymphoblastic leukemia confirm superiority of allogeneic transplantation over chemotherapy in the pre imatinib era: result from the international ALL Trial MCR UKALLXII/ECOG 2993.

[15] Ottman, O, & Pfeifer, H. Management of Philadelphia chromosome positive acute lymphoblastic leukemia (Ph+ALL) Hematology (2009). ASH Educational , 371-381.

[16] Shin, H, & Chung, J. S. and Cho Imatinib interim therapy between chemotherapeutic cycles and in vivo purging prior to autologous stem cell transplantation, followed by maintenance therapy is a feasible treatment strategy in Philadelphia chromosome-positive acute lymphoblastic leukemia. Bone Marrow Transplant. (2005). Nov;, 36(10), 917-8.

[17] Fielding, A. Current Managenemt Issues in Acute Lymphicityc Leukemia. ASH , 2011-231.

[18] Carpenter, P. A, Snyder, D. S, & Flowers, M. Prophylactic administration of imatinib after hematopoietic cell transplantation for high-risk Philadelphia chromosome-positive leukemia Blood (2007). , 2007, 109-2791.

[19] Wassmann, B, Pfeifer, H, & Stadler, M. Early molecular response to post transplantation imatinib determines outcome in MRD+ Philadelphia-positive acute lymphoblastic leukemia (Ph- ALL Blood. (2005). , 106, 458-463.

[20] Burke, J, & Trotz, B. Baker K allohematopoieic cell transplantation for Ph chromosome-positive ALL: impact of imatinib on relapse and survival.Bone Marrow Transplantation ((2009).

[21] Preudhomme, C, & Henic, N. Cazin B Good correlation between RT-PCR analysis and relapse in Philadelphia (Ph1)-positive acute lymphoblastic leukemia (ALL). Leukemia. (1997). Feb;, 11(2), 294-8.

[22] Ottmann, O. G, & Wassmann, B. Pfeifer H Imatinib compared with chemotherapy as front-line treatment of elderly patients with Philadelphia chromosome-positive acute lymphoblastic leukemia (Ph+ALL). Cancer. (2007). May 15;, 109(10), 2068-76.

[23] Lee, S, & Kim, D. W. Cho B Risk factors for adults with Philadelphia-chromosome-positive acute lymphoblastic leukaemia in remission treated with allogeneic bone marrow transplantation: the potential of real-time quantitative reverse-transcription polymerase chain reaction. Br J Haematol. (2003). Jan;, 120(1), 145-53.

[24] Yanada, M, Sugiura, I, & Takeuchi, J. Prospective monitoring of BCR-ABL1 transcript levels in patients with Philadelphia chromosome-positive acute lymphoblastic leukaemia undergoing imatinib-combined chemotherapy. Br J Haematol. (2008). Nov;, 143(4), 503-10.

[25] Pfeifer, H, & Wassmann, B. Pavlova A Kinase domain mutations of BCR-ABL frequently precede imatinib-based therapy and give rise to relapse in patients with de novo Philadelphia-positive acute lymphoblastic leukemia (Ph+ ALL). Blood (2007). Jul 15;, 110(2), 727-34.

[26] Soverini, S, & Vitale, A. Poerio A Philadelphia-positive acute lymphoblastic leukemia patients already harbor BCR-ABL kinase domain mutations at low levels at the time of diagnosis. Haematologica. (2011). Apr;, 96(4), 552-7.

[27] Nicola Gokbuget Recommendations of the European Working Group for Adult ALL 2011- 126

[28] Soverini, S, Colarossi, S, & Gnani, A. Resistance to dasatinib in Philadelphia-positive leukemia patients and the presence or the selection of mutations at residues 315 and 317 in the BCR-ABL kinase domain Hematologica (2007).

[29] Hu, Y, Liu, Y, & Pelletier, S. Buchdunger E Requirement of Src kinases Lyn, Hck and Fgr for BCR-ABL1-induced B-lymphoblastic leukemia but not chronic myeloid leukemia. Nat Genet. (2004). May;, 36(5), 453-61.

[30] Li, S. Src-family kinases in the development and therapy of Philadelphia chromosome-positive chronic myeloid leukemia and acute lymphoblastic leukemia. Leuk Lymphoma. (2008). Jan;, 49(1), 19-26.

[31] Fielding, A. K, Rchards, S. M, & Chopra, R. Outcome of 609 adults after relapse of acute lymphoblastic leukemia (ALL), an MRC UKALL12/ECOG 2993 study Blood (2007). Feb 1,109 (3) 944-50

[32] Ottmann, O, Dombret, H, Martinelli, G, et al. Dasatinib induces rapid hematologic and cytogenetic responses in adult patients with Philadelphia chromosome-positive acute lymphoblastic leukemia with resistance or intolerance to imatinib: interim results of a phase 2 study- Blood, (2007). , 2007, 110-7.

[33] Ishida, Y, Terasako, K, & Oshima, K. Dasatinib followed by second allegeneic hematopoietic stem cell transplantation for relapse of Philadelphia chromosome-positive acute lymphoblastic leukemia after the first transplantation Int J Hematol (2010). Oct,, 92(3), 542-6.

[34] Tiribelli, M, & Sperotto, A. Candoni A Mario TiribelliAlessandra SperottoAnna CandoniErica SimeoneSilvia ButtignolRenato FaninNilotinib and donor lymphocyte infusion in the treatment of Philadelphia-positive acute lymphoblastic leukemia (Ph+ ALL) relapsing after allogeneic stem cell transplantation and resistant to imatinib. Leukemia Research (2009). , 33(2009), 174-177.

Chapter 12

Alterations of Nutritional Status in Childhood Acute Leukemia

Alejandra Maldonado-Alcázar,
Juan Carlos Núñez-Enríquez,
Carlos Alberto García-Ruiz,
Arturo Fajardo-Gutierrez and
Juan Manuel Mejía-Aranguré

Additional information is available at the end of the chapter

http://dx.doi.org/10.5772/52715

1. Introduction

Nutritional status is the result of the interaction between environmental and genetic conditions in which a child lives, when these environmental conditions are favorable for life (physical, biological, nutritional and psychosocial), the genetic potential is expressed as an ideal state of nutrition, but when conditions are unfavorable such expression will be diminished, resulting in altered nutritional status, such as malnutrition, overweight and obesity, which among other things would cause the child did not respond to a disease or its treatment suitably at a given time. [1]

In different studies conducted in children with cancer, the authors have evaluated the impact of nutritional status, assuming that if a cancer patient is well nourished, have less toxicity caused by antineoplastic drugs, will have a greater immune resistance to processes serious infectious, and therefore have a better survival and quality of life than the patient who is not well nourished, so in this chapter we will mention the most important conclusions that have been made with respect to this issue. [2]

Malnutrition is the main nutritional disorder that occurs in children with cancer, and has been defined as a state in which a deficiency of energy, protein, and other nutrients, causes measurable adverse effects on the structure and functioning of organs and body tissues as well as the clinical course of a disease. In order to explain the mechanisms by which it causes malnutrition in children with cancer, three factors have been proposed: a) factors specific to the tumor (tumor growth factors released by the tumor cells as bombesin and adrenocorticotropic hormone) b) factors related to the patient (pediatric age, low socioeconomic status, poor nutrient intake, increased secretion of growth hormone and cytokines that are released by the body in response to tumor growth, among the most important are the tumor necrosis factor, interleukins 1 and 6), and last but not least, c) factors related to the treatment (type / dose of chemotherapy, site / dose of radiotherapy and surgery). It is also suggested that all these factors would cause an alteration in intermediary metabolism, with resultant decrease in appetite, which eventually lead to the patient to lose weight, creating a vicious cycle. [2-6]

1.1. Prevalence of malnutrition in children with cancer

It has been reported that children with cancer will develop signs and symptoms of malnutrition at some point in the disease by up to 50-60% of cases, however, this frequency may vary according to the type of neoplasm, and according to if the study was conducted in developed countries or in developing countries, where there has been an increased frequency of nutritional alterations. It should be mentioned, that the study of the prevalence of malnutrition in children with cancer is mainly determined by whether it is present at diagnosis, this is important because it also could establish their potential impact on the evolution of these patients before treatment started. [7,8]

In this regard, Brinksma A, et al., (2012) reported the prevalence of malnutrition at diagnosis for developed countries, through a systematic review which included patients with different types of childhood cancer, aged from 0-18 years of age for acute leukemias, the prevalence was 10%, 20-50% for neuroblastoma, and those classified as "other malignancies" was 0-30%, these prevalences are low when compared with those that have been estimated for developing countries where they are as high as 50% for all types of childhood cancers. [2,8,9]

2. Nutritional status assessment in children with acute leukemia

There are several clinical, biochemical and physiological indicators to diagnose malnutrition in children with cancer; such as the patient's age, the deficit of specific micronutrients and the presence or absence of infection. The severity of their malnutrition is determined mainly by anthropometric indicators, that are the indexes of weight-for-height (w/h) and weight-for-age (w/a), which indicates acute malnutrition (table 1), height-for-age (h/a) which indicate a delay in growth or chronic malnutrition; and the Body Mass Index (BMI), which is a figure that can diagnose a patient for being underweight, overweight or obesity. [10,11] (table 4)

http://dx.doi.org/10.5772/52715

Percentile	Diagnosis
<5	Malnourished
5-85	Normal
> 85 a < 95	Overweight
≥ 95	Obesity

Table 1. Diagnosis by percentile for the indexes weight-for-height, weight-for-age based on the World Health Organization (WHO) tables.

Waterlow´s Classification:

Denomination	Index	Classification
Wasting	Weight-for-height <5	Acute Malnutrition
Stunting	Height-for-age <5	delay in growth or chronic malnutrition

Table 2. Denomination of wasting and stunting with Waterlow´s classification. [12, 13]

Waterlow´s classifications:

Denomination	Index	Classification
Wasting, no stunting	Weight-for-height <5 , height-for-age Normal	Acute malnutrition
Wasting and stunting	Weight-for-height <5 , height-for-age <5	Exacerbated-chronic malnutrition
Stunting, no wasting	Weight-for-height Normal, height-for-age <5	Chronic malnutrition

Table 3. Combinations of nutritional diagnosis with Waterlow's classification. [12,13]

Percentil	Diagnosis
<5	Underweight - Malnourished
≥5 y <85	Normal
≥85- <94	Overweight
≥95	Obesity

Table 4. Diagnosis by percentile for the Body Mass Index (BMI) based on the World Health Organization (WHO) tables [10]

It's important to consider the body composition in children with cancer, with which we are able to determine the quantity of lean mass and body fat in their bodies, in order to see if there is muscular depletion. The anthropometric measures used to get body composition can be the Mid Upper Arm Circumference (MUAC), triceps (TSF), biceps, subscapularis and suprailiac skinfolds; [14] and in case of having the necessary equipment, the use of electric bioimpedance or D-XA (Dual X-Ray Absorptiometry) is recommendable.

With the mid upper arm circumference and the triceps skinfold, you can calculate the muscle and fat area by using the following formula:

Then comparing the score with the Frisancho tables where:

Percentile	Diagnosis
0 – 5	Wasted
5.1 – 15	Below average
15.1 – 85	Average
85.1 - 95	Above Average
>95	High muscle

Table 5. Diagnosis by percentile for upper arm muscle area based on Frisancho tables. [14]

Aside from those anthropometric indicators, there are biochemical indicators that are used to diagnose protein malnutrition, like albumin and pre-albumin which are the most important due to their hepatic synthesis, and total protein. [15,16]

The half- life of albumin is 20 days, therefore it can assess acute malnutrition and can be used as a morbidity and mortality prognosis factor.

Reference value	Diagnosis
3.5 - 5.5 g/dl	Well-nourished
2.8 - 3.5 g/dl	Malnourished Grade 1
2.1 - 2.7 g/dl	Malnourished Grade2
< 2.1 g/dl	Malnourished Grade 3

Table 6. Albumin reference values and diagnosis [15]

Prealbumin has a 2 days half life wich means it is a very sensible marker for acute malnutrition, but the result may be affected by inflammatory reaction, therefore is not useful to track changes on the nutritional status unlike albumin that can be a better marker for protein malnutrition. [16]

Reference value	Diagnosis
17 - 42 g/dl	Well-nourished
<17 g/dl	Malnourished

Table 7. Prealbumin reference values and diagnosis [17]

It is important to make a full assessment of nutritional status in these children as this can influence the patient's response to the treatment.

3. Impact of malnutrition in Acute Lymphoblastic Leukemia (ALL)

The study of the impact of malnutrition in children with cancer has been conducted primarily in patients with acute leukemia, specifically in (ALL) perhaps because it is the most common type of cancer in children worldwide. [18-21] In two papers published one by Underzo et al., and in another by Reilly J, et al., reported that the prevalence of malnutrition at diagnosis in patients with ALL was 7% for developed countries, and on the contrary, in different studies conducted in developing countries have reported higher prevalence of up to 21-23%, which confirms the statement that in countries with low economic development, malnutrition occurs more frequently, This could be a result of poverty. It is for this reason that for several years, these countries have made efforts to determine the true impact of malnutrition as a prognostic factor in patients with acute leukemia in children at different stages of treatment. [22-25]

3.1. Prognosis

As is known chemotherapy used in the treatment of patients with ALL has some serious effects that may endanger the life of patients at a given time. Among the most common side effects of QT are toxicity to various organs, infection, hemorrhage, tumor lysis syndrome (TLS), among others., which would be the cause of high morbidity and mortality. It is for this reason that the current chemotherapy protocols in children with ALL are based on a risk classification to reduce toxicity in low-risk patients as well as ensure that therapy is adequate and aggressive to those classified as high risk. [26,27]

In the group of patients with ALL who are malnourished at diagnosis, it was found that chemotherapy is more toxic and less effective compared to those found with adequate nutritional status, specifically haematological toxicity is the cause of most complications, such as an increased risk to present infections, bleeding and an increased risk of relapse, the above due to neutropenia, thrombocytopenia, and discontinuation of treatment, respectively.

The main effect of malnutrition on treatment, is due to an alteration of the biodisponibility of antineoplastic drugs, which is achieved through the following mechanisms: a) changes in absorption, eg for drugs like methotrexate and 6 mercaptopurine, b) the decreased drug transport by the reduction or lack of plasmatic proteins, and c) by decrease in hepatic metabolism of the antineoplastic mainly caused by a lack of enzymatic activity by cytochrome P450. [28-37]

Furthermore. highlight the importance of studying on the subject of how malnutrition affects the prognosis of patients with ALL, because in some of the studies did not allow conclusions to determine whether the association exists in some of these studies were given the limitations by factors such as inadequate sample size, the inconsistency in how to assess the nutritional status between studies, and also have not been studied other possible complications in the evolution of these patients, such as relapse, abandonment in the treatment, among others. [28,38-40]

3.2. Survival

Moreover, since 1980 the rates of event-free survival has improved in patients with ALL, currently reported survival at 5 years is 80% and 10-year survival is 60% in developed countries, however, in developing countries cure rates are less than 35%, so on a quest to determine the factors related to mortality in developed countries, but mainly in developing countries, has been studied by different authors on the role of malnutrition on survival of patients with ALL; remain controversial until now because while on the one hand, some authors have reported that survival rates are lower in malnourished patients compared with patients who are well nourished and of the same risk, in other studies, it has not been possible to confirm this association. [8,29,41] According to Reilly J, et al., There are three mechanisms that explain the direct influence of malnutrition on survival of patients with ALL: The first, means that if there is a greater severity of malnutrition, there will be a greater severity of leukemia this because as we know, malnutrition is a surrogate marker of the disease state, the second mechanism is related to immune system dysfunction that occurs in malnourished patients, which would cause increased susceptibility to potentially serious infections could lead to the death of the patient, and finally, a mechanism related to adipose tissue, which has as one of its main functions being a facilitator to take place the pharmacokinetics of many anticancer drugs, this tissue is functionally and structurally altered in malnutrition, resulting in a lower effective antineoplastic drugs and greater toxicity and that both could be potential factors sufficient to endanger the patient's life, however this mechanism has been studied by other authors who found no such effect. [23-39]

Therefore, it is believed that malnutrition alone is a major factor in poor prognosis and survival of patients with ALL, however, it is noteworthy that most of the studies performed, are from developed countries and / or where it is mainly evaluated the impact of malnutrition on long-term survival, so it is necessary to know whether the association also exists in developing countries, because these populations have certain characteristics, such as frequencies malnutrition and deaths occur primarily during the first year of treatment much higher, and it also has been reported as one of the main obstacles to improved survival rates in patients with ALL. [39,42-45]

http://dx.doi.org/10.5772/52715

3.3. Malnutrition and early mortality

Early mortality can be defined as death during the first year of treatment, and it includes treatments as chemotherapy of induction to remission, central nervous system prophylaxis and consolidation. In several cases around the globe, the early mortality rate for developed countries is significantly lower than the one presented in developing countries. Main causes for early mortality include complications during chemotherapy treatment, such as infections, hemorrhages and toxicity, since their presence often represent an interruption in the treatment.

A 1999 study conducted by Silverman and collaborators in the Dana-Farber Cancer Institute, United States; a mortality rate of 2% in the first stage of treatment was reported, mainly caused by infections. [46] Another study conducted in the UK in 1997 also measured the rate of early mortality in these patients, reporting a mortality rate of barely 1.2%, with infections still being the main cause of death; however, cases of brain hemorrhage and tumor lysis syndrome (TSL) were also detected. [47]

The country that reports the lowest percentage of mortality in early stages of treatment is Germany, which reported only a 1% death rate in their patients between 1984 and 1996; with most of the deceases caused by hemorrhages and tumor lysis. [41]

While that's the case in developed countries, where very low mortality rates are reported; a study conducted by Rivera Luna and collaborators in Mexico's Instituto Nacional de Pediatría (INP) threw results of a 15% mortality rate during the phases of induction to remission. [37] In other developing countries like Honduras, El Salvador, Brazil, and India mortality also shows a spike in rates compared to developed countries, with an early mortality rate of 20.8%, 12.5%, 14.9% and 17% respectively, as you can see in Graph 1. [48-51]

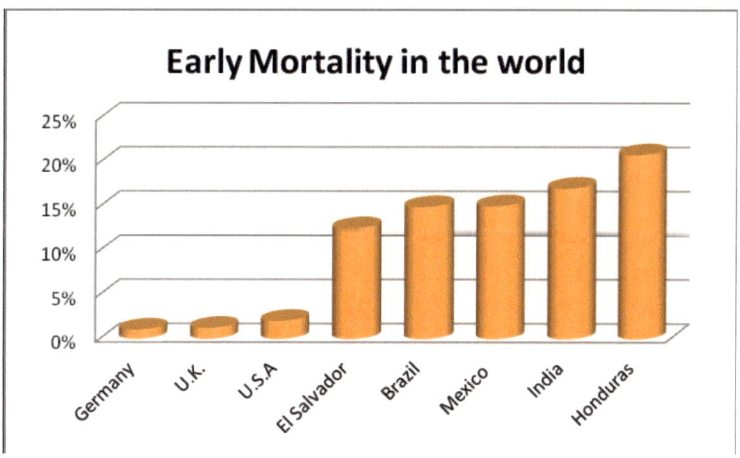

Germany	U.K.	U.S.A	El Salvador	Brazil	Mexico	India	Honduras
1%	1.20%	2%	12.50%	15%	15%	17%	21%

Graphic 1. Incidence of early mortality in patients with ALL around the world.

A possible explanation for this marked difference might be that malnutrition, poverty and lack of access to public health services are frequent problems in developing countries, unlike developed countries where children with leukemia have lower early mortality rates.

There have been several studies that try to correlate malnutrition with the evolution of patients with ALL. The first one was conducted in Mexico in 1989 by Lobato Mendiazabal et al., where there's a categorization of children with or without malnutrition based on weight-for-height indicators. It was found that, when measuring 5 year survival rate, 80% of children without malnutrition survived, while patients with malnutrition had a survival rate of barely 26% in the same period. [44]

As far as early mortality and relapses during the first year of treatment go, only 4% of children diagnosed with good nutrition suffered any of those events, while 63% of ill nurtured children experienced a relapse or death. This study was conducted in Puebla, with a sample size of 42 children of a single hospital facility (Hospital Universitario de Puebla). [44]

In a case and control study conducted by Mejia Aranguré and collaborators the state of nutrition of several patients with the weight-for-height indicator was tested and compared for diagnosis with the boards of Federico Gómez. For this study 93 cases of 2 hospital sources were taken; Hospital Infantil Federico Gómez and Hospital de Pediatría de Centro Médico Nacional S XXI. [35]

It was found that children with malnutrition at the moment of diagnosis were almost 2.6 times more likely to die in comparison to children without malnutrition. Therefore, it was concluded that malnutrition is a factor that increases the mortality rate of children with ALL, and an association directly proportional to the severity of the nutrition was established. [24]

In a prospective cohort conducted in 63 patients by Khan and collaborators, malnutrition was classified with the index of weight-for-height, and the result was that 46% of children with malnutrition at the moment of ALL diagnose completed their treatment; only 9.8% suffered a relapse and 45% died; meanwhile children without malnutrition experienced a 59% survival to their treatment, a 21% relapse rate and 19% died. Thus, malnutrition was considered as a bad prognosis factor for children with ALL. [36]

One of the most recent studies was conducted in Bangladesh by Hafiz MG and collaborators in 2008. This study only takes a sample of 66 patients from the Indian Pediatric Hospital, the index they used was the weight-for-height measurement, although they don't specify the tables that results were compared to in order to classify the state of nutrition.

They concluded that children that present malnutrition have 2 to 3 times the risk of infection in comparison to children without malnutrition. It was also observed that children with malnutrition needed more time for induction therapy since their dosage has to be lowered, or their treatment was interrupted for toxicity. [28]

http://dx.doi.org/10.5772/52715

Another study realized by Pedrosa F. and collaborators in 2000, took in account indicators as weight-for-height, height-for-age and weight-for-age; comparing them to WHO data. For this study they took in account patients with any type of leukemia and patients with solid tumors. This study was collaboration between two hospitals in El Salvador and Brazil, where they were able to include 443 patients. Of that number, 151 had an ALL diagnosis. At the beginning of the study children were classified as children with malnutrition and children without malnutrition, and children with malnutrition were provided with a dosage of albumin 2 weeks before starting chemotherapy. The study concluded that "malnourishment doesn't have a relevant association with these patients' survival". [38]

The most recent study published on this subject was conducted with patients of Mexico's Instituto Nacional de Pediatría, with 100 patients diagnosed with ALL. Their state of nutrition was determined with indicators of weight-for-height and height-for-age and compared to the NHANES tables of the CDC in the United States. This was a retrospective study where the follow up was done during the phases of induction to remission, and the results were as follow: 14.9% of children without malnourishment died during treatment phase, while 5.1% of patients without malnourishment perished in this stage of treatment Therefore, it was concluded that malnutrition didn't play an important role in early mortality in children with ALL. [37]

In a retrospective cohort done in El Salvador with 469 patients, besides BMI index, triceps skinfolds and Mid Upper Arm Circumference were taken into consideration. This study concluded that malnourishment had no association with mortality during treatment. [49]

A study conducted by Hijiya and collaborators demonstrated with a retrospective cohort of 621 patients of St. Jude's Hospital in United States concluded that BMI didn't affect the evolution of patients with ALL. This study took BMI as the main nutritional indicator and divided children in 3 groups: malnourished, normal and obese. The survival rates in these categories were similar, children with malnutrition presented a survivability rate of 86.1%, children with a normal nutrition state had an 86% survivability rate and in obese children the figure was of 85.9%. [39]

There's controversial information about the relationship between the effects of malnutrition in the evolution of patients with ALL, mostly because even with a wide range of studies, some conclude there's a significant relation between these factors [24,28,44] while others conclude that there's no relation. [37-39, 49]

One of the reasons is the bias in the classification of malnutrition, since in some studies like Pedroza and collaborators [38] the World Health Organization (WHO) charts are used, and in Rivera Luna and collaborators [37] they used the charts of the National Health and Nutrition Examination Survey (NHANES), while in the study conducted by Lobato Mendizabal and collaborators the charts of Ramos Galván were taken into account [44] and at last the study of Mejía Aranguré and collaborators used Federico Gómez' charts. [24]

In the studies mentioned, the sample was taken only from one or two hospital sources, so it's important to conduct a multicentre study that can show a wider panorama of the effects of malnourishment in the evolution of children with ALL.

Autor (Year)	**Lobato Mendiazabal et al. (1989)**	**Mejía Aranguré et al. (1999)**	**Pedrosa F. et al. (2000)**	**Rivera Luna et al. (2005)**
Country	Mexico	Mexico	El Salvador and Brazil	Mexico
Hospitals	Centro de Hematología Medicina Interna and Hospital Universitario de Puebla	Hospital de Pediatría S. XXI and Hospital Infantil de México Federico Gómez	Hospital de niños Benjamín Bloom and Instituto Materno-Infantil de Pernambuco	Instituto Nacional de Pediatría
Type of study	Prospective cohort	Case- control	Retrospective Cohort	Retrospective Cohort
Sample size	43 patients	93 patients, 17 cases and 76 controls	443 patients 151 with ALL	100 patients
Age	1-15 years	<16 years	0-17.8 years	0-15 years
Parameters used	Weight-for-age	Weight-for-height	Weight-for-age, Height-for-age Weight-for-height	Height-for-age, Weight-for-height
Classification	Ramos- Galvan's Tables	Federico Gómez Tables	WHO`s Tables	National Health and Nutrition examination survey NHANES
Results	5-year survival in well nourished versus malnourished patients: 83% in well nourished Vs 26% in malnourished. Death and relapses: 4% in well nourished vs. 63% malnourished. Reduction of chemotherapy treatment: 75% in well nourished Vs. 56% malnourished.	Children who had malnutrition at the time of diagnosis were 2.6 more likely to die than children without malnutrition; therefore malnutrition increases mortality in children with LLA.	Malnutrition has no association with survival of patients Note: A dose of Albumin was applied to malnourished children 2 weeks before they started treatment.	14.9% of well nourished children died during the induction to remission therapy; 15.1% of malnourished children died during the same stage of treatment, "Malnutrition does not play a role in early mortality in children with ALL".
Country	USA	Pakistan	Bangladesh	El Salvador
Hospitals	St. Jude´s Children Research Hospital	Shaukat Khanum memorial Hospital	Pediatric Hematology and Oncology	Hospital de niños Benjamín Bloom
Type of study	Retrospective cohort	Prospective cohort	Prospective cohort	Prospective Cohort
Sample size	621 patients	163 patients	66 patients	469 patients

http://dx.doi.org/10.5772/52715

Autor (Year)	Lobato Mendiazabal et al. (1989)	Mejía Aranguré et al. (1999)	Pedrosa F. et al. (2000)	Rivera Luna et al. (2005)
Age	1-16 years	<14 years	1-15 years	0-16 years
Parameters used	BMI	Weight-for-height	Weight for age	BMI, MUAC,(TSF)
Classification	CDC tables	Waterlow`s Classification	Not specified	CDC Tables
Results	Children were divided in 3 categories: <10° malnourished; >ó= 85° well nourished; > 85 < 95° overweight; >95 Obesity; Note: Chemotherapy dosage was not adjusted by BMI. Survival rate: 86.1%, 86.0%, 85.9% and 78.2% respectively BMI has no effect on the survival of LLA children.	Malnourished children: 46% complete treatment and were alive, 9.8% relapse and 45% died. Well nourished children: 59% complete treatment and were alive, 21.3% relapse and 19% died. " Malnutrition is a prognosis factor in LLA children"	Malnourished children are 3 times more likely to present infections tan well nourished ones. Malnourished children need more time of induction to remission treatment due to the dose reduction caused by toxicity.	Malnutrition has no association with early mortality in children with LLA.

Table 8. Studies about the effect of malnutrition at time of diagnosis and early mortality in children with ALL.

4. Overweight and obesity in survivors of childhood acute lymphoblastic leukemia

Concern about children who suffered from ALL is the long-term consequences that therapy may bring after the leukemia has been overcome. Various studies have shown that nutritional abnormalities like obesity and overweight are commonly found in ALL survivors, with a prevalence of 20-34% depending on the country where it has been studied. [52,53]

van Waas et al, conducted a study in 2004 in the Netherlands during the period from 2002 to 2007 in a single-center cohort of 500 survivors of childhood ALL. The ages of these patients at the time of the study ranged from 18 to 59 years, of which 288 were females and 212 were males, measured variables corresponded to the levels of total cholesterol, HDL cholesterol, systolic and diastolic blood pressure, BMI, and the authors finally concluded that patients who had been treated with cranial radiotherapy (CRT) had a higher frequency of overweight (59% versus 34%, P = 0.003) than those who had not received CTR. [54]

Obesity and overweight are defined are the result of varying degrees of abnormal or excessive accumulation of fat. The World Health Organization defines overweight as a BMI of 25 to 29.9, and obesity as a BMI of ≥30. The BMI modifications in survivors of childhood ALL are noteworthy because they are associated with insulin resistance, diabetes mellitus, hypertension, dyslipidemia and with an increased cardiovascular risk. [55]

4.1. Mechanisms involved in the development of overweight and obesity in ALL survivors

Because of this, the processes by which these nutritional abnormalities are developed by ALL survivors are being studied, though the exact mechanisms are still uncertain, nonetheless, there are some hypotheses that would explain metabolic deregulations leading to the development of altered BMI by the excessive accumulation of body fat. Here we will focus on the effects due to radiotherapy and corticosteroids. However, it is important to point out that exist other factors linked to these alterations. For example, long hospitalization periods because of inmunosuppression or vincristine-induced peripheral neuropathy may cause restricted physical activity in these patients. In addition to this, it should not be left out the usual risk factors for developing obesity of each population. [56]

4.1.1. Effects attributed to cranial radiation therapy

In one of the largest studies conducted so far related to the effect of radiotherapy for the development of overweight and obesity in ALL survivors by Oeffinger et al, (2003), reported that the dose and radiation site were the mainly cause. This study was conducted during the period from 1980 to 1994 the study population corresponded to 1765cases and 2588 controls aged 18-42 years old. Considering a radiation dose greater than 20Gy there was a risk factor for obesity in men with an OR 1.86 for ills (95% CI, 1.33 to 2.57, P<.001) and in women with an OR of 2.59 (95% CI, 1.88 to 3.55, P <0.001), without observing this nutritional disorder in patients who had received chemotherapy alone or had received cranial radiation doses of 10 to 19 Gy. [57]

Lackner H et al 1991and subsequently by Janiszewski et al., (2007), reported that the levels of growth hormone (GH), insulin-like factor (IGF1) and leptin levels were significantly lower in CRT than in non-CRT. [58,59]

The mechanism proposed to explain the growth hormone deficiency, holds that cranial radiotherapy (CRT) given at a young age to treat children suffering from ALL, damages the hypothalamus neurons, inducing growth hormone deficiency (GHD). [60] Deficiency in the secretion of growth hormone (GH) has been associated with the augmented percentage of body fat. Evidence that supports these hypothesis are the decreased levels of IGF-1 (also known as somatomedine C), which is a mediator of the GH action in target tissues.

Apart from their individual effects, there is evidence that relates leptin and GH. GH and IGF-1 are decreased in response to fasting. Impaired GH synthesis and secretion occurs along with a leptin deficiency or abnormality on its receptor. Leptin may also regulate GH via somatostatin synthesis inhibition and secretion, allowing GH to yield its actions over the targeted tissues. [61]

Among many other physiological functions of the GH, this hormone promotes utilization of fats as source of energy, inducing the liberation of fatty acids into the bloodstream. At the same time, it has anabolic protein effects which are traduced in an increase of lean body mass. [62]

Moreover, it has been recently suggested that only susceptible individuals will develop obesity when treated with CRT. This susceptibility has been tracked down to a polymorphism in the leptin receptor in the hypothalamus. This polymorphism (Arg/Arg) was found by Ross et al., to be associated to females having a BMI ≥25, treated with CRT. [63] Leptin is a hormone produced by adipocytes and it is involved in feeding behavior regulation and energy balance. Stored energy in adipose tissue is closely watched by the hypothalamus, through this hormone. An increase in adipose tissue will be traduced in increased leptin synthesis by adipocytes, and by negative feedback over the hypothalamus food intake will be inhibited. [64,65]

4.1.2. Corticosteroid therapy

Because corticosteroids are used to treat ALL, it is important to point out that they also promote leptin synthesis. However, conducted studies have only shown short-term effects on increasing body weight. However, these findings strongly suggest doing more research to determine if glucocorticoids induce long-term body weight via leptin synthesis or through other mechanisms. [66]

After it has been released to the blood stream, leptin reaches the central nervous system and binds to its receptors found in the hypothalamic neurons of the arcuate, ventromedial, and dorsomedial nuclei. The activation of the receptors, decreases the production of orexigenic (or appetite stimulant) substances such as neuropeptide Y and agouti-related peptide. It also activates the sympathetic nervous system, increasing the metabolic index and energy consumption. As for the insulin, leptin reduces its secretion, resulting in diminished energy storage. [62]

As it has been shown leptin insensitivity, would have repercussions in the regulation of body weight and metabolism. This leptin resistance can be attributed to abnormal receptors as well as malfunctioning intracellular signaling. [61] Either way, disruption of the leptin signaling, will eventually result in metabolic modifications that would lead to a raised BMI.

Furthermore, ALL survivors with CRT have higher risk of developing other components of the metabolic syndrome. [53] Gurney at al. encountered that ALL survivors who received CRT have increased total cholesterol levels, abnormally low HDL-C, altered triglycerides and LDL-C, compared to those who were not given CRT. [65]

5. Conclusions

As it has been shown, treatment for ALL predisposes patients to suffer from obesity and metabolic alterations, not only after, but also during it. Because of this, physicians should make patients being treated for ALL and those who have overcome ALL, aware of the possibility to develop these changes, and should strongly advise them to develop healthy life-styles, in order to counteract this increased risk. In addition, strict medical follow-up should be set for the early detection of this alterations, so that adequate medical intervention and/or habit shifts could take place before irreversible damage has occurred.

Acknowledgements

This work was funded by the Instituto Mexicano del Seguro Social through its program, Apoyo Financiero para el Desarrollo de Protocolos de Investigación en Salud en el IMSS(2005/1/I/078; FIS/IMSS/PROT/PRIO/11/017).

Author details

Alejandra Maldonado-Alcázar, Juan Carlos Núñez-Enríquez, Carlos Alberto García-Ruiz, Arturo Fajardo-Gutierrez and Juan Manuel Mejía-Arangué*

*Address all correspondence to: juan.mejiaa@imss.gob.mx

Research Unit in Clinical Epidemiology, Hospital of Pediatrics, National Medical Center 21st Century, Mexican Institute of Social Insurance, (IMSS), Mexico City, Mexico

References

[1] Krebs NF, Primak LE., Haemer M. Normal Childhood Nutrition & Its Disorders. In: Hay WW, Levin MJ, Sondheimer JM, Deterding RR, (eds.) CURRENT Diagnosis & Treatment: Pediatrics. New York: McGraw-Hill; 2011. Chapter 10. Available from http://www.accessmedicine.com/content.aspx?aID=6578685 (accessed August 19 2012)

[2] Brinksma A, Huizinga G, Sulkers E, Kamps W, Roodbol P, Tissing W. Malnutrition in childhood cancer patients: A review on its prevalence and possible causes. Critical reviews in oncology/hematology. 2012;83(2):249-75.

[3] Kramárová E, Stiller CA. The international classification of childhood cancer. International journal of cancer 1996;68(6):759-65.

[4] Draper GJ, Kroll ME, Stiller CA. Childhood cancer. Cancer surveys 1994;19-20:493-517.

[5] Reilly JJ, Odame I, McColl JH, McAllister PJ, Gibson BE, Wharton BA. Does weight for height have prognostic significance in children with acute lymphoblastic leukemia? The American journal of pediatric hematology/oncology 1994;16(3):225-30.

[6] Kuvshinnikov VA. The nutritional status characteristics and the protein metabolic indices of children with acute leukemia. Voprosy pitaniia 1990;(3):24-8.

[7] Tazi I, Hidane Z, Zafad S, Harif M, Benchekroun S, Ribeiro R. Nutritional status at diagnosis of children with malignancies in Casablanca. Pediatric blood & cancer 2008;51(4):495-8. ISSN:

[8] Sala A, Pencharz P, Barr RD. Children, cancer, and nutrition--A dynamic triangle in review. Cancer 2004;100(4):677-87.

[9] Barr RD, Ribeiro RC, Agarwal BR, Masera G, Hesseling PB, Magrath IT. Pediatric oncology in countries with limited resources. In: Pizzo PA, Poplack DG. (eds.) Principles and practice of pediatric oncology. Philadelphia: Lippincott, Williams and Wilkins; 2002. p1541–1552.

[10] Dávila-Rodríguez MI, Novelo-Huerta HI, Márquez-Solís R, Cortés-Gutiérrez E, Pérez-Cortés P, Cerda-Flores RM. [Nutritional indicators in children with acute lymphoblastic leukemia]. Revista médica del Instituto Mexicano del Seguro Social 2010 Nov-Dec;48(6):639-44.

[11] Zalina AZ Jr, Suzana S, A Rahman AJ, Noor Aini MY. Assessing the nutritional status of children with leukemia from hospitals in kuala lumpur. Malaysian journal of nutrition 2009 Mar;15(1):45-51.

[12] Waterlow JC. Classification and definition of protein-calorie malnutrition. British medical journal. 1972 Sep 2;3(5826):566-9.

[13] Waterlow JC, Buzina R, Keller W, Lane JM, Nichaman MZ, Tanner JM. The presentation and use of height and weight data for comparing the nutritional status of groups of children under the age of 10 years. Bulletin of the World Health Organization . 1977;55(4):489–498.

[14] Frisancho, A. R.; Tracer, S. P. Standards of arm muscle by stature for the assessment of nutritional status of children. American journal of physical anthropology 1987. 73(4):459-65

[15] Poskitt, E. Clinical nutritional assessant. Ed In: Practical Paediatric Nutrition. London; Butterworth, 1988

[16] Koskelo EK, Saarinen UM, Siimes MA. Low levels of serum transport proteins indicate catabolic protein status during induction therapy for acute lymphoblastic leukemia. Pediatric hematology and oncology 1991 Jan-Mar;8(1):53-9.

[17] Ingenbleel Y. DcVisscher M. DcNayeT P. Measurement of prealbumin as an index of protein-calorie malnutrition. Lancet 1972; 2(7768):106-9.

[18] Mejía-Aranguré JM, Bonilla M, Lorenzana R, Juárez-Ocaña S, de Reyes G, Pérez-Saldivar ML, González-Miranda G, Bernáldez-Ríos R, Ortiz-Fernández A, Ortega-Alvarez M, Martínez-García M del C, Fajardo-Gutiérrez A. Incidence of leukemias in

children from El Salvador and Mexico City between 1996 and 2000: population-based data. BMC Cancer 2005;5:33.

[19] Draper GJ, Kroll ME, Stiller CA. Childhood cancer. Cancer surveys 1994;19-20: 493-517.

[20] Mejía Aranguré JM, Ortega Alvarez MC, Fajardo Gutiérrez A. Acute leukemias epidemiology in children. Part 1. Revista médica del Instituto Mexicano del Seguro Social 2005;43(4):323-33.

[21] Pieters R, Carroll WL. Biology and treatment of acute lymphoblastic leukemia. Pediatric clinics of North America. 2008;55(1):1-20, ix.

[22] Uderzo C, Rovelli A, Bonomi M, Barzaghi A, Strada S, Balduzzi A, Pirovano L, Masera G. Nutritional status in untreated children with acute leukemia as compared with children without malignancy. Journal of pediatric gastroenterology and nutrition 1996 ;23(1):34-7.

[23] Reilly JJ, Weir J, McColl JH, Gibson BE. Prevalence of protein-energy malnutrition at diagnosis in children with acute lymphoblastic leukemia. Journal of pediatric gastroenterology and nutrition 1999;29(2):194-7.

[24] Mejía-Arangure JM, Fajardo-Gutíerrez A, Bernáldez-Ríos R, Rodríguez-Zepeda MC, Espinoza-Hernández L, Martínez-García MC. Nutritional state alterations in children with acute lymphoblastic leukemia during induction and consolidation of chemotherapy. Archives of medical research 1997;28(2):273-9.

[25] Delbecque-Boussard L, Gottrand F, Ategbo S, Nelken B, Mazingue F, Vic P, Farriaux JP, Turck D. Nutritional status of children with acute lymphoblastic leukemia: a longitudinal study. The American journal of clinical nutrition 1997;65(1):95-100.

[26] Pui CH, Campana D, Pei D, Bowman WP, Sandlund JT, Kaste SC, Ribeiro RC, Rubnitz JE, Raimondi SC, Onciu M, Coustan-Smith E, Kun LE, Jeha S, Cheng C, Howard SC, Simmons V, Bayles A, Metzger ML, Boyett JM, Leung W, Handgretinger R, Downing JR, Evans WE, Relling MV. Treating childhood acute lymphoblastic leukemia without cranial irradiation. The New England journal of medicine 2009;360(26): 2730-41.

[27] Pizzo PA, Poplack DG. Principles and Practice of Pediatric Oncology. Lippincott Williams & Wilkins;2011

[28] Hafiz MG, Mannan MA. Nutritional status at initial presentation in childhood acute lymphoblastic leukemia and its effect on induction of remission. Mymensingh medical journal 2008;17(2 Suppl):S46-51.

[29] Murry DJ, Riva L, Poplack DG. Impact of nutrition on pharmacokinetics of anti-neoplastic agents. International journal of cancer 1998;11:48-51.

[30] Longo DL. Approach to the Patient with Cancer. In: Longo DL, Fauci AS, Kasper DL, Hauser SL, Jameson JL, Loscalzo J, (eds.) Harrison's Principles of Internal Medicine.

New York: McGraw-Hill; 2012. Chapter 81. Available from http://www.accessmedicine.com/content.aspx?aID=9114033 (accessed August 18 2012).

[31] kumar R, Marwaha RK, Bhalla AK, Gulati M. Protein energy malnutrition and skeletal muscle wasting in childhood acute lymphoblastic leukemia. Indian pediatrics 2000;37(7):720-6.

[32] Koskelo EK, Saarinen UM, Siimes MA. Skeletal muscle wasting and protein-energy malnutrition in children with a newly diagnosed acute leukemia. Cancer 1990;66(2): 373-6.

[33] Lobato-Mendizábal E, Ruiz-Argüelles GJ, Marín-López A. Leukaemia and nutrition. I: Malnutrition is an adverse prognostic factor in the outcome of treatment of patients with standard-risk acute lymphoblastic leukaemia. Leukemia research 1989;13(10): 899-906.

[34] Shills ME, Young VR. Modern nutrition in Health and Disease. Philadelphia: Lea & Febiger;1988. p628.

[35] Mejía-Aranguré JM, Fajardo-Gutiérrez A, Reyes-Ruíz NI, Bernáldez-Ríos R, Mejía-Domínguez AM, Navarrete-Navarro S, Martínez-García MC. Malnutrition in childhood lymphoblastic leukemia: a predictor of early mortality during the induction-to-remission phase of the treatment. Archives of medical research 1999;30(2):150-3.

[36] Khan AU, Sheikh MU, Intekhab K. Pre-existing malnutrition and treatment outcome in children with acute lymphoblastic leukaemia. The Journal of the Pakistan Medical Association 2006;56(4):171-3.

[37] Rivera-Luna R, Olaya-Vargas A, Velásquez-Aviña M, Frenk S, Cárdenas-Cardós R, Leal-Leal C, Pérez-González O, Martínez-Avalos A. Early death in children with acute lymphoblastic leukemia: does malnutrition play a role? Pediatric hematology and oncology 2008;25(1):17-26.

[38] Pedrosa F, Bonilla M, Liu A, Smith K, Davis D, Ribeiro RC, Wilimas JA. Effect of malnutrition at the time of diagnosis on the survival of children treated for cancer in El Salvador and Northern Brazil. Journal of pediatric hematology/oncology 2000;22(6): 502-5.

[39] Hijiya N, Panetta JC, Zhou Y, Kyzer EP, Howard SC, Jeha S, Razzouk BI, Ribeiro RC, Rubnitz JE, Hudson MM, Sandlund JT, Pui CH, Relling MV. Body mass index does not influence pharmacokinetics or outcome of treatment in children with acute lymphoblastic leukemia. Blood 2006;108(13):3997-4002.

[40] Howard SC, Wilimas JA. Delays in diagnosis and treatment of childhood cancer: where in the world are they important? Pediatric blood & cancer 2005;44(4):303-4.

[41] Slats AM, Egeler RM, van der Does-van den Berg A, Korbijn C, Hählen K, Kamps WA, Veerman AJ, Zwaan CM. Causes of death--other than progressive leukemia--in childhood acute lymphoblastic (ALL) and myeloid leukemia (AML): the Dutch Childhood Oncology Group experience. Leukemia 2005;19(4):537-44.

[42] Lobato-Mendizábal E, López-Martínez B, Ruiz-Argüelles GJ. A critical review of the prognostic value of the nutritional status at diagnosis in the outcome of therapy of children with acute lymphoblastic leukemia. Revista de investigación clínica 2003;55(1):31-5.

[43] Weir J, Reilly JJ, McColl JH, Gibson BE. No evidence for an effect of nutritional status at diagnosis on prognosis in children with acute lymphoblastic leukemia. Journal of pediatric hematology/oncology 1998;20(6):534-8.

[44] Marín-López A, Lobato-Mendizabal E, Ruiz-Argüelles GJ. Malnutrition is an adverse prognostic factor in the response to treatment and survival of patients with acute lymphoblastic leukemia at the usual risk. Gaceta médica de México 1991;127(2): 125-31; discussion 131-2.

[45] Lobato Mendizábal E, Ruiz-Argüelles GJ. [Leukemia and malnutrition. III. Effect of chemotherapeutic treatment on the nutritional state and its repercussion on the therapeutic response of patients with acute lymphoblastic leukemia with standard risk]. Sangre 1990;35(3):189-95.

[46] Silverman LB, Gelber RD, Dalton VK, Asselin BL, Barr RD, Clavell LA, Hurwitz CA, Moghrabi A, Samson Y, Schorin MA, Arkin S, Declerck L, Cohen HJ, Sallan SE. Improved outcome for children acute lymphoblastic leukemia: results of Dana Farber Consortium Protocol 91-01. Blood 2001 Mar 1;97(5):1211-8.

[47] Hargrave DR, Hann II, Richards SM, Hill FG, Lilleyman JS, Kinsey S, Bailey CC, Chessells JM, Mitchell C, Eden OB; Medical Research Council Working Party for Childhood Leukaemia. Progressive reduction in treatment-related deaths in Medical Research Council childhood lymphoblastic leukaemia trials from 1980 to 1997 (UKALL VIII, X and XI) British journal of haematology 2001 Feb;112(2):293-9.

[48] Metzger ML, Howard SC, Fu LC, Peña A, Stefan R, Hancock ML, Zhang Z, Pui CH, Wilimas J, Ribeiro RC. Outcome of childhood acute lymphoblastic leukaemia in resource-poor countries. Lancet. 2003;362(9385):706-8.

[49] Gupta S, Bonilla M, Fuentes SL, Caniza M, Howard SC, Barr R, Greenberg ML, Ribeiro R, Sung L. Incidence and predictors of treatment-related mortality in paediatric acute leukaemia in El Salvador. British journal of cancer 2009;100(7):1026-31.

[50] Howard SC, Pedrosa M, Lins M, Pedrosa A, Pui CH, Ribeiro RC, Pedrosa F. Establishment of a pediatric oncology program and outcomes of childhood acute lymphoblastic leukemia in a resource-poor area. The journal of the American Medical Association 2004;291(20):2471-5.

[51] Advani S, Pai S, Venzon D, Adde M, Kurkure PK, Nair CN, Sirohi B, Banavali SD, Hawaldar R, Kolhatkar BB, Vats T, Magrath I. Acute lymphoblastic leukemia in India: an analysis of prognostic factors using a single treatment regimen. Annals of oncology 1999 Feb;10(2):167-76.

[52] Nathan PC, Jovcevska V, Ness KK, Mammone D'Agostino N, Staneland P, Urbach SL, Barron M, Barrera M, Greenberg ML. The prevalence of overweight and obesity in pediatric survivors of cancer. The Journal of pediatrics 2006 Oct;149(4):518-25.

[53] Skoczen S, Tomasik PJ, Bik-Multanowski M, Surmiak M, Balwierz W, Pietrzyk JJ, Sztefko K, Gozdzik J, Galicka-Latała D, Strojny W. Plasma levels of leptin and soluble leptin receptor and polymorphisms of leptin gene -18G > A and leptin receptor genes K109R and Q223R, in survivors of childhood acute lymphoblastic leukemia. Journal of experimental & clinical cancer research 2011 Jun 1;30:64.

[54] van Waas M, Neggers SJ, Pieters R, van den Heuvel-Eibrink MM. Components of the metabolic syndrome in 500 adult long-term survivors of childhood cancer. Annals of oncology 2010;21(5) 1121-6.

[55] World Health Organization. WHO: Obesity and Overweight. Fact Sheet N°311. May 2012 http://www.who.int/mediacentre/factsheets/fs311/en/(accessed 20 August 2012)

[56] Nathan PC, Wasilewski-Masker K, Janzen LA. Long-term outcomes in survivors of childhood acute lymphoblastic leukemia. Hematology/oncology clinics of North America 2009 Oct;23(5):1065-82, vi-vii.

[57] Oeffinger KC, Mertens AC, Sklar CA, Yasui Y, Fears T, Stovall M, Vik TA, Inskip PD, Robison LL. Childhood Cancer Survivor Study. Obesity in adult survivors of childhood acute lymphoblastic leukemia: a report from the Childhood Cancer Survivor Study. Journal of clinical oncology 2003;21(7) 1359-65.

[58] Lackner H, Schwingshandl J, Pakisch B, Knoblauch S, Mutz I, Urban C. [Endocrinologic function following cranial irradiation in acute lymphoblastic leukemia inchildhood]. Wiener klinische Wochenschrift 1991;103(19):581-4.

[59] Janiszewski PM, Oeffinger KC, Church TS, Dunn AL, Eshelman DA, Victor RG, Brooks S, Turoff AJ, Sinclair E, Murray JC, Bashore L, Ross R. Abdominal obesity, liver fat, and muscle composition in survivors of childhood acute lymphoblastic leukemia. The Journal of clinical endocrinology and metabolism 2007;92(10):3816-21.

[60] Diller L, Chow EJ, Gurney JG, Hudson MM, Kadin-Lottick NS, Kawashima TI, Leisenring WM, Meacham LR, Mertens AC, Mulrooney DA, Oeffinger KC, Packer RJ, Robison LL, Sklar CA. Chronic disease in the Childhood Cancer Survivor Study cohort: a review of published findings. Journal of clinical oncology 2009;27(14):2339-55.

[61] Ahima RS, Saper CB, Flier JS, Elmquist JK. Leptin regulation of neuroendocrine systems. Frontiers in neuroendocrinology 2000 Jul;21(3):263-307.

[62] Guyton AC, Hall JE. Pituitary hormones and their control by the hypothalamus. In: Textbook of Medical Physiology. Philadelphia: Saunders Elsevier; 2011. Chapter 75.

[63] Ross JA, Oeffinger KC, Davies SM, Mertens AC, Langer EK, Kiffmeyer WR, Sklar CA, Stovall M, Yasui Y, Robison LL. Genetic variation in the leptin receptor gene and obesity in survivors of childhood acute lymphoblastic leukemia: a report from the Childhood Cancer Survivor Study. Journal of clinical oncology 2004;22(17):3558-62.

[64] Garmey EG, Liu Q, Sklar CA, Meacham LR, Mertens AC, Stovall MA, Yasui Y, Robison LL, Oeffinger KC. Longitudinal changes in obesity and body mass index among adult survivors of childhood acute lymphoblastic leukemia: a report from the Childhood Cancer Survivor Study. Journal of clinical oncology 2008;26(28) 4639-45.

[65] Gurney JG, Ness KK, Sibley SD, O'Leary M, Dengel DR, Lee JM, Youngren NM, Glasser SP, Baker KS. Metabolic syndrome and growth hormone deficiency in adult survivors of childhood acute lymphoblastic leukemia. Cancer. 2006 Sep 15;107(6): 1303-12.

[66] Murphy AJ, Wells JC, Williams JE, Fewtrell MS, Davies PS, Webb DK. Body composition in children in remission from acute lymphoblastic leukemia. The American journal of clinical nutrition 2006;83(1):70-4.

Chapter 13

Acute Lymphoblastic Leukemia (ALL) Philadelphia Positive (Ph1) (Incidence Classifications, Prognostic Factor in ALL Principles of ALL Therapy)

Alicia Enrico and Jorge Milone

Additional information is available at the end of the chapter

http://dx.doi.org/10.5772/55095

1. Introduction

ALL is a malignancy of lymphoid cells occurring at any age. Almost 5000 cases are diagnosed annually in the USA. Cell-B subtypes account for 85–90% of cases in children and 75–80% of cases in adults; T-lineage ALL accounts for a small proportion of cases. It has a bimodal incidence occurring at 2–4 years of age followed by a gradual increase after the age of 50.

In the last years much progress has been made in understanding the biology of acute lymphoblastic leukemia which is now recognized as an expanding group of heterogeneous entities. Recognition of distinct gene expression patterns may identify patient subgroup with unique response to therapy and prognosis. Accurate definition of prognostic subgroups based on cytogenetic molecular marker has allowed institution of risk oriented therapies. [2] The Philadelphia (Ph1+) chromosome was first described in 1960 in a patient with chronic myeloid leukemia (CML). This is the product of the fusion of chromosomes 9 and 22, t (9;22), which results in a BCR-ABL hybrid gene. [2]

The incidence is approximately 20-30 % of adult patients with ALL who present the Philadelphia (Ph) Chromosome. Whereas Ph+ ALL is rare in children, comprising less than 5% of acute lymphoblastic leukemia, its incidence increases to approximately 40% in adults 40 years of age, with a 10% increment for every further decade of life with no sex difference. The majority of patients are diagnosed with de novo Ph+ ALL, although occasional cases of secondary Ph1+, ALL have been reported following chemotherapy or radiation therapy. [3, 4]. There are no known risk factors for Ph+ ALL. The associations with environmental socioeconomic infections and genetic events are being studied extensively in ALL. Few causal links have been established and the etiology of ALL remains obscure in most cases. The strongest associations to date exist with genetic factors and the role of Epstein Barr virus (EBV) and human immunodeficiency virus (HIV) in patients with mature B cell ALL [2].

2. Diagnosis

The characteristic findings of Ph1+ ALL is a reciprocal translocation t(9,22) (q34q11) that fuses the BCR gene from chromosome 22 to the ABL gene from chromosome 9. By standard cytogenetic analysis this becomes apparent as a shortened chromosome 22 referred to as the Philadelphia chromosome, which can also be visualized by fluorescent in situ hybridization (FISH) analysis. At the molecular level, the bcr/abl fusion transcript can be detected by RT-PCR. The location of the breakpoint within the BCR gene results in either the p190 $^{BCR/ABL}$ protein observed in Ph+ ALL (66.3% of the cases) or the p210 $^{BCR/ABL}$ protein common to patients with Ph+ CML which is present in ALL Ph+ (31,2%) The remaining cases are associated either with both transcript type or with atypical transcripts. [4]

Other additional chromosome aberrations were present in up to 79% of the cases in a large study of 209 patients (Moorman et al). Yanada et al. study involving 77 Ph+ ALL patients, additional aberrations with a frequency of greater than 10% included a second Ph chromosome (+der(22) t (9,22)) abnormalities involving the short arm of chromosome 9, monosomy 7, and trisomy 8. The presence of additional aberrations was associated with significantly shorter relapse free survival (RFS) and higher relapse rate. This was particularly pronounced for the +der (22)t(9,22) and abnormalities involving the short arm chromosome 9. In reference to this, standard karyotyping is mandatory to establish the initial diagnosis while FISH analysis may be used as a confirmatory technique. The major role of PCR analysis at diagnosis is determination of the type of fusion transcript, which becomes relevant during follow up studies of MDR. Using only PCR to establish the diagnosis is not acceptable, even more so as occasional patients harbor an aberrant fusion transcript that is not detected by standard primer combination [5,6.]

The white blood cell count is variable at diagnosis, hyperleukocytosis and/or splenomegaly may be present. Ph+ ALL is a B-precursor ALL which typically expresses the CD19 and CD10 antigens, and the CD34 antigen is expressed in 89% of cases. The most frequent immunologic subtypes are common ALL (78.2%) and pre-B ALL (19.9%), whereas only 1.9% of patients display the pro – B immunophenotype. Except for few case reports, the chromosome is not found in T linage ALL. Myeloid markers are frequently expressed, most notably the CD13 antigen (20%) and CD33 antigen (15%). CNS leukemia is infrequent (5%) at initial presentation, but there is an increased risk of developing meningeal leukemia during the course of treatment when compared with other B linage ALL. [7]

The main differential diagnosis at the begime,of the disease is chronic myelogenous leukemia (CML) lymphoblastic blast crisis (LBC). In the absence of a history of CML, myeloid hyperplasia, bone marrow basophilia, eosinophilia or excessive splenomegaly are suggestive of LBC-CML. While identification of the e1a2 fusion product (p190 $^{BCR-ABL}$) essentially rules out CML, the major BCR fusion transcript (p210 $^{BCR-ABL}$) is found in both Ph+ ALL and LBC-CML. This distinction is usually of no clinical significance. However, as newly diagnosed LBC-CML without a prior history of CML is generally treated in the same way as Ph+ ALL. [8]

3. Treatment of Ph 1+ ALL: The result with Imatinib and chemotherapy

Chemotherapy alone for adult with ALL Ph1+ is poor, with less than 10% probability. Long term survival. The development of tirosi kinase inhibitor, imatinib and its use with chemotheray for the induction obtained complete remission in ranged from 60-70%, moderately lower than 70-90 % achieved in Ph1+ negative ALL. The median CR duration was considerably inferior, however ranging from 9-16 month in patients treated only with chemotherapy with almost no long term survivor. Because of the poor outcome with chemotherapy, the allogeneic stem cell transplantation (SCT) is considered to be the treatment of choice in adult Ph+ ALL. [9]

Imatinib Mesylate (STI571 Glivec^{R}) (IM) was the first Tirosin Kinase inhibitor for CML treatment and now is the gold standard for the treatment of de novo CML in chronic phase. The BCR/ABL fusion gene encodes the chimeric BCR/ABL oncoprotein which has constitutively active tyrosine kinase activity. This results in dysregulated activity of additional signal transduction pathways located downstream of BCR/ABL. The strong pathophysiological similarity between Ph+ ALL and CML provided the rationale for exploring the clinical efficacy of IM. [10].

Druker et al. in one of the first evidence of clinical activity from a phase I study in 2001, in relapsed or refractory patients with Ph+ ALL which showed a significant number of hematological responses (70%) although only 20 % of the patients achieved a complete remission (CR). Later in 2002 these results were confirmed in phase II studies in which imatinib at daily doses of 400 mg to 600 mg induced a CR in 19% of the patients. These responses were not sustained however, and the estimated median survival in these studies was only 4.9 months. As a consequence, subsequent studies focused on the use of imatinib during front line therapy of Ph+ ALL, both as a single agent therapy and in combination with various chemotherapy regimens. A major goal of studies performed in younger patients was to increase the CR rate and improve the quality of response prior to hematopoietic stem cell transplantation (HSTC) in patients with a suitable donor. [12,13]. Several strategies have been evaluated to optimize the combination of imatinib and chemotherapy. Initial studies were based on schedules alternating imatinib and chemotherapy cycles followed by clinical trials that investigated schedules in which imatinib and chemotherapy were given concomitantly. The question of whether minimization of chemotherapy related toxicity by combining imatinib with less intensive chemotherapy or administering it alone yielded equivalent or superior results was also addressed. [11]

The current standard approach for patients in the combination of a chemotherapy protocol employing four to five cytotoxic agents typically used for ALL with imatinib at a daily dose of 400 mg to 800 mg (Table 1). Complete remission rates in these studies consistently exceeded 90%, the profile and incidence of severe toxicity were not different from those associated with the historic chemotherapy alone regimens. The overall survival (OS) in the different studies ranged from 36 to 76 %, although follow up is short (1-3 years) while the superiority of adding imatinib to conventional chemotherapy was strongly suggested by historical comparisons between the outcome of the patients using similar chemotherapeutic schedules with or without imatinib the impact of imatinib based regimen on long-term outcome is difficult to assess due to the higher rate of patients undergoing SCT in CR1, which became possible due to a lower incidence of early relapses. [10]

Subtype	Chemotherapy regimen	Imatinib dosing Induction (mg/d)	 Consolidation (mg/d)	 Mantenance (mg/d)	No	Results (%) CR	 Relapse	 DFS (at y)	 Survival (at y)
Adults									
Thomas el al	Hyper-CVAD	C(400)	C(400)	C(400)	39	92	14	83(3)	55 (3)
Yanada el al	JALSG ALL202	C(600)	A (600)	C(600)	80	96	26	60 (1) 51 (2)	76 (1) 58 (2)
Lee et al	Modified from Linker	C(600)	C(400)	C(400)	20	95	32	62 (2)	59 (2)
Wassmann et al	GMALL Alternating Concurrent	 None None	 A (400/600) C(600)	 NR NR	 47 45	 NA NA	 NR NR	 52 (2) 61 (2)	 36 (2) 43 (2)
de Labarthe el al	GRAAPH-2003	None	C(600)	NR	45	96	19	51 (1.5)	65 (1.5)
Ottmann et el al	GMALL Chemotherapy Imatinib	 None Only (600)	 C(600) C(600)	 C(600) C(600)	 28 27	 96 50	 41 54	 29 (1.5) 57 (1.5)	 35 (1.5) 41 (1.5)

C= concurrent; A= alternating; NR= not reported; NA= not applicable; JALSG = Japan Adult Leukemia Study Group; GMALL= German Multi-Centre Acute Lymphoblastic Leukemia; hyper-CVAD= fractionated cyclophosphamide, vincristine, doxorubicine, dexamethasone; GRAAPH= Group for Research on Adult Acute Lymphoblastic Leukemia; GIMEMA= Gruppo Italiano Malattie Ematologiche dell´Adulto; GRAALL=Group for Research in Adult Acute Lymphoblastic Leukemia; Pred= prednisone

C= concurrent; A= alternating; NR= not reported; NA= not applicable; JALSG = Japan Adult Leukemia Study Group; GMALL= German Multi-Centre Acute; Lymphoblastic Leukemia; hyper-CVAD= fractionated cyclophosphamide, vincristine, doxorubicine, dexamethasone; GRAAPH= Group for Research on Adult Acute Lymphoblastic Leukemia; GIMEMA= Gruppo Italiano Malattie Ematologiche dell´Adulto; GRAALL=Group for Research in Adult Acute Lymphoblastic Leukemia; Pred= prednisone

Table 1. Studies combining imatinib with chemotherapy for de novo Philadelphia chromosome positive (Ph+) ALL [10]

4. Approach in young patients

4.1. Imatinib in combination with chemotherapy in younger patients

The current standard approach for young patients is the combination of chemotherapy protocol employing four to five cytotoxic agent typically used for ALL with imatinib at a daily dose of 400 to 600 mg. Such an approach was pioneered by the MD Anderson Group. They combined sequential imatinib at 400 mg with 8 alternate hyper-CVAD and HD-MTX/AraC cycles (fractionated Cyclophosphamide, Vincristine, Doxorubicin and Dexamethasone alternating with cycles of high dose Methotrexate and Cytarabine) followed by imatinib maintenance at 600 mg/d. In this trial the CR rate was 93% with about 2 years of DFS rate of 75%. The molecular remission rate or negativity for bcr/abl transcript by RT-PCR and nested PCR approach 60%. [14]

Yanada et al. have likewise reported results in complete remission (CR) in 77 patient (96.2%), as well as polymerase chain reaction negativity of bone marrow in 71,3 % with the use a multidrug protocol plus imatinib. The authors described that the profile and incidence of severe toxicity were not different from those associated with our historic chemotherapy-alone regimen. Relapse occurred in 20 patient after median CR duration of 5,2 months. 49 patients underwent the allogeneic hematopoietic stem cell transplantation (HSCT), 39 of whom underwent transplantation during their first CR. The 1 year-event-free and overall survival (OS) rates were estimated to be 60.0% and 76.1%, respectively, which were significantly better than ourfortheir historic controls treated with chemotherapy alone. The probability of OS for this group of patients described by the author at 1 year was 73.3 % for those who underwent allogeneic HSCT and 84.8% for those who did not. [15]

Lee K-H et al. evaluated 20 patients with Ph+ ALL who were administered with induction chemotherapy daunorrubicin, vincristine prednisolone and L asparaginase along with imatinib 600 mg /day during remission induction and 400 mg /day during consolidation courses. 19 patients achieved complete remission (CR). In this trials, 15 underwent allogeneic hematopoietic cell transplantation (HCT) during first CR. After median follow up period of 799 days, 6 patients experienced recurrence. Eight died. Median CR duration was 821 days and median patient survival was 894 days. In the study the results were significantly longer by 2.9 and 2.3 fold respectively when compared to those of 18 historical patient treatments with same regimen of combination chemotherapy without imatinib. [16]

Wassmann et al. enrolled 92 patients with newly diagnosed Ph+ ALL in a prospective multicenter study to investigate sequentially 2 treatment schedules with imatinib administrated concurrent to or alternating with a uniform induction and consolidation regimen. Coadministration of imatinib and induction cycle2 (INDII) resulted in a CR rate of 95 % and polymerase chain reaction (PCR) negativity for BCR/ABL in 52 % of the patients compared with 19% in patients in the alternating treatment cohort. Remarkably, patients with and without a CR after induction cycle 1 (INDI) had similar hematologic and molecular responses after concurrent imatinib and INDII. 7 % of the patients underwent allogeneic stem cell transplantation (SCT), in first CR (CR1) both schedules of imatinib had acceptable toxicity and facilitated SCT in CR1 in the majority of patients but concurrent administration of imatinib and chemotherapy had greater antileukemic efficacy for this group. [17]

Labarthe et al. in 2007 published the results of 45 patients with Ph$^+$ ALL treated in the Group for Research on Adult Acute Lymphoblastic Leukemia (GRAAPH) 2003 study, where imatinib was started with HAM (mitoxantrone with intermediate-dose cytarabine) as consolidation therapy in good early responders (corticosensitive and chemosensitive ALL) or earlier during the induction course in combination with dexamethasone and vincristine in poor early responders (corticoresistant and/or chemoresistant ALL). Imatinib was then continuously administered until stem cell transplantation (SCT). Overall, complete remission (CR) and *BCR-ABL* real-time quantitative polymerase chain reaction (RQ-PCR) negativity rates were 96% and 29%, respectively. All of the 22 CR patients (100%) with a donor received allogeneic SCT in first CR. At 18 months, the estimated cumulative incidence of relapse, disease-free survival, and overall survival were 30%, 51%, and 65%, respectively. The authors described these 3 end points were favorable compared with results obtained in the pre-imatinib LALA-94 trial. [18]

Ottmann et al. recognized the potential benefit of administering imatinib simultaneously with chemotherapy rather than in an alternating manner which was investigated in two successive cohort of patients who were treated according to GMALL protocol and received imatinib either alternating with chemotherapy (first cohort) or simultaneously with induction and consolidation cycles (second cohort). The reported rate of complete molecular remission (CMR) was 19% and 52 % respectively, but this greater antileukemia efficacy did not translate into significant improvements in DFS or overall survival. [19] So far, the analyzed data showed the superiority of adding Imatinib to conventional chemotherapy and it was strongly suggested by historical comparison between the outcome of the patients using similar chemotherapeutic with or without imatinib. The magnitude of improvement was as high as 30% in the studies from MD Anderson and the GRAALL. These results were also confirmed by a pediatric study of Schultz et al. in which imatinib was given at 340 mg/m2 for an increasing number of days in combination with intensive chemotherapy. Early (1 year) EFS improved with increasing imatinib exposure from 70% to 95%. [20]

5. Imatinib-based therapy in elderly patients

5.1. Approach in older patients

While the strategy of combining imatinib with standard intensive chemotherapy protocol was explored primarily in younger patients, therapeutic approaches in elderly patients were focused more on reducing the intensity of chemotherapy. Vignetti et al. by GIMEMA (LAL0201) initiated a study with 30 patients who received a prephase with prednisone at increasing doses from 10 to 40 mg/m2/day followed by 45 day induction treatment with imatinib at the fixed dose of 800mg /day in combination with oral prednisone (40mg/m2/day) followed by maintenance with imatinib in all responding patients until occurrence of disease relapse or excessive toxicity. Complete remission was achieved in all patients (n=29). median survival from diagnosis was 20 month. In this study, the authors showed that elderly Ph(+) patients with ALL, often considered eligible only for palliative treatment strategies,may benefit from an imatinib-steroids protocol, which does not require chemotherapy or a long hospitalization; it is feasible, highly active, and associated with a good quality of life. [21]

Dalannoy et al., in another study from the GRALL (AFRO9 study), are currently testing a low intensity schedule (vincristine and dexamethasone), in combination with high dose imatinib (800mg/d) in elderly patients above 55 years (DIV regimen). Thirty patients were included in this study and were compared with 21 historical controls. Out of 29 assessable patients, 21 (72%9) were in CR after induction chemotherapy vs 6/21 (29%) in control. Five additional CRs were obtained after salvage with imatinib and four after salvage with additional chemotherapy in the control group. Overall survival (OS) was 66% at 1 year vs 43% in the control group. The

http://dx.doi.org/10.5772/55095

Subtype	Chemotherapy regimen	Imatinib dosing			No	Results (%)			
		Induction (mg/d)	Consolidation (mg/d)	Mantenance (mg/d)		CR	Relapse	DFS (at y)	Survival (at y)
Adults									
Vinetti el al	GIMEMA	+Pred (800)	Only (800)	Only (800)	30	100	48	48 (1)	74 (1)
Delannoy	GRAALL AFR09	None	C(600)	A (600)	30	72	60	58 (1)	66 (1)
Réa el al	GRAALL AFR07 pilot	C(800)	C(600)	C(600)	31	90	NR	48 (1)	60 (1)

Table 2. Studies combining imatinib with chemotherapy for de novo Philadelphia chromosome positive (Ph+) ALL in Elderly Patients [10]

1 year- relapse-free survival is 58 vs 11%. The author showed that the use of imatinib in elderly patients with Ph+ ALL is very likely to improve outcome, including OS. [22]

A pilot study of these combinations had shown promising results in relapsing and refractory Ph+ ALL with a CR rate of 90% in patients older than 55 years. This group, considers the hypothesis that Imatinib, combined with high-dose chemotherapy, is now becoming the gold standard for treatment of Philadelphia chromosome-positive acute leukemias. However, in all studies, imatinib dosage was tapered to 400–600 mg per day.) The group decided to initiate a clinical trial to evaluate an opposite strategy based on high-dose imatinib (800 mg per day) combined with a less intensive chemotherapeutic regimen (vincristine and dexamethasone), which we called the DIV induction regimen. Thirty-one patients (18 relapsing or refractory Ph + acute lymphoblastic leukemias and 13 lymphoid blast crisis chronic myelogenous leukemias) were enrolled. Complete remission (CR) was obtained in 28 out of 30 assessable patients. The median bcr-abl/abl ratio after the induction course was 0.1%. Median time to neutrophil recovery was 21 days. Nine out of 19 patients under 55 years old received allogenic stem cell transplantation after a median time of 78 days post-CR. Patients older than 55 experienced a 90% CR rate without additional toxicities, suggesting the DIV regimen may also be proposed as a front line therapy in older patients.[23]

6. Dasatinib in combination with chemotherapy

The combination of dasatinib with a variety of cytotoxic chemotherapy regimen both in younger and elderly patients with de novo or minimally pretreatment Ph+ ALL was explored in different groups of treatment. Ravandi et al. in one study phase II trial, showed patients with newly diagnosed Ph+ ALL who received dasatinib 50 mg PO BID (or 100 mg daily) for the first 14 days of each of 8 cycles of alternating hyperCVAD and high dose cytarabine plus methotrexate. Patients in CR continue to receive maintenance dasatinib 50 mg po BID (or 100 mg daily) and vincristine and prednisone monthly for 2 years followed by dasatinib indefinitely. With a median follow up of 10 months, 21 pts were alive and 18 were in CR; 2 died at induction, 3 pts died in CR; 1 from an unrelated cardiac event and 2 from infections. 5 pts relapsed (response durations were 54, 48, 47, 32, and 22 weeks) and 2 of them died. In 2 pts morphological relapse was preceded by flow and molecular relapse. Four relapsed pts developed new ABL mutations (3 T315I and 1 F359V). One patient underwent an allogeneic stem cell transplant. The author concluded that Dasatinib with HyperCVAD is effective in achieved molecular remission in patients with Ph+ ALL. They also found high incidence of T 315I ABL mutation among the relapsed patients. [24]

Reference	N (evaluated)	Age (range)	Dasatinib mg/d	ChThx regimen	Schedule of TKI and ChThx	CR%	PCR negative %	Induction death, n(&)	Relapse %	Outcome
Ravandi F 2008	28*	52(21-79)	100 QD	HyperCVAD	D1-14 of e/cycle	93	50	2(7)	5(18)	CR (10m):18 (64%) OS (10): 21 (75%
Rousselot P 2008	22	71 (61-83)	140 QD 100 QD	EWALL elderly	IND: parallel, then	95	28	1 (4.5)	1 (4.5)	na
Foa R 2008	48 (34)	54 (24-76)	70 BID	Steroid prephase then 12 w	Post-Induction therapy not	100	na	0	9 (27)	OS(10): 81%

*22 patients with de novo Ph+All, 6pts, with one prior treatment cycle

OS indicates overall survival; CR, complete remission; ChThx, chemotherapy; hyper-CVAD, fractionated cyclophosphamide, vincristine, doxorubicin, dexamethasone; IND, induction; na, not applicable; EWALL; European Working Group for Adult of the Europena LeukemiaNet

*22 patients with de novo Ph+All, 6pts, with one prior treatment cycle, OS indicates overall survival; CR, complete remission; ChThx, chemotherapy; hyper-CVAD, fractionated cyclophosphamide, vincristine, doxorubicin, dexamethasone; IND, induction; na, not applicable; EWALL; European Working Group for Adult of the Europena LeukemiaNet

Table 3. Studies with dasatinib for de novo Philadelphia chromosome + (Ph+) ALL.

In another study, Rousselot et al. evaluated that after a pre-phase with dexamethasone 10 mg/m^2 d-7 to d-3, dasatinib was administered at 140 mg QD (100 mg in patients over 70y) during the induction period in combination with IV injections of vincristine 1 mg and dexamethasone 40 mg 2 days (20 mg over 70y) repeated weekly for 4 weeks. Consolidation cycles consisted of dasatinib 100 mg/d administered sequentially with methotrexate 1000 mg/m^2 IV d1 (500 mg/m^2 over 70y) and L-asparaginase 10,000 UI/m^2 IM d2 (5,000 UI/m^2 over 70y) for cycles 1, 3 and 5 and cytarabine 1,000 mg/m^2/12h IV d1, d3, d5 (500 mg/m^2 over 70y) for cycles 2, 4 and 6. Maintenance phase consisted of dasatinib alternating with 6-MP and methotrexate orally every other month and dexamethasone/vincristine once every 2 months for up to 24 months. Median RFS and OS were 22.1 and 27.1 months, respectively. The group also showed dasatinib with low-intensity chemotherapy was highly effective in elderly patients with Ph+ ALL with a 90% CR and 22.1 months RFS. In concordance with Ravandi et al. the mutation T315I was associated with relapses. [25]

In these studies the CR rates were from 93 % until 100% independent of the regimen used, with molecular remission rates from 28% to 72%.

7. Dasatinib monotherapy

Dasatinib was used without chemotherapy. In this modality Foa el al by GIMEMA LAL1205 protocol, the patients with newly diagnosed Ph$^+$ ALL older than 18 (with no upper age limit) received dasatinib 70 mg BID IN induction therapy for 84 days combined with steroids for the first 32 days and intrathecal chemotherapy. Post-remission therapy was free. Fifty-three

http://dx.doi.org/10.5772/55095

patients were evaluable. All patients achieved a complete hematologic remission (CHR), 49 (92.5%) at day 22. At this time point, 10 patients achieved a BCR-ABL reduction to < 10^{-3}. At 20 months, the overall survival was 69.2% and disease-free survival was 51.1%. A significant difference in DFS was observed between patients who showed a decrease in BCR-ABL levels to < 10^{-3} at day 22 compared with patients who never reached these levels during induction. No deaths or relapses occurred during induction. Twenty-three patients relapsed after completing induction. A T315I mutation was detected in 12 of 17 relapsed cases. Treatment was well tolerated; only 4 patients discontinued therapy during the last phase of the induction when already in CHR. In adult Ph^+ ALL, induction treatment with dasatinib plus steroids is associated with a CHR in virtually all patients, irrespective of age, good compliance, no deaths, and a very rapid de bulking of the neoplastic clone.[26]

8. Maintenance therapy

To date there is no consensus as to what constitutes the most effective maintenance therapy in patients in whom allogeneic SCT is not possible. The recommendations of the European Working Group for Adult ALL provide no recommendations for maintenance therapy in patients not eligible for allogenic stem cell transplantation. Usually Imatinib is given either alone or in combination with classical ALL maintenance such as low dose methotrexate and 6-mercatopurine. However, data on the efficacy of these strategies is scarce. [22]

Potenza et al. in a study, with seven patients with Ph+ ALL who were in first complete remission and received maintenance therapy with imatinib alone, at 2 year progression free survival was 75%. The qPCR monitoring of BCR/ABL, persisting molecular complete response was associated with long lasting CR. The molecular relapse did not invariably mean hematological relapse and only the wide and rapid increment of BCR/ABL values was predictive of leukemia relapse. [27]

However, larger studies show less favorable results with Imatinib based maintenance.

M D Anderson employed more intensive maintenance therapy. They used imatinib 800 mg for 24 months with monthly vincristine and prednisone interrupted by 2 intensifications with Hyper-CVAD and imatinib, then imatinib indefinitely. [10]

The GMALL A and GRAAL presented an interesting approach in which imatinib is given concurrently with standard dose of Interferon or peg –Interferon. Wassmann et al. had a hypothesis that the experimental data suggested that interferon-α (IFN-α) enhances the antileukemic activity of imatinib. Therefore, the group combined imatinib and low-dose IFN-α in six patients with Ph+ ALL who were ineligible for stem cell transplantation. All patients had received imatinib for 0.5–4.8 months prior to IFN-α, for relapse or refractory Ph+ ALL or as an alternative to chemotherapy following severe treatment related toxicity. The results were encouraging, but longer follow up is needed to determine whether this strategy will translate into better relapse free survival. [28-29]

Longer follow up is needed to determine if this strategy will translate into better relapse-free survival. The European recommendation concluded that the standard approach to de novo Ph + ALL is the combination of intensive chemotherapy with imatinib (400 mg/d to 800/d) in young patients and reduced dose of chemotherapy with high dose imatinib (600 mg/d to 800 mg/d) for elderly patients. Allogeneic SCT is recommended to all eligible patients with a suitable donor and to continue imatinib with or without additional therapy in patients not undergoing SCT.[30]

9. Central nervous system (CNS) prophylaxis

Central nervous system leukemia is infrequent (5%) at initial presentation, but there is significant risk of developing meningeal leukemia during the course of treatment and the CNS directed prophylactic therapy should be considered mandatory in this patients.

Imatinib does not cross the blood brain barrier to an appreciable extent, levels in the cerebrospinal fluid have shown to reach approximately 1 - 2 % of serum level. This low degree of penetration into the CNS is most likely due to p-glycoprotein export pumps, and it is not increased in the setting of active meningeal leukemia. Therefore, active CNS directed prophylactic therapy is mandatory in all patients with Ph+ ALL. Both repeat intrathecal injection of chemotherapy e.g. methotrexate, alone or in combination with cytarabine and corticosteroid, and prophylactic cranial irradiation have been used successfully. There is currently no conclusive data whether for how long and at what interval intratecal chemotherapy should be continued in patients with sustained hematological even molecular remission and whether it may be prudent to administer some form of CNS prophylactic after SCT.[31,32]

Dasatinib showed in the clinical trials CA180006 better penetration of the CSF and achieved clinically active concentrations in small series of patients in whom stabilization and regression of CNS disease were achieved. The doses of Dasatinib 140 mg once a day or 70 mg twice a day. It remains to be determined whether the current approach to CNS directed prophylaxis can be modified in the context of dasatinib based treatment.[33]

10. Mechanism of resistance to therapy and progression

The mechanism of resistance to therapy is related to acquired genetic abnormalities in Ph+ ALL blast cells, which provide insights into pathogenesis and strongly influence prognosis. Cytogenetic abnormalities in addition to the Ph+ chromosome are present in approximately one third of cases of adult leukemia. Other Overexpression of bcr/abl fusion gene e.g. due to double Ph+ chromosome, activates a number of downstream signaling pathways involving the Ras/Raf/mitogen activated protein kinase and JAK-STAT (Janus Kinase signal transducer and transcription activator of transcription) development of growth factor independent malignant clones contributes to progression of the disease. [34]

http://dx.doi.org/10.5772/55095

11. Relapse associated with a BCR-ABL kinase domain point mutation

The development of clinical resistance to imatinib has now surfaced in several sites. Acquisitions of point mutations in the ABL tyrosine kinase domain (KD) that interfere with the binding of imatinib appear to be the most influential. ABL KD mutations generally are comprised of two categories. The first includes mutations that directly impede contact between imatinib and Bcr-Abl, such as the gatekeeper mutations T3151 or F317L. [35] The second involves mutations that alter the spatial conformation of the Bcr-Abl protein by affecting one of the two flexible loops: (1) the P-loop containing the ATP binding pocket, or (2) the activating loop. [36.37.38] To date, more than 50 ABL KD mutations have been identified. Although the prognostic significance of many of these remains unclear, the T315I mutation has been associated with a particularly adverse outcome since it disrupts a hydrogen bond critical for binding the TKI to the ATP- binding site. It has been identified in up to 20% of patients with imatinib-resistant Ph+ ALL, and also confers resistance to the second-generation TKIs nilotinib and dasatinib.[39]

In the GMALL study for elderly patients with Ph+ ALL, the incidence of ABL mutations by direct cDNA sequencing at the time of disease recurrence was 84%. In patients with ABL KD mutations, P-loop mutations predominated at a frequency of 57%, followed by the T315I mutation at 19%. The mutated clone comprised more than 50% of the ABL clones in all patients. [20] Pfeifer et al. also demonstrated that these ABL KD mutations were present in nearly 40% of the patients with de novo imatinib-naïve Ph+ ALL, with a distribution of P-loop mutations in 80% and the T315I mutation in 17%. However, the mutated ABL clone always comprised less than 2% of the sample, in contrast to the predominance of the mutated clone when associated with disease recurrence. These low-level ABL KD mutations in imatinib-naïve samples required more sensitive methods for detection (e.g., high-performance liquid chromatography). The presence of ABL KD mutations prior to imatinib did not correlate with known prognostic factors. There was no difference in the probability of achieving CR or molecular response based on the presence or absence of ABL KD mutations prior to imatinib therapy. No difference in remission duration was observed other than for those with the T315I mutation, which adversely affected outcome. In nearly all patients with an ABL KD mutation identified pretreatment, the same mutation was noted at the time of disease recurrence. Approximately 67% of the patients without an ABL KD mutation detected prior to imatinib had developed one at the time of disease recurrence. The discovery of novel acquired ABL KD mutations had also been reported in Ph+ ALL after sequential therapy with imatinib followed by the second-generation TKI dasatinib.[39]

Soverini et al. reported the development of the T315A and F317I (as opposed to the T315I or F317L) mutations that have inherent resistance to dasatinib. These ABL KD mutations could be suppressed by either imatinib or nilotinib given the lower IC50 with these compounds, although retreatment with imatinib after a prior failure would likely be ineffective due to the potential role of other coexisting mechanisms of resistance. Resistance screening with nilotinib, the other second-generation TKI, yielded only a limited spectrum of point mutations.[40] This suggests a lower rate of ABL KD mutations after Nilotinib therapy; however, additional analyses of ongoing clinical trials are needed to support this contention. [41]

Other mechanisms of resistance to imatinib and other TKIs include increased drug efflux, amplification of the BCR-ABL gene, and signaling independence of BCR-ABL after secondary transforming events (e.g., Src kinase pathway). Theoretically, dose escalation of imatinib or the use of more potent ABL inhibitors could circumvent the first two events, whereas use of novel Src inhibitors or multitargeted inhibitors would be required to restore sensitivity in the latter case [42]

12. Clinical implications of MRD

High levels of bcr-abl transcripts at different treatment stages indicate poor responsiveness to chemotherapy and to TKI, and intuitively could be considered a risk factor for disease recurrence. However, published data is not consistent. MRD levels determined at different time points prior to alloSCT were found to have prognostic relevance, with an early reduction in BCR-ABL transcript levels of at least 3 log appearing as the most powerful predictor of lower relapse rate and better DFS. The authors demonstrated the positive impact of imatinib on the outcome of allogeneic stem cell transplantation in adults with Philadelphia chromosome-positive acute lymphoblastic leukemia (Ph-positive ALL)and analyzed for risk factors that affect transplantation outcome, and they focused particularly on the prognostic relevance of minimal residual disease levels at each treatment stage. Prospective assessment of the extent of minimal residual disease reduction after the first 4-week imatinib therapy may allow the authors to identify subgroups of Ph-positive ALL transplants at high risk of relapse. [45] Stratification based upon MRD levels was also the principal prognostic parameter in two studies, Dombret H. et al. with 154 patients, and Pane F et al with 45 Ph+ ALL patients, respectively. [43,44,45,46]

In contrast, prospective MRD monitoring in 100 adult patients with Ph+ ALL treated with uniform imatinib- combined chemotherapy failed to establish an association between PCR negativity at the end of induction therapy and either relapse rate or relapse-free survival, although an increase in bcr-abl transcripts during hematologic CR was predictive of relapse in non-transplanted patients. [47]

Despite these discrepancies, these studies demonstrate that prospective monitoring of MRD has the potential to identify patients at risk of relapse, although the implication of different transcript levels and increments require validation within each therapeutic context or clinical study. These issues highlight the need for standardization and harmonization of methodologies used for bcr-abl quantification in Ph+ ALL. To achieve this aim at an international level, regular quality control rounds are jointly conducted by the European Working Group for Adult ALL (EWALL) of the European LeukemiaNet and the European Study Group for MRD Analysis in Acute Lymphoblastic Leukemia.

13. Treatment to relapse

Point mutations are the major mechanism of resistance to Imatinib therapy in Ph+ leukemia; different drugs active on mutant BCR/ABL or on its signal transduction pathway have been developed and tested at clinical level. Several second-generation ABL TKIs possess significant activity against imatinib-resistant BCR/ABL mutants, although their specificities vary.[48]

Dasatinib has been tested most extensively in Ph+ ALL and has been approved as second-line treatment of bcr-abl–positive leukemias in first time. Dasatinib (formerly BMS-354825) is a multitarget kinase inhibitor of Bcr-Abl, SRC family kinases, ephrin receptor kinases, PDGFR and KIT, among others. In a phase II study, dasatinib induces rapid hematologic and cytogenetic responses in adult patients with Ph+ ALL with resistance or intolerance to imatinib.[49]

Non-hematological side effects include diarrhea, nausea, headache, peripheral edema and pleural effusion. However, remission duration and PFS were short, due to resistance that was often associated with appearance of the T315I mutation. To enhance efficacy, dasatinib was combined with the hyperCVAD chemotherapy regimen in a phase II study with 14 patients, 3 of whom had CNS involvement. [50]

All patients responded; 71% achieved a CR, 64% achieved a major molecular response. With a median follow-up of 6 months, 7 patients remained in CR/CRp. Although toxicity was significant, with several episodes of gastrointestinal and subdural hemorrhage and pleural effusions, these preliminary results suggested that combination therapy should be preferred over single-agent therapy; alloSCT should be the goal if at all possible. To achieve a CR, mutation analysis should precede salvage therapy, and experimental treatment should be considered if the T315I mutation is detected, as this mutation confers resistance to all second generation ABL TKI. [50]

Small-molecule inhibitors developed to target Aurora kinases (AK), a family of serine-threonine kinases involved in the control of chromosome assembly and segregation during mitosis, have been found to possess activity against the T315I mutation. Several of these novel AK inhibitors have recently entered preclinical or clinical testing.. [51.52]

Another novel chemical class of compounds that bind to different structural pockets used by ABL kinase to switch between the inactive and active conformations, have recently been developed using structure-based drug design. Compounds have emerged that potently inhibit purified ABL in both the unphosphorylated and phosphorylated states via a non-ATP-competitive mechanism and impair proliferation and induce apoptosis of cells expressing a wide variety of BCR-ABL TKI-resistant mutants, including the T315I mutant, many P-loop mutants, and the dasatinib- resistant mutant F317L. [53]

14. New kinase inhibitors

Ongoing and future clinical trials will establish whether front-line therapy with second-generation ABL kinase inhibitors, ie, dasatinib, nilotinib, bosutinib and Inno-406, are superior to imatinib. Results may differ depending on their use as single-agents or as components for combination therapy. SCT-independent immunotherapeutic approaches are also evolving. Bispecific T cell–engager (BiTE) antibodies that transiently engage cytotoxic T cells for lysis of selected target cells are among the most interesting agents for immunotherapy of Ph+ ALL. The bispecific antibody construct called blinatumomab links T cells with CD19-expressing target cells, resulting in a non-restricted cytotoxic T-cell response and T-cell activation. A phase II dose-escalating study investigating the efficacy and safety of blinatumomab in ALL patients who are in complete hematological remission but remain MRD-positive is ongoing. Preliminary results indicate that treatment with blinatumomab is well tolerated and able to convert MRD- positive ALL into an MRD negative status. [54]

As a conclusion, our armamentarium of drugs that hold promise as active agents for treating Ph+ ALL is expanding substantially. Studies will need to focus on drug combinations, with specific attention to sequence and dosing of these agents. In designing trials, treatment algorithms should increasingly be based on molecular markers of disease and utilize quantitative assessment of MRD, and highly sensitive detection of mutations.[55]

15. Conclusion

The tyrosine kinase inhibitor (TKI) imatinib has become an integral part of front-line therapy for Ph+ ALL, with remission rates exceeding 90% irrespective of whether imatinib is given alone or combined with chemotherapy. Treatment outcome with imatinib-based regimens has improved compared with historic controls, but most patients who do not undergo allogeneic stem cell transplantation (SCT) (see the next chapter) eventually relapse. Acquired resistance on TKI treatment is associated with mutations in the bcr-abl tyrosine kinase domain in the majority of patients, and may be detected at low frequency prior to TKI treatment in a subset of patients. Second generation TKIs, eg, dasatinib and nilotinib, show activity against most of the bcr-abl tyrosine kinase domain (TKD) mutations involved in acquired imatinib resistance, but clinical benefit is generally short-lived. Accordingly, SCT in first complete remission (CR) is considered to be the best curative option. Molecular monitoring of minimal residual disease levels appears to have prognostic relevance and should be used to guide treatment. International standardization and quality control efforts are ongoing to ensure comparability of results. Mutation analysis during treatment relies increasingly on highly sensitive PCR techniques or denaturing and may assist in treatment decisions, e.g., in cases of molecular relapse. Results from current studies of second-generation TKI as front-line treatment for Ph+ ALL are promising and show high molecular response rates, but follow-up is still too short to determine their impact on remission duration and long-term survival. Strategies to improve outcome after SCT include the pre-emptive use of imatinib, which appears to reduce the relapse rate. In patients ineligible for transplantation, novel concepts for maintenance therapy are needed. These could involve novel immunotherapeutic interventions and combinations of TKI.

Author details

Alicia Enrico* and Jorge Milone

*Address all correspondence to: enrico@netverk.com.ar

Hematology Area Hospital Italiano de la Plata, Argentina

References

[1] Fadert S, Jeha S, Kantarjian H et al. The biology and Therapy of adult acute lymphoblastic leukemia. Cancer October 1 2003 volume 98 number 7 1337-1354

[2] Milone J, Enrico A -Treatment of Philadelphia chromosome-positive acute lymphoblastic leukemia

[3] The groupe francais de cytogenetique hematologique. Cytogenetic abnormalities in adult acute lymphoblastic leukemia; correlations with hematologic finding and outcome. A collaborative study of the groupe francaise de cytogenetique hematologique . Blood 1996; 87; 3135-3142

[4] Burmeister T, Schwartz S, Bartram CR, et al. Pacients age and BCR-ABL, frequency in adult B-precursor ALL: a retrospective analysis from the GMALL study group Boold 2008: 112:918-919

[5] Moorman AV, Harrison CJ, Buck GA et al. Adult leukemia Working Party Medical Research Council National Cancer Research Council National Cancer Research Institute. Karyotype is an independent prognosis factor in adult acute lymphoblastic leukemia (ALL) analysis of cytogenetic data from patients treated on the medical research council (MRC) UKALLXII/Eastern Cooperative Oncology Group (ECOG) 2993 trial Blood 2007; 109; 3189-97.

[6] Yanada M, Takeuchi J, Sugiura I et al. Japan Adult Leukemia Study Group Karyotype at diagnosis is the major prognostic factor predicting relapse-free survival for patients with Philadelphia chromosome-positive acute lymphoblastic leukemia treated with imatinib-combined chemotherapy Hematologica 2008;93:287-90

[7] Bene MC, Castolddi G et al. Proposal of the immunological calssifications of acute leukemias. European Group for the immunological characterizations of Leukemias (EGIL) Leukemia 1995, 10 1783-6.

[8] World Health OrganizationClassification of Tumor, Pathology and Genetics of Tumors of Haematopoietic and Lymphoid Tissues. 2001

[9] Ottmann G, and Wassmann B, treatment of Philadelphia chromosome positive Acute Lymphoblastic leukemia. American Society of Hematology 2005. Blood 118-122

[10] Druker BJ, Translation of the Philadelphia chromosome into therapy for CML Blood 2008; 50th anniversary review. 112:4808-4817.

[11] Ottmann O, Pfeifer. Management of Philadelphia Chromosome positive Acute Lymphoblastic Leukemia (Ph + ALL) Hematology 2009. Blood 371-381

[12] Druker B, Sawyers C, Kantarjian H et al. activity of a specific inhibitor of the BCR/ABL tyrosine kinase in the blastic crisis of chronic myeloid leukemia and acute lymphoblastic leukemia with the Philadelphia chromosome. NEJM vol.344, N°14-April5, 2001.

[13] Ottmann O , Druker B, Sawyers C, A phase 2 study of imatinib in patients with relapsed or refractory Philadelphia chromosome–positive acute lymphoid leukemias. Blood, 15 September 2002 Volume 100, Number 6

[14] Thomas D, Faderl S et al treatment of Philadelphia chromosome positive acute lymphocytic leukemia with hyper CVAD and Imatinib mesylate. Blood 15 June 2004 volume 103 number 12.

[15] Yanada M, Takeuchi J, Sugiura I et al. High complete remission rate and promising outcome by combination of imatinib and chemotherapy for newly diagnosied BCR/ABL positive Acute Lymphoblastic Leukemia: A Phase II study by japan adult leukemia study group. J of CO.2006 Volume 24 number 3, January 20

[16] Lee K, Lee h, Choi s Clinical effect of imatinib added to intensive combination chemotherapy for newly diagnosed Philadelphia chromosome positive acute lymphoblastic leukemia. Leukemia 2005 19, 1509 1516.

[17] Wassmann B, Pfeifer H, Goekbuget N et al. Alternating versus concurrent schedules of imatinib and chemotherapy as front-line therapy for Philadelphia-positive acute lymphoblastic + leukemia (Ph ALL)

[18] de Labarthe A, Rousselot P, Huguet-Rigal F et al. Imatinib combined with induction or consolidation chemotherapy in patients with de novo Philadelphia chromosome–positive acute lymphoblastic leukemia: results of the GRAAPH-2003 study blood, 15 February 2007 volume 109, number 4

[19] Ottmann O, Wassmann B, Pfeifer H et al. GMALL Study Group . Imtinib compared with chemotherapy as front line treatment of elderly patients wit philadephia positive acute lymphoblastic leukemia Cancer 2007, 109,2068-2076

[20] Schultz K, bowman P, Aledo A, et al. Improved early event free survival with Imatinib in Philadelphia positive chromosome Acute leukemia lymphoblastic a children oncology group study. Journal of Clinical Oncology. Vol. 27 number 31 November 1 2009.

[21] Vignetti M, Fazi P, Cimino G et all- Imatinib plus steroids induces complete remissions and prolonged survival in elderly Philadelphia chromosome –positive patients with acute lymphoblastic leukemia without additional chemotherapy: results of the

Gruppo Italiano Malattie Ematologiche dell'Adulto (GIMEMA) LAL0201-B protocol Blood 1May 2007 Vol 109, N9.)

[22] Delannoy A , Delabesse E, Lheritier V et al. Imatinib and methylprednisolone alternated with chemotherapy improve the outcome of elderly patients with Philadelphia-positive acute lymphoblastic leukemia: results of the GRAALL AFR09 study Leukemia (2006) 20, 1526–1532 & 2006

[23] Rea D, Legros L, Raffoux E, et al. High-dose imatinib mesylate combined with vincristine and dexamethasone (DIV regimen) as induction therapy in patients with resistant Philadelphia-positive acute lymphoblastic leukemia and lymphoid blast crisis of chronic myeloid leukemia. Leukemia (2006) 20, 400–403 & 2006

[24] Ravandi F, Thomas D, Kantarjian H, Phase II Study of Combination of hyperCVAD with Dasatinib in Frontline Therapy of Patients with Philadelphia Chromosome (Ph) Positive Acute Lymphoblastic Leukemia (ALL) Blood (ASH Annual Meeting Abstracts) 2008 112: Abstract 2921

[25] Rousselot R, Cayuela J, Hayette S- Dasatinib (Sprycel®) and Low Intensity Chemotherapy for First-Line Treatment In Elderly Patients with De Novo Philadelphia Positive ALL (EWALL-PH-01): Kinetic of Response, Resistance and Prognostic Significance Blood (ASH Annual Meeting Abstracts) 2010 116: Abstract 172

[26] Foà R, Vitale A, Vignetti M. Dasatinib as first-line treatment for adult patients with Philadelphia chromosome–positive acute lymphoblastic leukemia blood dec 15 2011 vol 118, num 25 6521-6528

[27] Potenza L, Luppi M , Riva G et al. Efficacy of imatinib mesylate as maintenancetherapy in adults with acute lymphoblastic leukemia in first complete remission. Hematologica/ The Hematology Journal- 2005;90(9) 1275

[28] Wassmann B, Scheuring U, Pfeifer U -Efficacy and safety of imatinib mesylate (Glivect) in combination with interferon-a(IFN-a) in Philadelphia chromosome-positive acute lymphoblastic leukemia (Ph+ ALL)LEUKEMIA 2003- 17, 1919-1924

[29] 29-Rousselot P, Huguet F, Vey N, et al. Maintenance Therapy by Gleevec and Pegasys in Patients with Philadelphia Chromosome Positive Acute Lymphoblastic Leukemia Not Eligible for hematopoietic stem cell transplantation. Blood (ASH Annaul Meeting Abstracts) Nov 2007; 110:2812

[30] Ottmann O, Rousselot P, Martinelli G- Treatment of ALL -Recommendations of the European Working Group for Adult ALL- ELN European Leukemia Net- 2011-116.

[31] Bujassoum S, Rifkind J, Lipton J, isolated central nervous system relapse in lymphoid blast crisis chronic myeloid leukemia and acute lymphoblastic leukemia in patients in imatinib therapy – Leuk Lymphoma 2004,45:401-403.

[32] Pfeizer H, Wassmann B, Hofmann W et al. Risk and Prognosis of Central Nervous System Leukemia in Patients with Philadelphia Chromosome-Positive Acute Leukemias Treated with Imatinib Mesylate-clinical cancer res 2003,9,4674-81

[33] Porkka K, Koskenvesa P , Lundán T- Dasatinib crosses the blood-brain barrier and is an efficient therapy for central nervous system Philadelphia chromosome –positive leukemia – Blood 2008, 112:1005-1012.

[34] Buscar

[35] Azam M, Latek RR, Daley GQ. Mechanisms of autoinhibition and STI-571/imatinib resistance revealed by mutagenesis of BCR-ABL. Cell. 2003;112:831-843

[36] Gorre ME, Mohammed M, Ellwood K, et al. Clinical resistance to STI-571 cancer therapy caused by BCR-ABL gene mutation or amplification. Science. 2001;293:876-880.

[37] Hochhaus A, Kreil S, Corbin AS, et al. Molecular and chromosomal mechanisms of resistance to imatinib (STI571) therapy. Leukemia. 2002;16:2190-2196.

[38] Shah NP, Nicoll JM, Nagar B, et al. Multiple BCR-ABL kinase domain mutations confer polyclonal resistance to the tyrosine kinase inhibitor imatinib (STI571) in chronic phase and blast crisis chronic myeloid leukemia. Cancer Cell. 2002;2:117-125.

[39] Pfeifer H, Wassmann B, Pavlova A, et al. Kinase domain mutations of BCR-ABL frequently precede imatinib-based therapy and give rise to relapse in patients with de novo Philadelphia-positive acute lymphoblastic leukemia (Ph+ALL). Blood. 2007;110:727-734

[40] Soverini S, Martinelli G, Colarossi S, et al. Second-line treatment with dasatinib in patients resistant to imatinib can select novel inhibitor-specific BCR-ABL mutants in Ph + ALL. Lancet Oncol. 2007;8:273-274

[41] Jabbour E, Cortes J, Giles F, O'Brien S, Kantarijan H. Drug evaluation: Nilotinib - a novel Bcr-Abl tyrosine kinase inhibitor for the treatment of chronic myelocytic leukemia and beyond. IDrugs. 2007;10:468-479.

[42] Thomas J, Wang L, Clark RE, Pirmohamed M. Active transport of imatinib into and out of cells: implications for drug resistance. Blood. 2004;104:3739-3745.

[43] Dombret H, Gabert J, Boiron JM, et al. Groupe d'Etude et de Traitement de la Leucémie Aiguë Lymphoblastique de l'Adulte (GET-LALA Group). Outcome of treatment in adults with Philadelphia chromosome-positive acute lymphoblastic leukemia results of the prospective multicenter LALA-94 trial. Blood. 2002; 100: 2357-2366

[44] Shin HJ, Chung JS, Cho GJ. Imatinib interim therapy between chemotherapeutic cycles and in vivo purging prior to autologous stem cell transplantation, followed by maintenance therapy is a feasible treatment strategy in Philadelphia chromosome-positive acute lympho- blastic leukemia. Bone Marrow Transplant. 2005; 36: 917-918.

[45] Lee S, Kim YJ, Chung NG, et al. The extent of minimal residual disease reduction after the first 4-week imatinib therapy determines outcome of allogeneic stem cell

transplantation in adults with Philadelphia chromosome-positive acute lymphoblastic leukemia. Cancer. 2009; 115:561-570.

[46] Pane F, Cimino G, Izzo B, et al. Significant reduction of the hybrid BCR/ABL transcripts after induction and consolidation therapy is a powerful predictor of treatment response in adult Philadelphia-positive acute lymphoblastic leukemia. Leukemia. 2005;19: 628-635

[47] Yanada M, Sugiura I, Takeuchi J, et al. Japan Adult Leukemia Study Group. Prospective monitoring of BCR-ABL1 transcript levels in patients with Philadel- phia chromosome-positive acute lymphoblastic leukaemia undergoing imatinib-combined chemo- therapy. Br J Haematol. 2008; 143: 503-510.

[48] Redaelli S, Piazza R, Rostagno R, et al. Activity of bosutinib, dasatinib, and nilotinib against 18 imatinib- resistant BCR/ABL mutants. J Clin Oncol. 2009;27:469-471.

[49] Ottmann O, Dombret H, Martinelli G, et al. Dasatinib induces rapid hematologic and cytogenetic responses in adult patients with Philadelphia chromosome positive acute lymphoblastic leukemia with resistance or intolerance to imatinib: interim results of a phase 2 study. Blood. 2007;110:2309-2315.

[50] Jabbour E, O'Brien S, Thomas DA, et al. Combination of the HyperCard regimen with dasatinib is effective in patients with relapsed Philadelphia Chromosome Ph positive acute lymphoblastic leukemia (ALL) and lymphoid blast phase chronic myeloid leukemia (CML-LB) [Abstract] Blood. 2008; 112: 2919.

[51] Carpinelli P, Moll J. Aurora kinases and their inhibitors: more than one target and one drug. Adv Exp Med Biol. 2008;610:54-73.

[52] Gautschi O, Heighway J, Mack PC, et al. Aurora kinases as anticancer drug targets. Clin Cancer Res. 2008;14:1639-1648.

[53] Gumireddy K, Baker SJ, Cosenza SC, et al. A non-ATP- competitive inhibitor of BCR-ABL overrides imatinib resistance. Proc Natl Acad Sci U S A. 2005;102:1992- 1997

[54] Bargou R, Leo E, Zugmaier G, et al. Tumor regression in cancer patients by very low doses of a T cell- engaging antibody. Science. 2008;321:974-977.

[55] Topp M, Goekbuget N, Kufer P, et al. Treatment with Anti-CD19 BiTE antibody blinatumomab (MT103 / MEDI-538) is able to eliminate minimal residual disease (MRD) in patients with B-precursor acute lymphoblastic leukemia (ALL): first results of an ongoing phase II study [abstract]. Blood. 2008;112:672

Chapter 14

Invasive Fungal Infections in ALL Patients

Roman Crazzolara, Adrian Kneer,
Bernhard Meister and Gabriele Kropshofer

Additional information is available at the end of the chapter

http://dx.doi.org/10.5772/54990

1. Introduction

The success rate of acute lymphoblastic leukemia (ALL) therapy has gradually increased over the past decades. With more than 80% long-term survivors, treatment of ALL in children is undoubtedly one of the great success stories of innovative study-controlled modern medicine [1]. Attempts to boost cure rates for those who do not respond to therapy or relapse with more intense chemotherapy including allogeneic hematopoietic stem cell transplantation have further improved the outcome of patients, particularly for prognostic unfavorable subgroups [2]. However, intensification of treatment can substantially increase morbidity, the risk for life-threatening sequelae and mortality [1].

Several studies address this important issue and report on the emergence of fungi. A retrospective review of ~ 5.600 patients who underwent hematopoietic stem cell transplantation at the Fred Hutchinson Cancer Research Center (Seattle) from 1985 to 1999 reports a constant increase of 3.5% in the one-year cumulative incidence of probable and proven invasive fungal infections [3]. Investigation of autopsies, skin, and lung biopsies, and bronchoalveolar lavage fluid analyses reveal that non-fumigatus Aspergillus species, such as Fusarium and Zygomycetes have increased, especially in patients, who have received multiple transplants. These observations are particular worrisome given the increasing importance of amphothericin-B resistant organisms, resulting in a very poor one-year survival rate of ~ 20% [4]. For those who do survive, length of hospital stay and total hospital charges are increased, compared with immunocompromised patients without fungal infection [5].

Despite much effort has been taken to improve therapeutic treatments and strategies, there still remains much uncertainty and controversy regarding the best method to diagnose, prevent and treat fungal infections [6]. Practicing physicians approach this uncertainty by treating suspected infections empirically. However, researchers that conduct clinical trials tend to accept only cases in which the diagnosis is certain in order to improve clarity and uniformity of clinical trials. Therefore, members of the European Organization for Research and Treatment of Cancer / Invasive Fungal Infection Study Group (EORTC) and the National Institute of Allergy and Infectious Disease (NIAID) Mycoses Study Group (MSG) formed a consensus study group to define standard definitions of invasive fungal infections for clinical research [7]. Practice guidelines are intended to limit practice variations towards movements such as evidence-based medicine and are primarily suggested by the European Conference of Infections in Leukemia (ECIL; http://www.ebmt.org/Contents/Resources/Library/ ECIL/ Pages/ECIL.aspx). For the clinical purpose there is still a need to develop more effective prevention and treatment strategies. Such strategies may rely on newer antifungal agents that are active against amphothericin B resistant moulds and are well tolerated. Because of limited number of affected patients, multicenter collaborative trials are required.

This case-based review examines the current literature to explore basic concepts on epidemiology, diagnosis and treatment of invasive fungal infections in ALL patients. A case report will be used to illustrate these specific issues.

2. Methods

A systematic review of the literature for an explicit identification of major problems related to the heterogeneity of patients with acute lymphoblastic leukemia who have invasive fungal infections was undertaken. *Pneumocystis* infections were not considered. In brief, the abstracts of 711 articles published from 1985 through 2012 were screened. Of these, 41 articles were finally selected because these report clinical research on patients with ALL who also had deep-tissue fungal infections. The minimum diagnostic criteria used to include patients in the study were extracted from definitions devised by the investigators. Likewise, the criteria used to express different degrees of diagnostic probability were summarized, as were the terms most often used to express these levels of uncertainty.

3. Case study: A sixteen-year old patient with Ph+ ALL

A sixteen-year old adolescent was referred to the outpatient oncologic clinic with suspicion of a proliferative disease of the hematopoietic system. Two weeks prior the admission, the patient suffered from sub febrile temperatures and fatigue. At the time of the visit to the general physician scarlet was ruled out and the patient discharged. At admission, the patient's general condition was slightly deteriorated; his physical examination revealed petechial rash over the extremities, pallor and hepatosplenomegaly. Laboratory findings showed ALL with a positive BCR/ABL result and an absolute count of 398.000 blasts per μL. He was subjected to treatment with the ALL BFM 2000 program for high-risk patients. He responded well to chemotherapy and achieved complete morphological remission on day ten of treatment. Following day fifteen, the tyrosine-kinase inhibitor Imatinib Mesylate was added to the standard treatment.

On the thirtieth day of induction chemotherapy the patient developed fever of 39.2°C. Physical examination was unremarkable. The laboratory tests showed leucopenia (0.5 x 10^9/L) with an absolute neutrophilic count of 19/µL, but no elevation of inflammatory proteins (CRP <0.06 mg/dL).

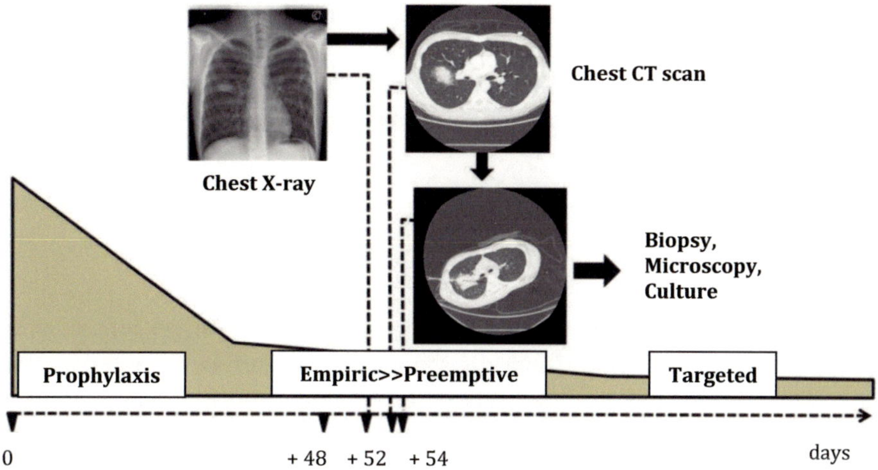

Figure 1. Time course of diagnosis and treatment of fungal infection in a Philadelphia chromosome-positive acute lymphoblastic leukemia (Ph+ALL) patient. Fungal infection was suspected by a chest X-ray on day thirty four of induction chemotherapy for Ph+ ALL. Prophylactic treatment with Fluconazole was switched to pre-emptive therapy with liposomal Amphothericin. Five days later histology of the fungal mass obtained by computed tomography (CT)-guided percutaneous biopsy confirmed the diagnosis of invasive mould infection. Culture revealed Aspergillus flavus, susceptible to Voriconazole.

Empirical antibiotic regimen was initiated with a carbapenem (Meropenem) and an aminoglycoside (Gentamycin). Because of relapsing fever four days after the initiation of antibiotics, vancomycin was added. Both blood and urine cultures were aseptic.

A chest X-ray showed a distinctive and peculiar mass in the middle of the right lung. Because the radiological image was ambiguous the diagnostics were extended by a chest CT scan, which showed a large mass in the right upper lobe, surrounded by a wide zone of ground-glass attenuation demonstrating the halo sign. On the ground of the radiologic examinations, fungal infection was suspicioned and pre-emptive antifungal therapy was initiated. Fluconazole, included in the treatment as a prophylactive measure, was replaced by liposomal Amphothericin administered at a dose of three mg/kg once daily. On the next day CT-guided biopsy was planned to obtain a definitive diagnosis. Biopsy was performed with only a single puncture using a 20 G cutting needle. No pneumothorax or hemorrhage was noted after the procedure. Histological examination yielded dichotomously branching septated hyphae consistent with Aspergillus species, confirming the diagnosis of invasive fungal infection. Culture demonstrated a growth of Aspergillus flavus. Antifungal susceptibility testing with the agar-based MIC test showed good activity for Voriconazole, Posaconazole and Caspofungin, but high MIC^{90} for liposomal Amphothericin.

Accordingly antifungal therapy was switched to Voriconazole (6 mg/kg) for eight weeks intravenously and then orally until the twelfth week. CT imaging studies that followed confirmed a gradual recession of the lesion. The patient underwent right sided thoracotomy with wedge resection of the fungal mass. Histopathology revealed Aspergilloma with surrounding chronic granulomatous inflammation, fibrosis and sheets of macrophages. Post-operative course was uneventful and no recurrence of fungal infection over twenty four months follow up was observed. He underwent allogeneic hematopoietic stem cell transplantation and has been in complete molecular remission since.

4. Epidemiology

Worldwide surveys evaluating the epidemiology of invasive fungal infections have been conducted in large center studies in North America [8]. In European countries data is most commonly derived from single-center reports or regional reports from single countries [8]. Though local epidemiology is a cornerstone of clinical decision making, efforts are now undertaken worldwide to start multi-national surveys on fungal infections in order to improve uniformity of clinical trials.

Until 2 decades ago, infections by Candida were the most common fungal pathogen in patients treated for ALL. However, with the introduction of Fluconazole as primary antifungal prophylaxis and the application of more aggressive treatment protocols, including allogeneic hematopoietic stem cell transplantation, a notable shift towards the advent of invasive aspergillosis has been noted [9]. Whereas almost all of the fungal infections were attributable to candidiasis (11/11) in autopsy studies of the late seventies, mould infections were responsible for 62% of IFIs (16/26) two decades later [9]. Concordantly, a large multi-centre report from the SEIFEM-2004 study (Sorveglianza Epidemiologica Infezioni Fungine nelle Emopatie Maligne) confirms this trend, indicating, that over half of all fungal infections (346/538) were caused by moulds, in most cases Aspergillus species (310/346) [10]. Most importantly, such infections have become a prime cause of death in patients with hematologic malignancies. The IFI-attributable mortality rate was 39% (209/538). The highest IFI-attributable mortality rates were associated with zygomycosis (64%) followed by fusariosis (53%), aspergillosis (42%), and candidemia (33%) [10].

Along with the increased incidence of mould infections caused by Aspergillus species, other emerging mould opportunistics, such as Zygomycetes and Fusarium species, have progressively been noted; interestingly, frequency varies by geographical location [8]. Another trend in changing the face of epidemiology is that infections caused by non-albicans Candida species (e.g. Candida glabrata, C. krusei, C. tropicalis, C. parapsilosis) have steadily increased, particularly in patients with ALL [11].

http://dx.doi.org/10.5772/54990

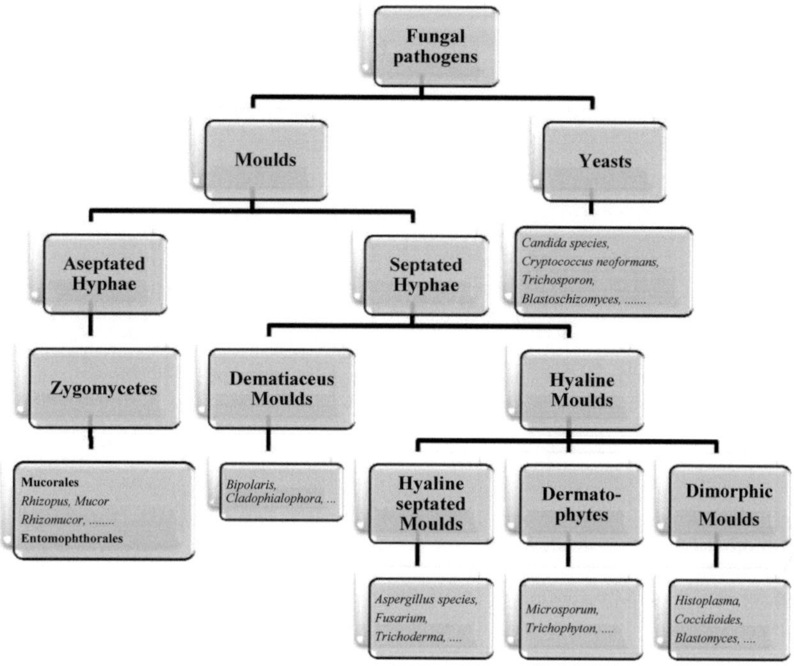

Figure 2. Pathogenic fungi that cause disease in acute lymphoblastic leukemia (ALL) Patients. A schematic classification depending on phylogenetic properties of fungal pathogens encountered in ALL patients is presented.

Yeast like pathogens enter the body via the gut or skin and mostly follow the pattern of fungemia and disseminated infection known from Candida species. Rarely the central nervous system, cardiovascular system or other tissues represent sites of dissemination [12].

Besides invasive infections of the skin and subcutaneous tissues, moulds involve, as airborne pathogens, the sino-pulmonary tract; the emerging opportunistic moulds have a higher propensity for dissemination, in particular into the central nervous system. Because of the lack of specific clinical, radiographic and histological features and the absence of diagnostic surrogate markers in blood, the diagnosis depends on the identification of the organism by means of culture based methods [12].

5. Diagnostics

In general, diagnostic testing should begin with non-invasive methods and only approach invasive steps if needed. Diagnostic options include conventional or high-resolution CT (this has less radiation exposure and was performed in this case report), positron emission tomography (PET), magnetic resonance imaging (MRI), GM assay, 1,3-ß-D-Glucan test, Polymerase chain reaction (PCR), bronchoalveolar lavage, blood culture and tissue biopsy. At this time,

MRI and PET are more research-oriented than commonly used clinical approaches. The utility of standard blood cultures is limited because of a high percentage of false-negative results, particularly in patients with disseminated aspergillosis. Of the listed options, the GM and 1,3-ß-D-Glucan serum assay, PCR and the CT scan will be described in detail.

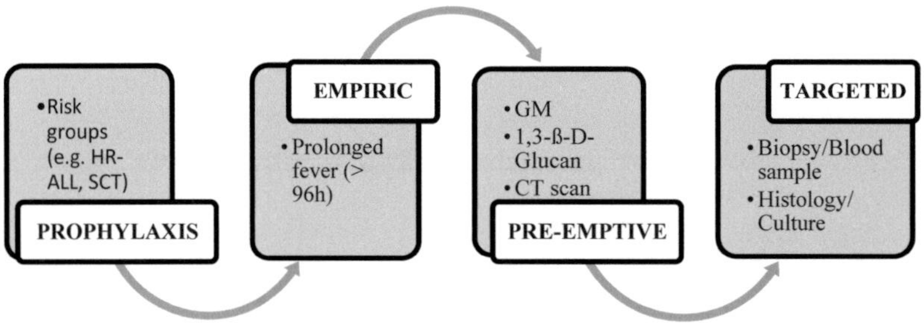

Figure 3. Simplified view of antifungal strategy in acute lymphoblastic leukemia (ALL) patients. Clinical practice (not EORTC criteria) in the management of IFIs depends on the population at risk (e.g. genetics, clinical), availability/value of diagnostic tests and availability/effectiveness of antifungal drugs. HR-ALL: high risk – acute lymphoblastic leukemia; SCT: stem cell transplantation; GM: Galactomannan; CT: computed tomography.

5.1. Galactomannan (GM)

GM testing with the Platelia Aspergillus Enzyme Immunoassay (EIA; Biorad Laboratories, Redmond, WA) has been approved by the U.S. Food and Drug Administration (FDA) for Aspergillus diagnostics and is included as a mycological criterion in the revised definitions of invasive fungal disease from the EORTC/MSG consensus group [6]. The test is based on detection of a component of the Aspergillus cell wall, Galactomannan (GM), which is released in the surrounding environment by growing Aspergillus species. Concentration of serum GM correlates with fungal burden in animals with experimental pulmonary aspergillosis – and, according to the 2011 ECIL clinical practice guidelines may be considered as surrogate marker for detection of invasive aspergillosis (http://www.ebmt.org/Contents/Resources/Library/ECIL/Pages/ECIL.aspx). Recent data suggest that sequential measuring of GM serum levels may be used for therapeutic monitoring in children and adults with pulmonary aspergillosis. The guidelines from the Infections Disease Society of America (IDSA) state, that duration of antifungal therapy must not only rely on disappearance of GM levels, but also on resolution of clinical and radiological findings [13].

The GM EIA has been most studied in hematologic malignancy and bone marrow transplantation populations. Both the specificity and sensitivity of the GM EIA for invasive aspergillosis are high for infected, neutropenic adult patients from these populations. Comparison of 5 studies which use EORTC/MSG criteria and give adequate information for individual patients with results of a formal meta-analysis, indicate sensitivity, specificity of 76% to 73%, 86% to 90% in children and adults respectively [14]. Controversy of GM testing exists about the interpretation of the assay cutoff level (0.5, 1.0), which was originally set at 1.5 and was applied in Europe but which was lowered to 0.5 after review by the FDA. Studies have shown that using an index cutoff for positivity of 0.5 versus greater indices substantially increases sensitivity, with only minimal loss in specificity [15]. Factors, which increase false positivity and influence the specificity of the assay, include a low level of cut-off (<0.5), colonization with Bifidobacterium bifidum in the intestinal flora, which mimics the epitope recognized by the EB-A2 in the enzyme-linked immunosorbent assay kit [16] and invasive infections with other fungi, such as Penicillium spp., histoplasmosis, and blastomycosis [13]. Moreover, cross-reactivity of the assay has been shown with the use of piperacillin/ tazobactam or amoxicillin/ clavulanate antibiotic therapy and in infants with the nutrition of milk-based formulas [17].

The IDSA guidelines currently recommend using the GM EIA in conjunction with CT scans for early, noninvasive diagnosis of invasive aspergillosis in high-risk patients [13]. The test should be performed serially, at least twice per week through the periods of highest risk, whether the periods involve neutropenia or active GVHD [13].

When GM in serum is used for screening for invasive mold infection in children with hematological malignancies/undergoing HSCT, data should be interpreted with caution, since the assay has a number of limitations in the sensitivity and specificity profile. Prospective monitoring of GM in serum every three to four days in children at high risk for IFD is reasonable for early diagnosis of invasive aspergillosis. Although the optimal cut-off value of GM in the serum of children is not well defined, published data support the use of a threshold of an optical density index 0.5 (http://www.ebmt.org/Contents/Resources/Library/ ECIL/Pages/ ECIL.aspx).

5.2. 1,3-ß-D Glucan

1,3-ß-D Glucan (BG) is a fungal cell wall component circulating in the blood of patients with invasive aspergillosis, candidemia, but also Fusarium, Trichosporum, Saccharomyces, and Pneumocystis jirovecii. Moreover, BG is also detected in patients with infections due to bacteria such as Streptococcus pneumoniae, Pseudomonas aeruginosa and in healthy individuals. However, BG is absent in patients with cryptococcosis and zygomycosis [18]. Antibiotics such as cefepime, piperacillin/tazobactam or meropenem may cause positive BG levels. Investigations using different BG assays in 2979 patients (594 with proven or probable IFI) have reported a pooled sensitivity of 76.8% and specificity of 85.3% [19]. Differences in study design (population studies versus case-control, variation in the number of proven or probable IFIs, proportions of patients with candidemia and aspergillosis, case-mix of neutropenic and non-neutropenic patients, and previous antifungal prophylaxis) highlight the need for further investigations. In children, data is very limited: elevated levels of BG were reported in a case-control study of only four children with IFI (3 patients with candidemia, one patient probable aspergillosis) [20].

The Fungitell assay (Associates of Cape Cod) for detection of 1,3-ß-D Glucan is approved by the FDA for the diagnosis of invasive mycoses, including aspergillosis [13] and is included as mycological criterion in the revised definitions of invasive fungal disease from the EORTC/MSG consensus group [6]. Unfortunately, there is no recommendation from ECIL or IDSA for clinical practice. However, BG testing in adults is considered as having good diagnostic accuracy for early diagnosis of IFD; in children, data are too limited to make any recommendations (http://www.ebmt.org/Contents/Resources/Library/ ECIL/Pages/ ECIL.aspx).

5.3. PCR

Detection of antifungal DNA has been advocated as a promising, rapid and more sensitive diagnostic tool, but false-positive results can occur, and a standardized commercial method is not yet available. Several PCR assays to detect fungal DNA have been described, but most have shown that the global performance was too low to be of clinical interest. Different situations have been reported: PCR either has high sensitivity and NPV, while specificity and PPV is low, or, conversely, high specificity and PPV with low sensitivity and NPV [21-24]. These discrepancies can be due to the different technical approaches used. Indeed, a major difference is the type of PCR method used in these studies, i.e., nested PCR, PCR–enzyme-linked immunosorbent assay, or RT-PCR [22;24]. Also, the superiority of large serum volumes (> 1 ml) in comparison with conventional serum samples (100 µl to 200 µl) has clearly been shown [23]. In view of changing epidemiology a panfungal PCR might be advantageous to permit the detection of a wide range of fungal pathogens. Its sensitivity of 96%, negative predictive values of 98%, whereas the specificity and positive predictive value were 77% and 62%, respectively is far superior to single PCR measurements [25].

In summary, despite ISDA and ECIL do not give any recommendations, combining non-culture based diagnostics is an important research direction that may improve the overall predictive value of these systems [26].

5.4. Chest CT scan

Systematic chest CT scan allows early diagnosis of invasive pulmonary aspergillosis, is more sensitive and specific than traditional chest radiographs and is a clinical criterion in the revised definitions of invasive fungal disease from the EORTC/MSG consensus group. Characteristic findings consist of nodules surrounded by the 'halo sign', an area of haziness or ground-glass opacity, or pleura-based, wedge-shaped areas of consolidation [27]. These findings correspond to areas of hemorrhagic infarcts. In severely neutropenic patients, the halo sign is highly suggestive of angioinvasive aspergillosis. However, a similar appearance has been described in a number of other conditions, including infections with herpes virus or cytomegalovirus, Kaposi sarcoma, Wegener granulomatosis, and bronchiolitis obliterans organizing pneumonia [12]. The air crescent sign, a crescent-shaped area of radiolucency in a region of nodular opacity, is usually seen during convalescence in angioinvasive aspergillosis (i.e., 2–3 weeks after initiation of treatment and concomitant with resolution of the neutropenia) [28]. Of note, some studies suggest that cavitation and the air-crescent sign are more likely to be observed in adults, and may frequently be absent from CT scans obtained from young children with pulmonary invasive aspergillosis [29]. When obtaining serial CT scans, it is also important to realize that irrespective of antifungal therapy, the pattern is characterized by an initial rise in number and size of lesions, followed by a plateau in lesion size, and gradual reduction [12]. Moreover, is time until complete radiologic remission and outcome independent of initial or maximum

http://dx.doi.org/10.5772/54990

lesion size and number in patients with invasive pulmonary aspergillosis [30]. The appearance of cavities on serial CT scans (frequently accompanied by the appearance of the air-crescent sign as neutropenia resolves) may be indicative of patient recovery. Similarly, if antifungal therapy is initiated and subsequent scans show an increase in the number or size of lesions, this is more likely a reflection of the typical progression of disease rather than failed therapy. According to the ECIL recommendations, in high-risk patients with persistent febrile neutropenia that persists beyond 96 hours or with focal clinical findings, imaging studies (e.g., CT-scan of the lung or adequate imaging of the symptomatic region) should be performed. Further diagnostic work-up (e.g., BAL, biopsy) should be considered and mold-active antifungal treatment should be initiated.

6. Treatment

Antifungal strategies include prophylaxis, empiric antifungal therapy, pre-emptive antifungal therapy and treatment of established invasive fungal infection (Figure 3). For individual patient populations, each strategy needs to consider the patients risk, the local epidemiology, the availability of diagnostic tools and the availability and effectiveness of antifungal agents. Last, but not least a cost – benefit analysis (i.e. toxicity, financial aspects) is mandatory. For the purpose of this textbook spectrum, potency, mode of action, and clinical indication of antifungal agents will be discussed.

6.1. Amphotericin B

Amphotericin deoxycholate (DAMB) and its lipid formulations, including amphotericin B colloidal dispersion (ABCD), amphotericin B lipid complex (ABLC), and liposomal amphotericin B (LAMB,) have a wide range of activity against most fungal pathogens. Only Aspergillus terreus and Fusarium species are less susceptible (Table 1.) [31].

In comparison to DAMB, nephrotoxicity is rarely seen with the use of the lipid formulations; infusion-related reactions, such as fever, chills and rigor are substantially less frequent with LAMB. Mild increases in bilirubin and alkaline phosphatase are associated with all three lipid formulations, elevation of transaminases with LAMB only. Currently, DAMB is licensed for neonatal invasive candidiasis and induction therapy for cryptococcal meningitis; LAMB is approved as first line empirical treatment of suspected invasive aspergillosis and candidiasis; ABCD is licensed for second-line treatment of patients with invasive aspergillosis, and ABLC for second-line treatment of patients with invasive Candida or Aspergillus infections [34].

The recommended therapeutic dosages are 0.7 to 1.0 mg/kg/day for DAMB, 3–4 mg/kg/day for ABCD, 5 mg/kg/day for ABLC, and 3 (to 5) mg/kg/day for LAMB, respectively. The available evidence does not suggest pharmacokinetic differences of LAMB between adults and children including preterm and newborn infants [33].

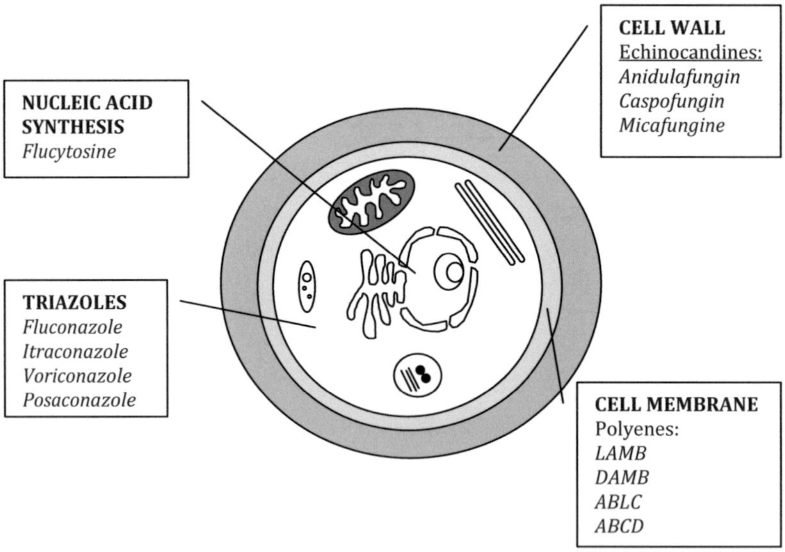

Figure 4. Schematic overview of current antifungal agents in regard to its target. Flucytosine inhibits RNA and DNA synthesis, Triazoles inhibit ergosterol biosynthesis, polyenes bind to sterols in the plasma membrane and echinocandines inhibit beta [1,3]-D-Glucan-synthesis. LAMB: liposomal Amphotericin B; DAMB: Amphotericin B deoxycholate; ABCD: Amphotericin B colloidal dispersion; ABLC: amphotericin B lipid complex.

6.2. Fluconazole

Fluconazole has a very narrow fungal susceptibility against Candida species (Candida glabrata and krusei have a high MIC index) and lacks activity against Aspergillus species and zygomycetes (Table 1.). Fluconazole is not metabolized and mainly renally excreted, and drug levels correlate with strictly with renal function [33]. It is licensed for prophylactic use in patients at risk for IFIs and for targeted treatment of candidiasis. For pediatric patients (they show a more rapid excretion and shorter half-life), the recommended dosage is higher than for adults, 8 to 12 mg/kg/day versus 5 mg/kg/day, respectively [34].

6.3. Itraconazole

The compound is active against most Candida and Aspergillus species, but the susceptibility against Candida glabrata and C. krusei is limited (Table 1). There is no activity against zygomycetes. The pharmacokinetics is characterized by inter-individual variability of gastrointestinal absorption and hepatic metabolism [35]. Accordingly, measurement of drug levels is necessary and results of meta-analysis suggest that the trough plasma level should be higher than 0.5 μg / mL [36]. Concerns have arisen on the interaction with drugs such as vincristine and cyclosporine, which are major components of both induction ALL therapy and prevention of GvHD in ALL transplanted patients. Moreover, 10% of patients experience gastrointestinal adverse effects, such as nausea and diarrhea, which limits its acceptance [34]. According to the

http://dx.doi.org/10.5772/54990

	Amphothericn B	Fluconazole	Voriconazole	Posaconazole	Itraconazole	Caspofungin	Micafungin
Candida albicans	+	(+)	+	+	+	+	+
C. parapsilosis	+	+	+	+	+	+/-	+/-
C. lusitaniae	-/+	+	+	+	+	+	+
C. tropicalis	+	-/+	+	+	+	+	+
C. glabrata	+	-	-/+	+	-/+	+	+
C. krusei	+	-	-/+	+	-/+	+	+
Asp. fumigatus	+	-	+	+	+	+	+
Asp. flavus	(+)	-	+	+	+	+	+
Asp. terreus	-	-	+	+	+	+	+
Asp. niger	+	-	(+)	+	(+)	+	+
Zygomycetes	+	-	-	(+)	-	-	-
Fusarium spp.	(+)	-	-	-	-	-	-

+ = high activity rate; (+) = little reduced activity rate; -/+ = higher resistant rates in some areas; - = mostly resistant [11;32;33].C.: Candida; Asp.: Aspergillus; spp.: species.

Table 1. Susceptibility of important fungal pathogens against some common antifungal agents.

ECIL and IDSA guidelines, Itraconazole should be used as second-line therapy in the prevention of IFIs.

6.4. Voriconazole

Voriconazole has similar activity as Itraconazole and is active against most Candida and Aspergillus species, but not zygomycetes, Candida glabrata and C. krusei (Table 1.). The effectiveness of this compound has been demonstrated in large clinical trials in both adults and children, and has led to its approval for empirical and pre-emptive antifungal therapy [31]. Because of its wide use, breakthrough infections with zygomycetes have been reported [37]. Additionally, breakthrough infections with susceptible strains have been noted in patients with low plasma levels, necessitating the monitoring of through plasma levels [38]. In children, Voriconazole is more rapidly metabolized, suggesting a higher dosage of 7-8 mg/kg/b.i.d. than in adults (4-5 mg/kg/b.i.d.) [33]. Relevant side effects of Voriconazole include elevations of liver enzymes, visual disturbances and photosensitivity skin reactions, particularly if combined with nucleoside analoga, which are commonly used in the treatment of ALL. In addition, the interaction of Voriconazole with a number of drugs (e.g. Vincristine, Cyclosporine A, and Omeprazole) has to be considered [33].

6.5. Posaconazole

This compound has a potent and broad-spectrum activity against most clinically important fungal infections, including zygomycetes, distinguishing it from the other azoles [33]. According to the ECIL/ IDSA guidelines it is recommended as second-line treatment of aspergillosis, fusariosis, chromoblastomycosis and coccidioidomycosis. In addition, Posaconazole is approved for prophylaxis in high-risk patients older than 13 years of age with ALL and in hematopoietic stem cell transplant patients with graft-versus-host disease [31;39]. The dosage for prophylaxis is 200 mg three times daily, for salvage treatment the dose is increased to 400 mg two times daily. Similar to Voriconazole, interference with cytochrome P450 dependent metabolites (e.g. Cyclosporine) need to be considered [34].

6.6. Caspofungin

Caspofungin is active against Candida spp. and Aspergillus spp., but resistant against Cryptococcus species and zygomycetes (Table 1.). It is licensed for adult and pediatric patients, including neonates, for empirical antifungal therapy in persistently febrile neutropenic patients, for second-line pre-emptive therapy of suspected aspergillosis and for primary therapy in non-neutropenic patients with invasive Candida infections. The recommended dose regimen in adults consists of a single 70-mg loading dose on day 1, followed by 50 mg daily thereafter [34]. A dosage of 1 mg/kg for children has been suggested [31]. A favorable safety profile has been described, the most common drug-related adverse events were fever, increased ALT, and rash; few events were serious or required treatment discontinuation [40].

6.7. Micafungin

Micafungin was recently licensed for neonates, children and adults for prophylaxis and treatment of invasive candidiasis in patients with prolonged neutropenia and after hematopoietic stem cell transplantation [41]. The spectrum of activity is similar to that of Caspofungin (Table 1). The recommended dosage is 100 mg/day for invasive candidiasis (≤40 kg body weight: 2 mg/kg) with the option of dose escalation to 200 mg/day or 4 mg/kg/day; and 50 mg/day (≤40 kg: 1 mg/kg) in the preventive indication [34]. The most frequent adverse events include vomiting, high fever, diarrhea, nausea, and hypokalemia [41].

7. Conclusion

Although various guidelines on antifungal management have been published, we suggest using a simple approach, which is guided by local factors, such as the pattern of resistance and the availability of diagnostic tools. As newer strategies might soon be implemented, we are unable to assess the efficacy of our approach to date. Our report underlines that many

http://dx.doi.org/10.5772/54990

questions regarding antifungal treatment have to be addressed in future studies, such as the duration of treatment or the benefit of costly combination antifungal therapy.

Acknowledgements

We thank Kinderkrebshilfe Tirol und Vorarlberg for funding.

Author details

Roman Crazzolara*, Adrian Kneer, Bernhard Meister and Gabriele Kropshofer

*Address all correspondence to: roman.crazzolara@i-med.ac.at

Department of Pediatrics, Medical University of Innsbruck, Austria

References

[1] Pui, C, Relling, M. V, & Downing, J. R. Mechanisms of disease: Acute lymphoblastic leukemia. New England Journal of Medicine (2004)., 1535-1548.

[2] Arico, M, Valsecchi, M. G, Camitta, B, Schrappe, M, Chessells, J, Baruchel, A, et al. Outcome of treatment in children with philadelphia chromosome-positive acute lymphoblastic leukemia. New England Journal of Medicine (2000)., 998-1006.

[3] Marr, K. A, Carter, R. A, Crippa, F, Wald, A, & Corey, L. Epidemiology and outcome of mould infections in hematopoietic stem cell transplant recipients. Clinical Infectious Diseases (2002)., 909-917.

[4] Mcneil, M. M, Nash, S. L, Hajjeh, R. A, Phelan, M. A, Conn, L. A, Plikaytis, B. D, et al. Trends in mortality due to invasive mycotic diseases in the United States, Clinical Infectious Diseases (2001)., 1980-1997.

[5] Zaoutis, T. E, Heydon, K, Chu, J. H, Walsh, T. J, & Steinbach, W. J. Epidemiology, outcomes, and costs of invasive aspergillosis in immunocompromised children in the United States, 2000. Pediatrics (2006). EE716., 711.

[6] de PBWalsh TJ, Donnelly JP, Stevens DA, Edwards JE, Calandra T et al. Revised definitions of invasive fungal disease from the European Organization for Research and Treatment of Cancer/Invasive Fungal Infections Cooperative Group and the National Institute of Allergy and Infectious Diseases Mycoses Study Group (EORTC/MSG) Consensus Group. Clin Infect Dis (2008)., 1813-1821.

[7] Ascioglu, S, Rex, J. H, De Pauw, B, Bennett, J. E, Bille, J, Crokaert, F, et al. Defining opportunistic invasive fungal infections in immunocompromised patients with cancer and hematopoietic stem cell transplants: An international consensus. Clinical Infectious Diseases (2002). , 7-14.

[8] Lass-florl, C. The changing face of epidemiology of invasive fungal disease in Europe. Mycoses (2009). , 197-205.

[9] Koch, S, Hohne, F. M, & Tietz, H. J. Incidence of systemic mycoses in autopsy material. Mycoses (2004). , 40-46.

[10] Pagano, L, Caira, M, Candoni, A, Offidani, M, Fianchi, L, Martino, B, et al. The epidemiology of fungal infections in patients with hematologic malignancies: the SEIFEM-2004 study. Haematologica-the Hematology Journal (2006). , 1068-1075.

[11] Pfaller, M. A, & Diekema, D. J. Epidemiology of invasive candidiasis: a persistent public health problem. Clinical Microbiology Reviews (2007). , 133.

[12] Franquet, T, Muller, N. L, Gimenez, A, & Guembe, P. de La TJ, Bague S. Spectrum of pulmonary aspergillosis: histologic, clinical, and radiologic findings. Radiographics (2001). , 825-837.

[13] Walsh, T. J, Anaissie, E. J, Denning, D. W, Herbrecht, R, Kontoyiannis, D. P, Marr, K. A, et al. Treatment of aspergillosis: clinical practice guidelines of the Infectious Diseases Society of America. Clin Infect Dis (2008). , 327-360.

[14] Pfeiffer, C. D, Fine, J. P, & Safdar, N. Diagnosis of invasive aspergillosis using a galactomannan assay: A meta-analysis. Clinical Infectious Diseases (2006). , 1417-1427.

[15] Marr, K. A, Balajee, S. A, Mclaughlin, L, Tabouret, M, Bentsen, C, & Walsh, T. J. Detection of galactomannan antigenemia by enzyme immunoassay for the diagnosis of invasive aspergillosis: Variables that affect performance. Journal of Infectious Diseases (2004). , 641-649.

[16] Mennink-Kersten MASHKlont RR, Warris A, Op den Camp HJM, Verweij PE. Bifidobacterium lipoteichoic acid and false ELISA reactivity in aspergillus antigen detection. Lancet (2004). , 325-327.

[17] Steinbach, W. J. Invasive aspergillosis in pediatric patients. Current Medical Research and Opinion (2010). , 1779-1787.

[18] Senn, L, Robinson, J. O, Schmidt, S, Knaup, M, Asahi, N, Satomura, S, et al. Beta-D-glucan antigenemia for early diagnosis of invasive fungal infections in neutropenic patients with acute leukemia. Clin Infect Dis (2008). , 1, 3.

[19] Karageorgopoulos, D. E, Vouloumanou, E. K, Ntziora, F, Michalopoulos, A, Rafailidis, P. I, & Falagas, M. E. beta-D-Glucan Assay for the Diagnosis of Invasive Fungal Infections: A Meta-analysis. Clinical Infectious Diseases (2011). , 750-770.

[20] Mularoni, A, Furfaro, E, Faraci, M, Franceschi, A, Mezzano, P, Bandettini, R, et al. High Levels of beta-D-Glucan in Immunocompromised Children with Proven Invasive Fungal Disease. Clinical and Vaccine Immunology (2010). , 882-883.

[21] Hummel, M, Spiess, B, Roder, J, Von Komorowski, G, Durken, M, Kentouche, K, et al. Detection of Aspergillus DNA by a nested PCR assay is able to improve the diagnosis of invasive aspergillosis in paediatric patients. Journal of Medical Microbiology (2009). , 1291-1297.

[22] Lass-florl, C, Gunsilius, E, Gastl, G, Bonatti, H, Freund, M. C, Gschwendtner, A, et al. Diagnosing invasive aspergillosis during antifungal therapy by PCR analysis of blood samples. J Clin Microbiol (2004). , 4154-4157.

[23] Suarez, F, Lortholary, O, Buland, S, Rubio, M. T, Ghez, D, Mahe, V, et al. Detection of Circulating Aspergillus fumigatus DNA by Real-Time PCR Assay of Large Serum Volumes Improves Early Diagnosis of Invasive Aspergillosis in High-Risk Adult Patients under Hematologic Surveillance. Journal of Clinical Microbiology (2008). , 3772-3777.

[24] Cesaro, S, Stenghele, C, Calore, E, Franchin, E, Cerbaro, I, Cusinato, R, et al. Assessment of the lightcycler PCR assay for diagnosis of invasive aspergillosis in paediatric patients with onco-haematological diseases. Mycoses (2008). , 497-504.

[25] Landlinger, C, Preuner, S, & Baskova, L. van GM, Hartwig NG, Dworzak M et al. Diagnosis of invasive fungal infections by a real-time panfungal PCR assay in immunocompromised pediatric patients. Leukemia (2010). , 2032-2038.

[26] Lass-florl, C, Resch, G, Nachbaur, D, Mayr, A, Gastl, G, Auberger, J, et al. The value of computed tomography-guided percutaneous lung biopsy for diagnosis of invasive fungal infection in Immunocompromised patients. Clinical Infectious Diseases (2007). EE104., 101.

[27] Taccone, A, Occhi, M, Garaventa, A, Manfredini, L, & Viscoli, C. Ct of Invasive Pulmonary Aspergillosis in Children with Cancer. Pediatric Radiology (1993). , 177-180.

[28] Franquet, T, Muller, N. L, Oikonomou, A, & Flint, J. D. Aspergillus infection of the airways: computed tomography and pathologic findings. J Comput Assist Tomogr (2004). , 10-16.

[29] Thomas, K. E, Owens, C. M, Veys, P. A, Novelli, V, & Costoli, V. The radiological spectrum of invasive Aspergillosis in children: a year review. Pediatric Radiology (2003). , 10.

[30] Brodoefel, H, Vogel, M, Hebart, H, Einsele, H, Vonthein, R, Claussen, C, et al. Long-term CT follow-up in 40 non-HIV immunocompromised patients with invasive pulmonary aspergillosis: Kinetics of CT morphology and correlation with clinical findings and outcome. American Journal of Roentgenology (2006). , 404-413.

[31] Groll, A. H, & Tragiannidis, A. Update on antifungal agents for paediatric patients. Clin Microbiol Infect (2010). , 1343-1353.

[32] Lass-florl, C. Invasive fungal infections in pediatric patients: a review focusing on antifungal therapy. Expert Review of Anti-Infective Therapy (2010). , 127-135.

[33] Lehrnbecher, T, Mousset, S, Sorensen, J, & Bohme, A. Current practice of antifungal prophylaxis and treatment in immunocompromised children and adults with malignancies: a single centre approach. Mycoses (2009). , 107-117.

[34] Groll, A. H. Efficacy and safety of antifungals in pediatric patients. Early Hum Dev (2011). Suppl 1:SS74., 71.

[35] Chiou, C. C, Walsh, T. J, & Groll, A. H. Clinical pharmacology of antifungal agents in pediatric patients. Expert Opin Pharmacother (2007). , 2465-2489.

[36] Glasmacher, A, Prentice, A, Gorschluter, M, Engelhart, S, Hahn, C, Djulbegovic, B, et al. Itraconazole prevents invasive fungal infections in neutropenic patients treated for hematologic malignancies: Evidence from a meta-analysis of 3,597 patients. Journal of Clinical Oncology (2003). , 4615-4626.

[37] Trifilio, S, Singhal, S, Williams, S, Frankfurt, O, Gordon, L, Evens, A, et al. Breakthrough fungal infections after allogeneic hematopoietic stem cell transplantation in patients on prophylactic voriconazole. Bone Marrow Transplantation (2007). , 451-456.

[38] Trifilio, S, Pennick, G, Pi, J, Zook, J, Golf, M, Kaniecki, K, et al. Monitoring plasma voriconazole levels may be necessary to avoid subtherapeutic levels in hematopoietic stem cell transplant recipients. Cancer (2007). , 1532-1535.

[39] Groll, A. H, & Walsh, T. J. Antifungal efficacy and pharmacodynamics of posaconazole in experimental models of invasive fungal infections. Mycoses (2006). , 49, 7-16.

[40] Walsh, T. J, Viviani, M. A, Arathoon, E, Chiou, C, Ghannoum, M, Groll, A. H, et al. New targets and delivery systems for antifungal therapy. Medical Mycology (2000). , 38, 335-347.

[41] Lehrnbecher, T, & Groll, A. H. Micafungin: a brief review of pharmacology, safety, and antifungal efficacy in pediatric patients. Pediatr Blood Cancer (2010). , 229-232.